ACUPUNCTURE

The Past and the Present

Kee Chang Huang

VANTAGE PRESS
New York

FIRST EDITION

Published by Vantage Press, Inc.
516 West 34th Street, New York, New York 10001

Manufactured in the United States of America
ISBN: 0-533-11678-3

Library of Congress Catalog Card No.: 95-90683

0 9 8 7 6 5 4 3 2 1

- To Peter K. Knoefel, M.D., Professor Emeritus and former Chairman of the Department of Pharmacology & Toxicology, University of Louisville, for his valuable advice and inspiration over the last four decades;
- To my colleagues and co-workers, for their enthusiastic support and cooperation throughout these years;
- And, not least of all, to my wife, Shou-Shan; my children, Kou Chu, Anna, and Karen; and my grandchildren, whose encouragement and love I have cherished throughout the years.

Contents

Foreword

Western culture has incorporated and adopted many important ideas and products from the Orient since the days where silk and spices first reached the crossroads of East and West. In the fourteenth century, Marco Polo brought to the Western World knowledge from China of such marvels as pasta, gunpowder, rockets, and printing with movable type. In the West, however, acquaintance with Oriental medicine and science has been delayed, in part, by a paucity of professionals who could integrate the essence of Chinese philosophy as it appears in medicine and science with similar disciplines in Western culture.

Kee Chang Huang—teacher, scientist, philosopher and physician—embodies the melding of East and West. "K.C.," as he is fondly known by his friends and colleagues, was born and educated in Canton, Southern China, receiving his M.D. at Doctor Sun Yat-sen University, Medical Faculty. After his graduation he worked at the NIH in China as a Research Fellow and taught Pharmacology in Shanghai Medical College. In 1953 he received his Ph.D. in Physiology from Columbia University in New York. For over 50 years K.C. has taught and conducted pharmacological and physiological research in medical schools in the United States, Middle East, and China.

In this book, K.C. has supplied Westerners with a carefully researched and distilled resource on acupuncture, a procedure used in China over 4,000 years. This is not, however, a book of techniques; rather, he has provided a review of the use of acupuncture in various diseases and disorders as its techniques have been modified and its applications expanded in response to the ebb and flow of interest and popularity over the centuries.

Throughout his work the author has presented an even-handed review of accepted Western explanations for physiologic actions and, where possible, has suggested explanations within the parameters of Western thought for electrical and chemical changes observed in response to acupuncture. Every effort has been made to produce an unbiased review of the practice of acupuncture.

A valuable and succinct overview of Chinese scientific and medical philosophy prepared with the cooperation of Professor De-An Tang in China, has been included in chapter two. In this review, acupuncture, as a method of medical therapy, is placed within the framework of the Chinese philosophy of the Yin and Yang, Qi, and the Five Elements.

This book is an achievement in scholarship which brings to the Western physician, and scientist, a valuable source of information on acupuncture and should assist him as well in understanding the basics of Chinese philosophy applied to medicine and science.

Eugene H. Conner, M.D.
Former Professor and Chairman,
Department of Anesthesiology,
University of Louisville
1995

Preface

As a child in China I watched a traveling practitioner sit at the market corner piercing needles into peasants' ears before extracting a bad tooth or relieving chronic back pain. Children tend to be more credulous than adults, but even then I was curious to know how this method worked. Now, after studying in Western medicine and having more than forty years of research experience in human physiology, this question still remains.

The Chinese have practiced the art of acupuncture as early as the Stone Age, but in the many centuries since then, no real scientific explanation of the effective mechanisms of acupuncture has emerged. Because traditional Chinese medicine is not based on the rigorous scientific principles and methods required by Western medicine, many non-Chinese (and Western-trained Chinese) view acupuncture as either a form of quack charlatanry or as a mystic New Age ritual. Yet it cannot be denied that physicians in Europe and America, as well as in China, have had success in using acupuncture as an inexpensive and effective treatment of a variety of diseases. Since 1958, acupuncture anesthesia has replaced general anesthesia in many Chinese hospitals and clinics, with documented use in cases ranging from cranial to open-heart surgery, from abdominal laparatomy to Cesarean section. In addition, it is claimed to be the treatment of choice in China for over one hundred different diseases.

This book attempts to address the question of how acupuncture triggers changes in the physiological functions of the body, examining empirical data made available by Chinese clinics over the past several decades. The book has two major sections. The first explores how the Chinese developed various acupuncture techniques over the years, how they derived the Meridian Principles, where the acupoints are located, their interconnection, and the principal therapeutic uses. The second reviews practical clinical applications of acupuncture currently in use. While all material is presented in a fashion intended to be accessible by the educated layman and of interest to practitioners, it is hoped that this work will stimulate the Western medical profession to explore acupuncture's effective mechanisms more vigorously. Of particular interest is understanding how acupuncture can promote the defense mechanisms of the body, and whether acupuncture can induce changes in the molecular biological system, most notably the receptor-binding or enzymatic functions.

I would like to express my gratitude for the contributions of the following people:

W. Michael Williams, M.D., Ph.D., Professor of Pharmacology and Toxicology, University of Louisville, for his valuable discussions and suggestions throughout the preparation of this manuscript;

Professor De-An Tang, Department of Physiology, Tianjin Traditional Chinese Medical College, Tianjin, People's Republic of China, for his contribution to the chapter on the history of acupuncture;

Shi-Yu Wu, Ph.D., Professor of Physics, University of Louisville, for his inspiring discussions on the subject of laser principles and applications;

The librarians of the University of Louisville Medical Science Library and the Tianjin Medical University Library (Tianjin, PRC) for their generous help in the search for relevant literature;

The various authors who have kindly allowed reproduction of figures and tables from their texts;

And special thanks to my youngest daughter, Karen, who patiently edited portions of the manuscript prior to publication.

ACUPUNCTURE

1
Introduction

Throughout man's history, philosophical understanding of life and the study of medicine have developed simultaneously. Sickness and death are unavoidable, and the science of medicine stems naturally from man's desire to both enjoy and give greater meaning to life. Every culture develops some form of medicine as a tool for survival, but this knowledge rarely lasts long if it is based on superstition rather than observable empirical evidence and a fundamental understanding of physiology and pathology.

Acupuncture, one of the oldest forms of Chinese medicine, has withstood the test of time, having been practiced across China for more than four thousand years. Archaeological findings show that the practice of acupuncture may actually have started in the Stone Age, as indicated by the discovery of the so-called Blan Shi, or needle-shaped stone. The first written record of the technique, however, comes to us from the *Huang Ti Nei Chian,* or the *Yellow Emperor's Classic of Internal Medicine,* which was written by unknown authors around 100 B.C. and is purported to be the work of the Yellow Emperor, who ruled China between 2697 and 2597 B.C. Huang Ti and his chief administrative advisors were said to be interested in the study of medicine and commissioned a comprehensive written record of diagnostic technique, treatments with herbs, and acupuncture. The resulting work is one of the earliest writings on Chinese culture and science.

Acupuncture stands as one of the chief achievements of Chinese science, comprising knowledge gained from centuries of clinical experience and explained by a macrocosmic philosophy that is not yet completely understood or accepted by Western scientific standards. It has been used not only to alleviate pain, being applied as an anesthetic for tooth extractions or minor surgical operations, but also as a healing method for a variety of illnesses. Despite the introduction of Western medical methods in China over the last two hundred years, acupuncture shows no signs of becoming obsolete or abandoned.

Yet acupuncture itself is perceived by many Westerners as a form of voodoo medicine. The term *acupuncture* comes from the words *acus,* or needle, and *puncture,*to pierce. It is an ancient Chinese system of medicine in which a fine needle is inserted into the body at an exact point, or acupoint. Practitioners of acupuncture claim that acupoints reside along "meridians" within the body and are used in a precise fashion dictated by the disease requiring treatment. Western studies, however, have not yet found a convincing physiological basis for these meridians.

Chinese medical literature places acupuncture and moxibustion together under a single subject called Zhen Djiu. Moxibustion is a technique that employs thermal stimulation at the acupoint instead of a needle, but is based on the same principles and theories as acupuncture. Acupuncture, or Zhen Djiu, was selectively used by Chinese *tai-fu* (scholarly physicians) or *sen-sei* (travelling practitioners) to treat patients experiencing chronic pain or to assist in surgical operations. It is said that Hua Tau (A.D.145–203), a great Chinese surgeon during the Han Dynasty, was a master of acupuncture and successfully used the technique to treat many patients (5). Legend has it that when

Hua Tau fell ill and required cranial surgery, he used acupuncture on himself as an anesthetic, remaining conscious to give advice to the physicians performing the operation.

The techniques of acupuncture and other Chinese medicine were imported into Japan between the seventh and eighth centuries and were rapidly assimilated into Japanese science. However, acupuncture was not known in Europe even after Marco Polo returned from his landmark visit, and acupuncture was first mentioned in European literature only in the sixteenth century by Fernand Mendex Pinto. Later, the term *acupuncture* came into medical use after two surgeons from the Dutch East India Company published their studies on the subject.

It wasn't until the nineteenth century, however, that European and American physicians turned their attention to the field, becoming fascinated with the possibilities of the technique. In *Principles and Practices of Medicine* (Philadelphia, 1892), Sir William Osler listed acupuncture as treatment for lumbago (p. 282) and sciatica (p. 820). He and a colleague, Dr. Harvey Cushing, attempted to use acupuncture in treating their patients, admitting that they lacked a complete understanding of the technique, but noting that "it is a popular procedure of the day" (4).

In 1939, *L'acupuncture Chinoise* was published by George Soulie de Morant, a French diplomat who wrote this text based on his observations during a long tour of duty in China. Although not a physician himself, de Morant was instrumental in bringing the technique into many hospitals and clinics throughout Europe, creating a special breed of Sino-Western doctors and scholars of distinction.

Ironically, while Western physicians were beginning to explore the possibilities of this ancient technique, Chinese physicians were beginning to turn away from this practice. The introduction of opium and the development of other new potent analgesic agents, both narcotic and nonnarcotic, saw an abatement in the use of acupuncture in the late nineteenth and early twentieth centuries.

Necessity forced the Chinese to reexamine the potential of this practice after the Communist revolution in 1949. By 1957, China had become isolated from the West once again, and her people were deprived of Western medicines and equipment necessary for treating illnesses. In response, the Chinese government revived traditional Chinese medicine, establishing more than one dozen traditional medical colleges and institutes to train doctors and perform research.

Physicians and surgeons in China have now made acupuncture the treatment of choice for more than two hundred different diseases. Acupuncture anesthesia, a term once unheard of, has become common in Chinese hospitals and clinics, replacing general anesthesia in procedures ranging from cranial to open heart surgery, from abdominal laparotomy to cesarean section. With the reopening of diplomatic relations between China and the United States after Pres. Richard Nixon's historic 1972 visit, these achievements gained prominence in Western media. China was flooded with delegations and missions sent to study acupuncture. In the United States, committees were organized to exploit and investigate the subject. New texts were published in both Chinese and English, dealing with its uses and applications (2,3,7).

Voodoo Medicine or Science?

Between 1968 and 1977, over eight thousand papers concerning the clinical uses and successes of acupuncture were published in China alone, covering more than three hundred different diseases (1). The accumulation of data showing the efficacy of acupuncture has forced Western scientists to acknowledge that acupuncture is not a myth. However, few are willing to grant it status as a "science." Outside of China, acupuncture has not been listed as a specific course in recognized medical curricula.

Among licensed physicians in the West, acupuncture is gaining some acceptance, albeit very slowly. According to recent medical reports, nearly 10 percent of all European doctors have experimented with acupuncture in treating patients, though only 2 percent devote their entire practice to acupuncture therapy. In many cases, acupuncture therapy has been pursued at the request of the patients, particularly in cases of resistance to medication.

One of the major sources of skepticism about acupuncture stems from the lack of reliability in selecting the correct acupoint, or focus. The *Huang Ti Nei Chian* lists 361 acupoints on the surface of the body, each with its own name; that number was increased to 647 in Wa Shou's *The Exposition of Fourteen Meridians* (A.D.1304–1386 Ming Dynasty). Assuming that the surface area of an adult is approximately 2.0 square meters, (m^2) this works out to be one acupoint for every 20 square centimeters (cm^2) area. A child of 80 centimeters height and 30 kilograms weight has a surface area of approximately 0.68 square meters; the acupoint distribution in this child would be 1 acupoint for every 10 square centimeters!

Acupoints are very crowded in certain areas, particularly in the ear, the wrist, and the ankle. It is difficult to point out the exact location of one acupoint versus another. Furthermore, an average acupoint has a diameter of 0.2 to 0.3 centimeters, located right on the pathway of its corresponding meridian. Because the location of acupoints will differ slightly from patient to patient, the only means of determining the successful selection and needling of an acupoint is by the subject judgment of the patient, who should feel *tae qi*, a propagational sensation along the acupoint's channel or meridian when the needle is exactly on the acupoint.

Locating an acupoint is not like finding a vein for intravenous injection, an intravertebral aperture for intrathecal injection, or a nerve trunk for nerve blocking. There is no anatomical structure to pinpoint the acupoint. Some investigators have claimed that acupoints differ electrophysiologically from nonacupoints, displaying lower electrical resistance. Various electronic instruments have been developed that claim to be able to show where the "acupoint" is located; however, they have not been proven completely successful.

How Does It Work?

One fundamental question remains in every scientist's mind: How does acupuncture work? While ample evidence is available to demonstrate that acupuncture can produce desired effects, how can we explain the mechanisms by which acupuncture triggers changes in the physiological functions of the body?

One of the dozens of Western practitioners of acupuncture, Felix Mann, used a mixture of traditional Chinese philosophy and Sir Charles Scott Sherrington's neurological phenonema to explain the mechanisms of acupuncture, interpreting his clinical data on acupuncture-induced healing based on the relationship of five elements (6). But the discovery and isolation of opioid peptides in the central nervous tissue in 1975, together with a new understanding of the correlation and interaction between different neurotransmitters during stimulation and activation, now gives us a different viewpoint for examining acupuncture.

Our current understanding indicates that acupuncture promotes a defensive mechanism in the body. It is not a hypnotic trick, nor a psychological cohesion. In ancient times, acupuncture was probably only used to relieve pain, particularly chronic pain, migraine headaches, lumbago, and dysmenorrhea when opium was not available or other analgesic herbs were ineffective. By accident, the Chinese also discovered that acupuncture can produce other therapeutic effects besides analgesia. Data show that many almost-miraculous healing effects can occur during acupuncture.

For example, acupuncture can improve immunity, suppress hypersensitivity, and increase serum immunoglobins levels. Furthermore, acupuncture can abolish abstinent symptoms due to cigarette smoking or alcohol consumption. Does this action involve an influence of certain enzymatic reactions or a change of receptor binding? The exact causes are still not understood.

Acupuncture has a high effective rate in the treatment of impotency and difficult ejaculation in men. Is it possible that acupuncture might increase biosynthesis and/or the release of nitric oxide (NO) in the penile vascular muscles, which result in penile erection and ejaculation? This is a purely speculative assumption. At the present time, we don't have an ideal animal model to test such a hypothesis.

Adding to the mystery surrounding acupuncture is the nature of its application. Like Western medicine, much of traditional Chinese medicine advocates a symptomatic treatment of many diseases, e.g., treating the head for headaches, healing the foot when it is hurt. However, this is not the case in acupuncture. In the treatment of headaches, the acupuncturist pierces a needle at the remote area, such as the leg or the ear. For thyroidectomy or gynecological operation, the patient can be placed under anesthesia by puncturing a needle at the HoKu (LI 4) acupoint of the hand, or the Sanyinjiao (Sp 6) acupoint on the leg. Furthermore, an acupuncture effect can produce quite different vascular responses and skin temperature changes depending upon whether the needle is applied on the ipsilateral or on the contralateral side of the body. The neurophysiological interpretation as shown in Sherrington's integrative action of the nervous system is thus far the best explanation we have of such action.

The extent to which acupuncture is effective is also in question, as much of the clinical data currently available from China was not collected in the rigorous fashion expected by Western scientists. For instance, some astonishing clinical data have shown that an 80-percent success rate has been obtained via acupuncture therapy in the treatment of deaf mutism, especially in cases of deafness induced by drug intoxication; the clinical assessment of these patients prior to treatment is largely incomplete, raising doubts about the accuracy of the reports. Although animal and human experimentation has shown that acupuncture does cause an increase in the level of opioid peptides and their release in the nervous tissues (including the brain stem and spinal cord), it is unknown whether acupuncture also affects the special sense center organs, such as auditory or olfactory senses. It is hoped that researchers in otology and neurophysiology will be sufficiently stimulated by the presentation of these data in this book to search for a possible answer to this question.

This book is not a manual for acupuncture therapy. It does not dwell on the details of technique or practice. Nor is it intended to glorify acupuncture as a miracle cure for certain intractable illnesses or to promote it in place of other medical procedures, e.g., general anesthesia. Indeed, having been educated and trained primarily in Western medicine and science, the author embarked upon this project with considerable skepticism.

Instead, this book examines new studies from animal experimentation to try to explain how acupuncture works. Chapter 3 introduces the concept of meridian channels as the Chinese practitioners visualize and describe in detail most old Chinese texts on acupuncture and moxibustion. Chapter 4 lists, for practical reasons, only the most commonly used acupoints for acupuncture therapy. Chapters 5, 6, and 7 explain how pain sensation occurs and the significant role of opioid peptides and other neurotransmitters in acupuncture-induced analgesia. Most data used comes from two teams in China—one from Beijing and one from Shanghai. Clinical application of acupuncture and its effectiveness are described separately in chapters 8 to 23.

Acupuncture provides a way to detect abnormalities in bodily functions. As the early work of Y. Nakatani of Kyoto University of Japan describes, acupoints can serve as alarm outposts for internal organs, indicating when organs become sick and useful as a virtual diagnostic tool on some pathological functional changes. Acupuncture can also cause a change in body immunity, directly or indirectly, via a transformation of T lymphocytes. It has been speculated that acupuncture may activate interferon formation in the body and may synergize with other systems or drugs to modify or promote the biosynthesis of certain specific enzymes in the body; this may be useful in the treatment of some specific illness such as smoking and alcoholism.

Prospectively, it is also postulated that acupuncture may act on cellular membrane, particularly nerve membrane and specific receptors on the membrane, causing a change in their affinity or binding to a neurotransmitter or ligand.

This opens a whole new horizon to medicine. It makes use of various forms of physical stimulation—pressure, heat, sound, electricity, electromagnetic forces, lasers—to imply that interactions with these field energies can effectively produce a balancing and harmonizing action beneficial to our bodies.

Although we don't completely understand the mechanisms of action by which acupuncture works, there is sufficient evidence to support a very reasonable scientific basis for this ancient art within Western medicine. Recent technological advances in acupuncture show great promise in promoting it in the directions of preventive medicine, immunology, and molecular biology.

References

1. Chang, C. T., et al. The Research on Acupuncture Anesthesia (in Chinese). Beijing: The Science Publisher, 1986.
2. Chen, J. Y. P. Acupuncture Anesthesia in PRC. U.S. Department of Health Education and Welfare. DHEW 75–769, 1975.
3. Chung, I. Y., ed. An Outline of Chinese Acupuncture. Oxford: Pergamon Press, 1975.
4. Conner, E. H. Personal communication. 1994.
5. Huang, K. C. Pharmacology of Chinese Herbs. Boca Raton CRC Press. p. 13.
6. Mann, F. Acupuncture, the Ancient Chinese Art of Healing. New York: Random House, 1971.
7. Tan, L. T., et al. Acupuncture Therapy, Current Chinese Practice. Philadelphia: Temple University Press, 1973.

2
A Brief History of Acupuncture*

For thousands of years, Chinese civilization flourished in isolation, locked away from Western eyes. China's ingenious developments in the arts and sciences were largely unknown to the Western world prior to the late nineteenth century, with only faint, almost-mystical rumors seeping out via irregular spice and silk trade.

Thus, when Prof. Joseph Needham of Cambridge University embarked on a tour of China during the World War II, he left England with only vague expectations of an ancient yet backwards culture. To his surprise, he found evidence of extensive technological and scientific achievements, many of which were paradoxically superior to European methods, yet at the same time more primitive and less understood.

Needham returned to England determined to launch a crusade to integrate Chinese science and culture with modern Western methods. He and his colleagues subsequently wrote more than twenty volumes on Chinese science and culture, forming a solid foundation for Western understanding of Chinese history and civilization. Of particular interest is Needham's study of Chinese medicine and acupuncture, in which he writes: "It is surely a very hopeful circumstance that Europeans are now giving up their rather self-satisfied parochialism and are eager to look at other systems of medicine . . . especially Chinese medicine, which comes from a highly continuous and complex civilization paralleling our own. . . . " (3)

Skepticism about acupuncture generally centers not around the technique itself, but the accompanying philosophy in which medicine and science are discussed. All Chinese traditional medicine is based on the philosophy of yin and yang; the balance between these two forces; blood and Qi; and the interaction of the five elements.

Yin-Yang Doctrine

The Chinese believe that the universe is governed by two opposing forces, both at macrocosmic and microcosmic levels. These two forces, the Yin and the Yang, were first described in the *Huang Ti Nei Chian* to explain how sickness occurs; since then, the Chinese have tried to apply this doctrine to all phases of life and activity.

Yin represents nature's feminine side. It is the dark aspect of the universe, comprising tranquility, depth, cold, and wetness; the Earth, the moon, and water are Yin elements. Yang represents

*Prof. De-An Tang of Tianjin Traditional Chinese Medical College, Tianjin, People's Republic of China, coauthors this chapter.

nature's masculine side. It is the bright aspect of the universe, comprising activity, height, heat, and dryness; the sun, heaven, and fire are Yang elements.

Westerners tend to interpret Yin as a negative force, balancing the positive force of the Yang, but the Chinese view the two as complementary forces that cannot exist without each other. When Yin and Yang are in harmony, the body is normal and healthy; disruption of that harmony results in pathological symptoms. Successful treatment of an illness depends on harmonizing Yin and Yang, to return the body to a state of balance.

Taoism has extended the Yin and Yang doctrine explicitly into all stages of life, as well as into day and night. These two forces are materialized in the human body and encircle it in equal terms, as shown in figure 2-1.

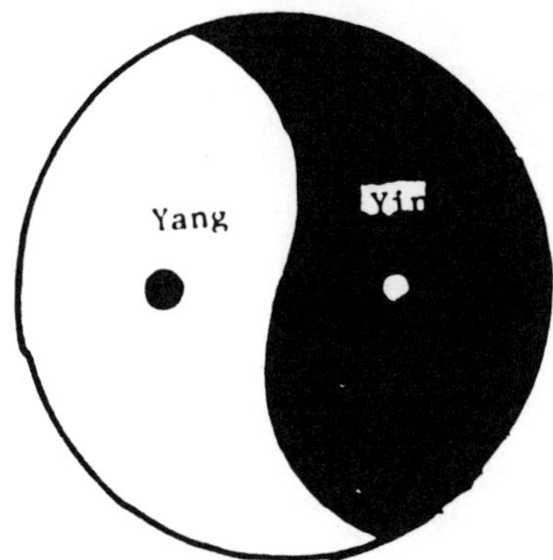

Figure 2-1. The Yin and Yang (The Tai-Ji-Tu, or Universe)

In the human body, the skin or external parts belong to the Yang, while the interior belongs to the Yin. The anterior side is Yin while the dorsal side is Yang. The flexor side of the extremity is Yin while the extensor side is Yang. Of the organs, the "solid" organs (lungs, spleen, heart, kidneys, liver, and pericardium) called *zhan* are Yin, while the "hollow" organs or viscerals (the stomach, small intestine, large intestine, urinary bladder, gallbladder, and "Triple burner"), called *fu,* are Yang.

Qi

Qi is one of the fundamental concepts of Chinese thought. The term literally means gas or vapor and refers to the energy of life or vital force of the body. Qi circulates in the body in a similar fashion as blood, though without use of a specific anatomical structure.

According to the *Nei Chian,* Qi is a combination of what is received from the heavens and the Qi inherent in water and food; it permeates the whole body. Chuang Tze (369–286 B.C.), one of ancient China's greatest philosophers and a disciple of Taoism, claimed that "life is the follower of death, and death is the predecessor of life. Man's life is due to the conglomeration of Qi, and when the Qi are dispersed, death occurs." The martial art of Qi-Gong is based on the principle that Qi also controls the movement of blood: "Qi is the general of the blood; if Qi moves, then the blood moves."

There are two types of Qi circulating in the body—the Nourishing Qi and the Protecting Qi. The Chinese believe that Qi comes from water and food, entering via the stomach and from there being transmitted to the lungs and other organs. The purer portion of food (after digestion and absorption) serves as the Nourishing Qi, circulating together with blood within the Chien-Loh, or meridians, and the blood vessels. The Protecting Qi receives the less pure portion of food and remains outside of the Chien-Loh and blood vessels, serving to warm the subcutaneous tissues, moisten the skin, and control the opening and closing of the pores. The Nourishing Qi is a Yin component, while the Protecting Qi is yang.

The *Nei Chian* states: "If Qi and blood are not evenly balanced, the Yin and the Yang will oppose each other. Qi will rebel against the Protecting Qi, blood against the Nourishing Qi. Blood and Qi will be separated, one being full and the other empty."

The Five Elements

In addition to the Yin and the Yang, Chinese philosophy divides the world into five elements, and everything belongs to one or more of these elements. These elements are wood, which represents the liver and gallbladder; fire, representing the heart and small intestine; earth, representing the spleen and stomach; metal or gold, representing the lungs and large intestine; and water, representing the kidney and bladder.

As shown in figure 2-2, the laws governing the movement of the five elements specify that each element creates and promotes its partner elements but controls and counteracts an opposing element. For example, wood promotes fire and restrains earth, while each promotes metal and restrains water.

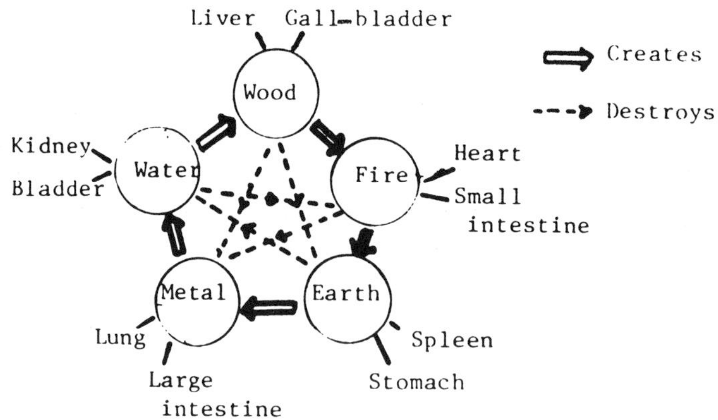

Figure 2-2. The Five Elements and Their Interaction

The philosophy of the five elements is applied to traditional Chinese medicine to explain some of the physiological functions of the solid and hollow organs (*zhan* and *fu*) and their interconnections. Each element controls or restrains a particular set of organs, and the occurrence of diseases or pathological changes in organs and tissues is said to involve disorders in the mutual control elements.

The Chinese theorized that by knowing which element is associated with each organ, it would be possible to apply acupuncture at the exact foci on meridian channels controlled by those elements to exert either a synergetic or counteracting action on the organs. The results of such treatment is dose-dependent, depending on the duration and frequency of the stimulation.

The Origin of Acupuncture Therapy and Its Early Experiments

According to the archaeological findings in China, acupuncture originated in the prehistoric Stone Age Era, long before any written records existed. Primitive commune society had no knowledge of medicine or the use of herbs. As an automatic reflex to pain, people would press their fingers on the injured area for temporary relief. Subsequently, they found that using a sharp stone was more effective—a skill that some experts think may have been learned from observing wild animals in their surroundings (2). News of successful experiences with the technique was passed from person to person, from father to son and grandson, and then spread from tribe to tribe either orally or by factual exhibition. This was not only beneficial to the people but also a way to preserve the knowledge for later generations.

By the New Stone Age, approximately eight thousand years ago, men had mastered the technique of grinding stone and begun to manufacture different utensils and tools to meet their particular needs. Stones sharpened into a needle shape were used to perforate furuncles and clean putrefied tissue. The Blan Shi was one such needlelike stone being used in that period. Figure 2-3 shows a Blan Shi that was excavated in Inner Mongolia, dating back approximately eight thousand years; similar stones have also been found in China's Shangtong Province.

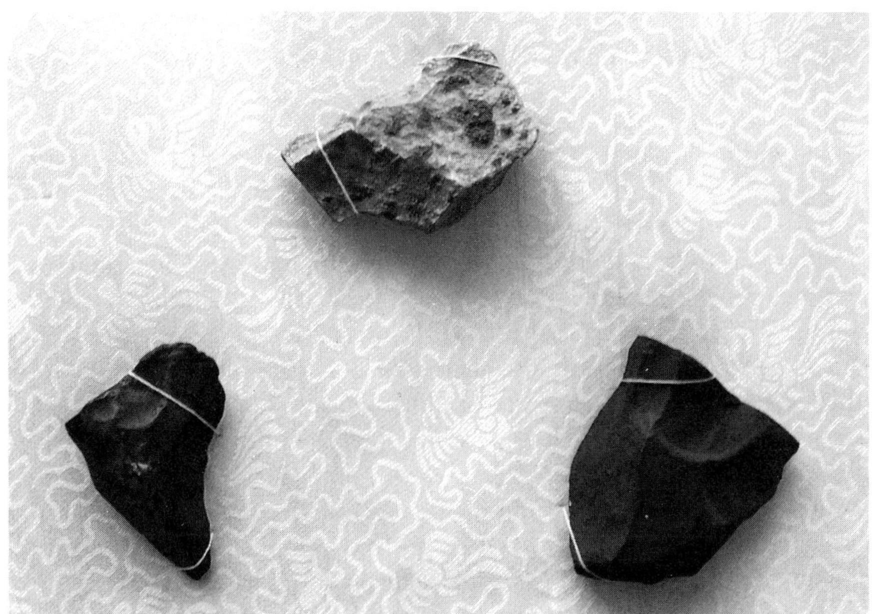

Figure 2-3. The Blan Shi (Evacuated from a Tomb Located in Inner Mongolia, China)

Blan Shi is not the only evidence of the early origins of acupuncture. Other archaeological findings in China show that needles made of other materials were also used in prehistoric times, such as the pottery Tao Zhen and the bone Giu Zhen.

It is believed that acupuncture originated from tribespeople who husbanded horses and cattle in northern China. Due to the cold climate and their habit of eating raw meat, the people frequently suffered from indigestion and abdominal pains. They found that warming themselves near fire reduced their suffering greatly. Recognizing the healing value of heat, they learned to treat pain through thermal stimulation, initiating the method of heat massage and heated stones to pierce the skin. This was the beginning of the practice of moxibustion.

But a systematic practice of acupuncture did not develop until after 2697 B.C., when Huang Ti, the famed Yellow Emperor, ascended to the Chinese throne. Huang Ti is said to have discussed methods of diagnosis and the treatment of ailments with his administrative advisors, Gi Po and Lei Kung; these advisors were probably scholars as well as politicians, well versed in medicine and philosophy. Huang Ti and his advisors taught medical practitioners how to perform acupuncture techniques and developed an elaborate science to explain the mechanisms of action. They introduced the term *Chien Loh,* or the channels of meridian and collaterals, whereby acupuncture effects are transmitted.

These teachings were recorded in writing by unknown authors nearly two thousand years later, around 100 B.C., in the *Huang Ti Nei Chian,* or the *Yellow Emperor's Classic of Internal Medicine.* The *Nei Chian* contains 162 chapters in eighteen volumes and is divided into two parts: the "Su Wen" section, "Questions and Answers," and the "Ning Chiu" section, known commonly as "Needle Classic." This latter section discusses the theory of Chien-Loh, or meridians and collaterals as used in the practice of acupuncture in diagnosis and treatment. The original version of the *Nei Chian* contained nine volumes for each section; a newer, more popular edition divides the "Su Wen" into twenty-four volumes and the "Ning Chiu" into twenty volumes.

Figure 2-5 shows a page in volume 1 of the "Ning Chiu" that discusses the use of needles. Here the Yellow Emperor tells his advisor Gi Po:

> It sorrows me to see my people living in great hardship and suffering all kinds of ailments. To treat their diseases, I will not depend on herbs, nor on the Blan Shi. Instead, I intend to use a fine metal needle to pierce into the body and open up the obstructed Chien Mah [the meridian and pulse], harmonizing the Qi with the blood and bringing the body's balance back into equilibrium. . . . .

The "Ning Chiu" is considered by most Chinese scholars to be the foundation of acupuncture, dealing explicitly with the theory and technique of that practice. It classifies the uses of acupuncture according to types of ailments with clear, precise description and systematically assembles knowledge of acupuncture, summarizing the theory and its clinical practice based on prior experiences. It has contributed greatly to the study of health and medicine in China for thousands of years.

Further studies on acupuncture were supposedly included in a book titled *Huang Ti Nan Chien,* or the *Yellow Emperor's Difficult Classics.* That work has been lost but is referred to by other writings of the same and later periods.

After the Era of the Yellow Emperor, China gradually moved into a feudal society, in which the social structure was relatively stable. For several hundred years there was no war or famine. The economy grew steadily larger and more affluent. Peace and prosperity made life easy, and people had more time to devote to scholarly activities. They paid more attention to their personal welfare and longevity, actively pursuing various means of sustaining and enjoying life.

This was the time of the Sha, Shang, and Zhou Dynasties (circa 2,000 to 400 B.C.), in transition to the Bronze Age. Utensils of copper and bronze have been found from this era, including bronze acupuncture needles. However, the stone Blan Shi was still the major tool for treating disease at this time, as metal remained too precious for widespread use. Also, a needle made by animal bone was widely used (see figure 2–6).

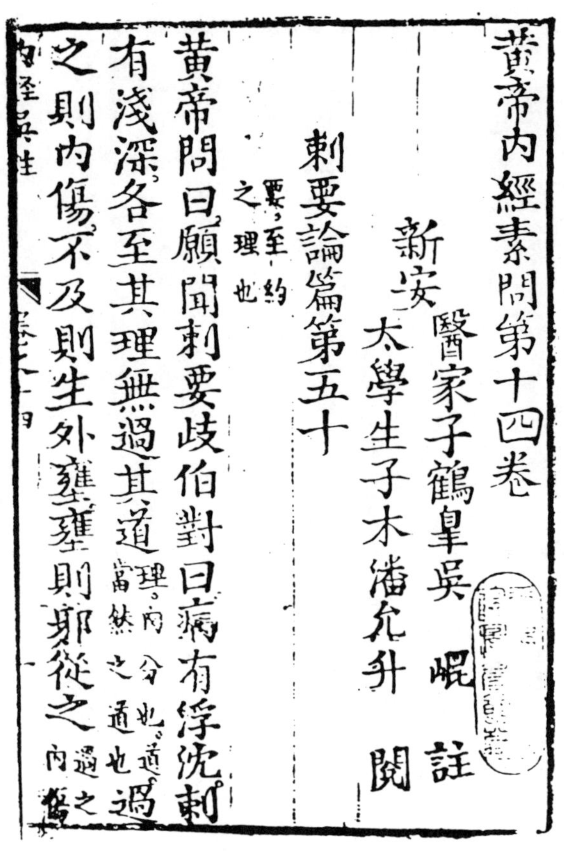
黃帝內經素問第十四卷

新安 醫家子鶴皋吳崐 註
太學生子木潘允升 閱

刺要論篇第五十 要，至約之理也

黃帝問曰：願聞刺要。岐伯對曰：病有浮沈，刺有淺深，各至其理，無過其道。理，內分也。道，當然之通也。過之則內傷，不及則生外壅，壅則邪從之。過之內傷

Figure 2-4. A Page from "Su Wen" of *Huang Ti Nei Chian*

Translation: *Huang Ti Nei Chian,* "Su Wen," vol. 14

Sen-An:
Physician Scholar Wu Kon of Schor-Fun edited
Scholar Pun Yuen-sin of Jie-Moo checked

Chapter 50: "The Importance of Puncture"

Q. (Huang Ti): I would like to learn the importance of puncture.

A. (Gi Po): Illness can be mild or severe, puncture can be shallow or deep. Each has to be applied according to its cause, should not be overdosaged nor underdosaged. Overdosage will injure the internal, underdosage will let the invasion from the outside, resulting in a stagnation and followed by disease . . .

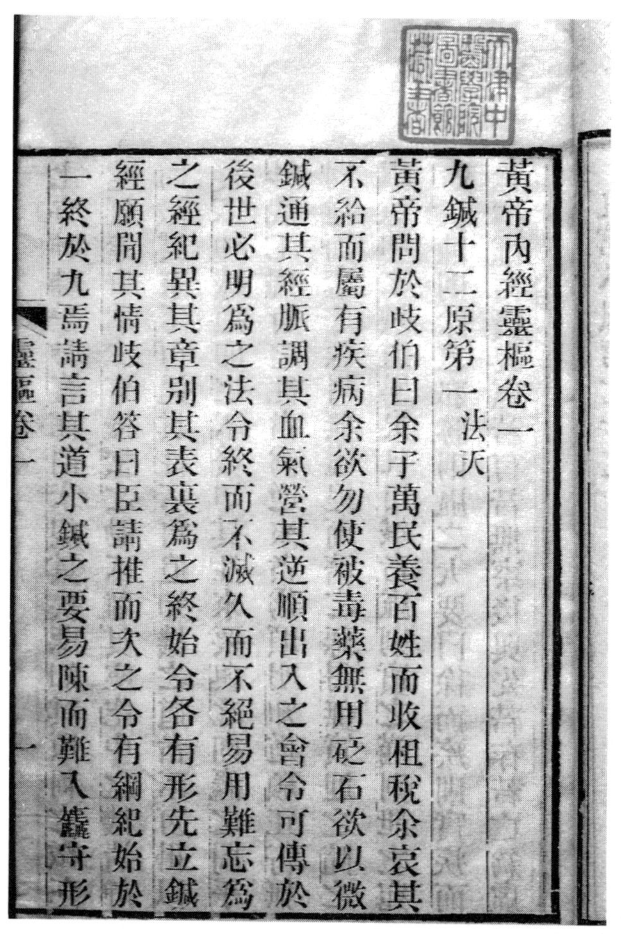

黃帝內經靈樞卷一
九鍼十二原第一 法天
黃帝問於岐伯曰余子萬民養百姓而收租稅余哀其
不給而屬有疾病余欲勿使被毒藥無用砭石欲以微
鍼通其經脈調其血氣營其逆順出入之會令可傳於
後世必明爲之法令終而不滅久而不絕易用難忘爲
之經紀異其章別其表裏爲之終始令各有形先立鍼
經願聞其情岐伯答曰臣請推而次之令有綱紀始於
一終於九焉請言其道小鍼之要易陳而難入麤守形

靈樞卷一　一

Figure 2-5. A Page from "Ning Chiu" ("Needle Classic") of *Huang Ti Nei Chian*

Translation: *Huang Ti Nei Chian,* "Ning Chiu," vol. 1

"Nine Needle Twelve Origins" Chapter 1 (Fa-Tien)

Huang Ti asked Gi Po: I govern my constituents and tax the population. I sorrow over their insufficiency and poor health. I wish not to use the toxic herbs, nor the Blan Shi, using a small needle to open the meridian and circulation, to regulate the blood and Qi, counter the hostile and make my patient recover quickly.

I would like to transfer this method to my next generations; it would not be forgotten and will be kept permanently.

To begin with, I would write the "Needle Classic" first and want to know the details.

Gi Po answered: Let me expand the subjects and classify them from one to nine. First I would like to talk about the small needle and how it would get into the Ning (the essence) . . .

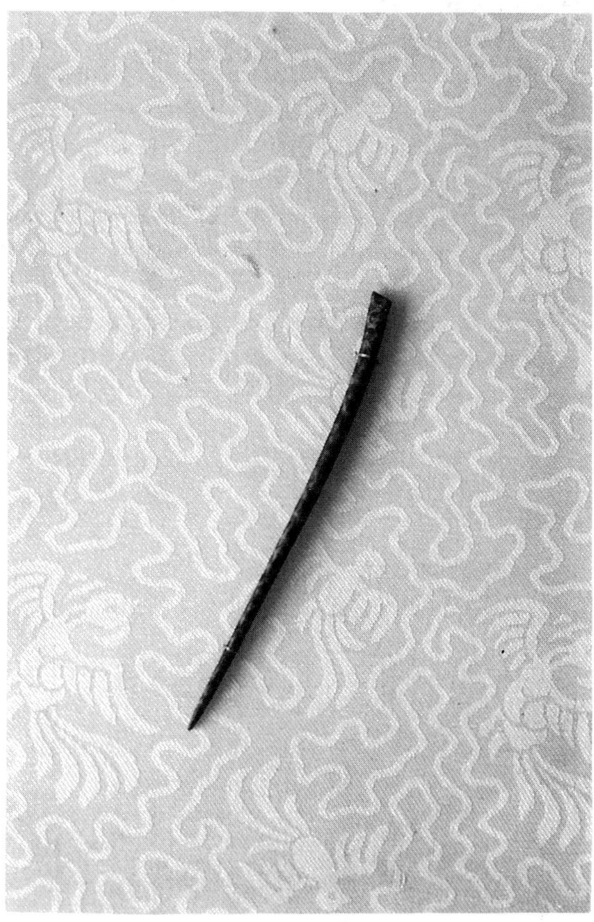

Figure 2-6. The Bone Needle (Evacuated from a Tomb in Zhou Hou Din, China)

By the end of the Bronze Age, the Chinese had accumulated much knowledge of medicine and health protection, and a number of important writings on acupuncture and medicine were handed down. The Chinese began to recognize the differences between medical treatment and witchcraft—the former being an art of healing based on experience and practice, while the latter was couched in superstition and mystic rites. A famous physician of the late Bronze Age/early Iron Age, Pin Choi (407–310 B.C.), was particularly vigorous in denouncing the use of witchcraft to treat illnesses, advocating more scientific methods. Knowledge of medicine, including acupuncture, was preached energetically and advanced rapidly among both the scholarly aristocracy and the common people.

It is believed that the doctrine of Yin and Yang and the philosophy of the five elements were first established in this period. For the first time medicine was explained in terms of "the harmonization of the body in Heaven and Earth." Man's pulse, blood, spirit, and mental state were discussed avidly by scholars, and various concepts of Chinese natural philosophy were developed, including Qi and Fon ("wind"). Notable scholars and medical practitioners mastered the techniques of acupuncture and moxibustion for use in healing. For example, the famed veterinarian Sun Yang, or Sun Pai-loh, practiced acupuncture on horses and cattle, recording his experiences in *Pai-loh's Needle Classic.*

The Theory and Practice of Acupuncture

Between 475 and 24 B.C., Chinese culture advanced to the Iron Age. People learned how to utilize fire and high temperatures to purify iron and apply alchemic techniques to make alloys. Metal implements became more common, and the stone Blan Shi was replaced by needles made from iron, silver, or gold. Acupuncture therapy advanced rapidly as the method of choice in treating many diseases; the application of the nine needles described in the "Ning Chiu" was expanded substantially. Moxibustion also became a formalized technique, with the burning of a "moxa wool" in the form of a cone or stick, to be applied on certain acupoints. These techniques were possibly used a long time ago by the caveman who placed heat directly on the area where the pain was located.

Figure 2-7 shows a copy of Nine Needle illustrated in the book of Ning Chiu.

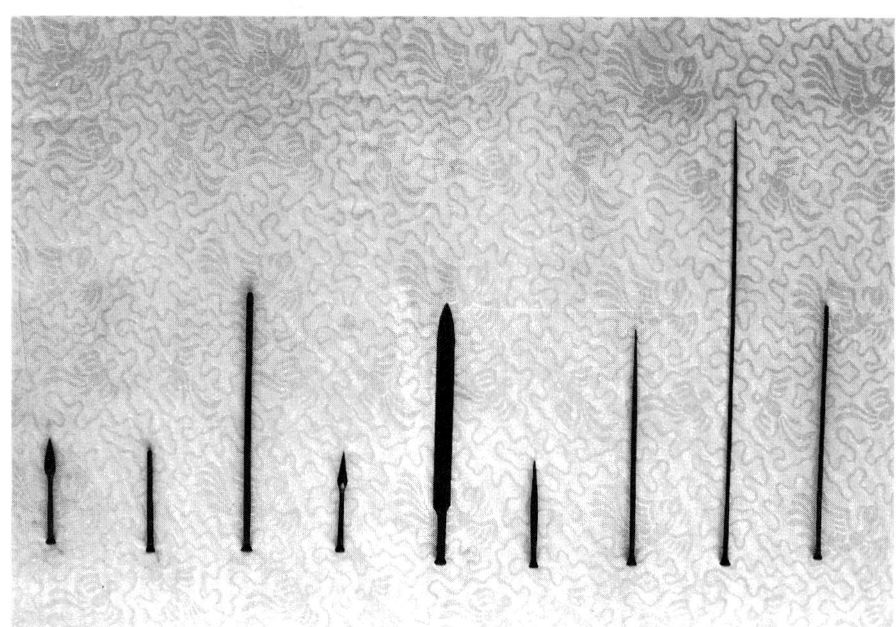

Figure 2-7. The Nine Needles (From "Ning Chiu" of Huang Ti Nei Chian)

Ironically, while years of peace allowed the initial development of acupuncture techniques, war provided the impetus for further development in the theory and application of that art. China witnessed a period of almost constant warfare between 475 and 24 B.C., as powerful warlords battled for control of the country. War was followed by hardship and diseases, and the study of acupuncture advanced rapidly as physicians were called on to treat a wider range of ailments.

The *Si Gi,* written by See Ma Chin during the Han Dynasty, reports that Pin Choi's chief successes in healing patients occurred during his travels around China in the service of first one warlord and then another. Pin Choi employed a variety of healing techniques, including decoctions of herbs, massage, acupuncture, and thermal acupuncture with burning sticks. The *Si Gi* also noted the work of Chuen Yu-Yi (circa 180 B.C.), an acupuncture specialist who recorded twenty-five medical cases with detailed names, addresses, symptoms, date of treatment, and the kind of herbs or acupuncture used in each case; these are considered to be the earliest medical records known to man.

From A.D.265 to 581, China was engaged in civil war, and the people starved as they fled from the path of battle. Acupuncture was deemed to be the simplest and most convenient form of medical treatment, requiring no elaborate setups and thus ideal for physicians forced to practice in temporary shelters. One physician of the time, Guo Hong, wrote a book titled *Emergency Treatment with Acupuncture,* which summarized many of his experiences. Other writings from the same period include the *Atlas of Ming Tong Acupuncture,* by Hsu Hi, which describes the exact location of each acupoint, and a six-volume work titled *Techniques for Pacifying the Sick,* by Gar Si-shi, in which the veterinary use of acupuncture and heat cauterization are first mentioned.

History has passed down references to many other writings on acupuncture, nearly all of which were lost during the wars. The 1973 evacuation of the No.3 Ma Wang Tu Han's tomb in Changsha, Hunan Province, brought to light several scrolls dated back to around 250 B.C., during the Qin Dynasty. Among these were two descriptions of the lost *Chien Mah,* or *Classics on Pulse,* reflecting the scope and thinking of early Chinese scholars on medicine and natural science.

The wars subsided somewhat during the East Han and Three Kingdoms Era (A.D.15–265), and the teaching and theory of acupuncture were expanded. Among the most important endeavors of this time was the work of Huang Fu-mi (A.D.215–282). Huang Fu-mi revised the *Huang Ti Nei Chian* into a more readable format, combining it with information from the *Management of Min Ton Acupuncture and Therapy* to elaborate techniques, and eliminated erroneous data. The resulting work clarified the principles of acupuncture in easy to understand terms and simplified the techniques. Huang Fu-mi's book, *Acupuncture ABCs,* also brought together the basic theories of traditional Chinese medicine and acupuncture, formulating a unique system. The *Acupuncture ABCs* contains twelve volumes, a total of 128 chapters, and is classfied according to "Zhan-Fu", "Qi and Blood," "Chien-Loh," "Shue-Yue," "Pulse and Diagnosis," "Technique of Acupuncture and Moxibustion," and "Clinical Applications." This work is still in use by acupuncturists and scholars as one of the chief reference materials on the subject. It raised the standing of Huang Ti Ming Tong acupuncturology, influencing the future understanding and development of acupuncture greatly (4, 5, 6, and 7).

Prosperity and peace reigned once again during the Tsuai and Tang Dynasties (A.D.580–906). During this time, the Tsuai emperor appointed the physician Tin Yuen to head a committee for the task of revising the *Atlas of Ming Tong Acupuncture.* The committee collected records of the clinical experiences of outstanding physicians and practitioners of past centuries, drawing one of the earliest colored atlases on acupuncture in Chinese history. This atlas was named the *Ming Tong Three Persons Atlas* but was, unfortunately, lost over the years.

In the same period, Sun Si Yi wrote *The Thousand Major Recipes Used for Emergency* and *The Thousand Accessory Recipes.* Yang Shan-shin's *Huang Ti Nei Chian Ming Tong* was a revision of acupuncture technique based on Huang Ti Ming Tong studies.

The writings on veterinary medicine are included in *Collection of Si Ma An's Cattle,* by Li Shi, and *The Atlas of Acupoint Nominations, Atlas of Po-Loh's Moxibustion and Cauterization Techniques, and Song and Poem on Moxibustion and Cauterization,* by other authors.

It was also during the early Tang Dynasty that the practice of acupuncture was raised to high honor. The imperial court created ranks of "Master of Acupuncture" and "Master of Moxibustion" to honor specialists in these professions. The court also established a commission to govern medical education in four fields of medicine as well as in herbal lore and apothecary sciences; acupuncture was one of the four branches of medicine recognized. Subsequently, the commission recommended the adoption of additional ranks for physicians, including "Doctor of Acupuncture," "Assistant in Acupuncture," "Master of Acupuncture," "Aide in Acupuncture," and "Apprentice in Acupuncture."

Expansion of Acupuncture Practice and Schools of Thought

During the period known as the Five Nations Era and the Yuan and Ming Dynasties (A.D.907–1636), the invention of the printing press helped to preserve literature and historic records. Dissemination of knowledge in the fields of medicine and acupuncture was facilitated and subsequently exported to surrounding Asian countries; Chinese texts on acupuncture were also found as far distant as India and Eastern Europe.

Other aspects of the acupuncture technique were enhanced during this time. Under the auspices of the governments, Wang Wei-E (A.D.987–1067) revised the *Huang Ti Ming Tong* and wrote a new text titled *An Illustrated Manual of Acupoints Using Bronze Figures,* which was designed to accompany bronze figures indicating acupoint locations. Engraved on these full-size bronze models of the human body were the location of the 361 acupoints and the fourteen meridians. Inside the models were shown the solid organs (*zhan*) and the viscerals (*fu*). The bronze models were used chiefly for teaching and examining purposes.

Three hundred years later, during the Southern Song Dynasty, Wong Gi-chong wrote an important work titled *A Classic of Acupuncture and Its Uses for Sustaining Life,* which unified the theory and teaching of the Chien-Loh doctrine and the principle of acupoint location. Subsequently, during the Yuan Dynasty, Wah Shou (A.D. 1304–86) published *An Exposition of Fourteen Meridians,* which further interpreted the ideas and practices of the *Huang Ti Ming Tong's* theory on meridians and collaterals. Wah was also the first physician known to identify and diagnose measles (although it was not known at that time that it was the result of a viral infection) by spotting a bluish-white spot that appeared on the mouth mucosa (1).

It was at this time that a number of schools of thought arose to debate various philosophies and interpretations of acupunctural practices. The classic school of *Huang Ti Ming Tong* practices was represented by Wang Wei-E and Wah Shou; the Pin Choi school of thought was represented by Hsu Hi of the Song Dynasty; and the "Ancient and Present Conciliatory" school was represented by Wong Gi-chong. In addition, there were groups specifically interested in acupuncture methods (Jia Hong of the South Song Dynasty), groups interested in moxibustion (Tao Shao of South Song Dynasty), groups interested specifically on the precise location and chronology of acupoints selection (He Yao-Yu and Yan Kong-Ming of the Jiang Dynasty), and groups interested in the anatomy of acupuncture (Yang Gai and Zheng Gi of the Song Dynasty). Refinement of acupuncture techniques led to such diverse practices as Tao Han's idea of the need to apply pressure on an exact acupoint at an exact time in order to achieve optimal effect, to Ma Tine Yang's studies on a few important foci for treatment of all ailments.

The rivalry between these schools reached their peak during the Ming Dynasty (A.D. 1368–1644). For example, the actual physical maneuver used to apply acupuncture needles evolved into twenty different types of applications, involving complex multiple steps. Studies of moxibustion also increased, with competing techniques ranging from the use of moxa cones versus simple sticks, lukewarm heat versus burning, and "Thunder Fire" needling versus "Tia-Yao" needling.

It was during this period that the number of acupoints increased tremendously. Each practitioner who considered himself an expert in the subject attempted to propose new acupoints as a means of promoting his own expertise, adding to the body of work on the technique. By the time Wah Shou published *An Exposition of the Fourteen Meridians,* the total number of acupoints had nearly doubled, to 647!

The use of acupuncture in veterinary medicine developed in parallel during this period. Wang Yue wrote a book titled *A Collection of Recipes in Treating Cattle,* which devoted one chapter to uses of acupuncture, while Yu Bo-yuen and Yu Bo-han wrote *The Yuen Hang Complete Atlas of Cows, Horses, and Camels,* in which acupuncture and moxibustion application on domestic animals was discussed; in the latter, symptoms and various diseases observed in cows, horses, and camels were discussed, together with types of medication and acupuncture techniques necessary for healing. Other writings included *Ming Tong and Moxibustion Techniques for Horses* and *A Discussion on Healing Cattle,* which concentrated on the methods of acupuncture and moxibustion.

The Decline of Traditional Medicine

The practice of traditional Chinese medicine ebbed during the Chin Dynasty (A.D.1657–1911), as the imperial court fell under Western influences. Acupuncture was viewed as a superstition, and the Royal Medical College closed down its Department of Acupuncture in 1822; the practice of acupuncture was banned. After the Opium War of 1844, Western medicine became particularly prevalent in China.

But the official ban on acupuncture did not stop the common people from continuing to seek out the services of acupuncturists. To the rage of the imperial court, scholars and acupuncture experts established a society that published manuscripts and journals on the subject, thus underscoring the government's increasingly poor control of the country. These acts of rebellion built a foundation for the education of future acupuncturists, preserving the historical origins of the field and introducing its techniques to the West. In 1899, *Eastern and Western Concepts on the Bronzeman's Atlas* was published by Liu Chong-han, representing the first Chinese work to promote scientific interchange between Eastern and Western medicine.

The Chin Dynasty was overthrown in 1911 in a revolution led by Dr. Sun Yat-sen, a Western-educated physician. Chinese traditional medicine and acupuncture fell into greater disfavor under the Kou Ming Tong regime. The only noteworthy writing on acupuncture to come out of that period was Tong Shi-chin's *Investigation of Electro-acupuncture* (1934), which was the first evidence that the Chinese have made use of electrical stimulation in acupuncture therapy.

A New Renaissance

Years of war soon resumed, first with the fight between the Kou Ming Tong and the Communists, followed by the Japanese invasion of China and World War II. As a representative of the common people, the Communist army promoted traditional medicine and acupuncture, reversing earlier bans. Many Western-trained physicians who espoused the Communist cause came to join the traditional acupuncturists, learning the technique and using it to treat their patients.

In 1945, an acupuncture clinic was opened in the Bethune International Peace Hospital in the city of Yen-An—wartime headquarters of the Communist government—a first step toward the actual integration of traditional Western medicines. In 1947, the Health Department of Jenan Territory issued a manuscript on practical Acupuncturology, while the School of Public Health of the Health Department of North China People's Government added classes in acupuncture to their curriculum.

After the 1949 revolutionary victory, the new government began to reemphasize the importance of traditional medicine and acupuncture. The number of studies of acupuncture increased overwhelmingly, and the stature of acupuncturists was raised to that of other professionals. Between 1951 and 1955, the central government established several acupuncture institutes and research laboratories to study the field. Local provincial governments also established research institutes, while most Western-style hospitals in China set up separate departments and wards for acupuncture practice. All traditional Chinese medical colleges now include a Department of Acupuncture, offering both master's and Ph.D. degrees in acupuncture. Even the Western-styled medical colleges list acupuncture in their curricula and research.

It continues to be a priority of the Chinese government to restore the practice of acupuncture as an inherent part of the Chinese heritage while promoting modern scientific studies of the basic mechanisms of action. Over the last forty years, a tremendous volume of clinical data on acupuncture therapy has accumulated, showing the efficacy of its action as a form of natural therapy that does not interfere with normal physiological functions. In recent years, the technique has been extended into the fields of anesthesia, electro-acupuncture (EAP), laser irradiation, electromagnetism, and microwave irradiation.

The field of acupuncture has itself been categorized into separate areas of scientific investigation. A few of these include the medical history of acupuncture, the meridianology, the science of acupoints, the science of acupuncture and moxibustion, diagnosis by meridians, acupuncture prescription and acupuncture therapeutics, acupuncture anesthesiology, practical acupuncture dosimetry, and microcirculation in acupuncture. Clearly, this ancient science has been inaugurated into a new scientific field, advancing in modern technology. It no longer lies in obscurity or isolation.

Toward an International Science

Chinese acupuncture technology began to spread to other parts of Asia during the sixth century A.D. In A.D. 541, Emperor Liang Mu-ti sent a delegation of medical practitioners and technicians to Po-Chi, the ruler of Korea, who subsequently established a school to train acupuncturists. Twenty-one years later, the emperor sent a copy of the "Ning Chiu," the "Needle Classic," to Japanese emperor Yin-ming. Gi-chong of Jiangsu Province traveled to Japan to teach medicine, bringing with him 164 volumes of medical literature, including the *Ming Tong Atlas*. At the same time, Japan sent several delegations to China to study the traditional Chinese medicine, including acupuncture, establishing a special commission on acupuncture. Both Japan and Korea have since assimilated Chinese medicine, including acupuncture, into their own traditional culture and systems.

During the eighth to tenth centuries, a commercial route was opened between Southwest Asia and the Persian Gulf. Chinese seapower was at its peak at this time. As a result, Chinese medical literature, including pulse diagnosis and *materia medica*, were translated into Arabic. In addition, Chinese practitioners were invited to Vietnam to treat the royal family, with such great success that the Chinese were called "angel physicians" by the Vietnamese.

In the Western world, acupuncture was not known until the sixeenth century. It was first brought in as a kind of folk medicine, treated chiefly as an Oriental curiosity. The first serious Western study on acupuncture occurred in 1671, when the Reverend Father Harview published a treatise titled *Les Secrets de la Medicine des Chinois*. Other works soon followed, including a 1683 dissertation written by William Rhye, a physician attached to the Dutch East Indian Company, and a German book by Engelbert Kampfer.

For a brief while in the nineteenth century, acupuncture enjoyed wide acceptance and popularity among the French. The Academie des Sciences appointed a commission to study the field, and many famous French clinicians devoted considerable time to investigating the subject. Later, during the early twentieth century, interest was revived by the writing of George Soulie de Morant, who spent twenty years as a diplomat in China and observed the treatments of Chinese patients by acupuncture. Although not a physician himself, he was convinced that acupuncture held great value for the West. Upon returning to France, he published *A Synopsis of the True Chinese Acupuncture* (1934) and the two-volume work *L'acupuncture Chinoise* (1939). These books inspired the widespread use of major hospitals and clinics and promoted formal teaching and research in acupuncture at French medical schools. De Morant is generally credited with igniting a renaissance in the field of acupuncture in the West.

The international exchange of information on acupuncture increased tremendously after the 1949 Communist Revolution in China. Cooperation between Communist Bloc countries included ideas on science and medicine, and acupuncture became more widely used in Eastern Europe and the Soviet Union. The non-Communist world became more aware of the technique after the resumption of diplomatic relations between the United States and China, with acupuncture moving into the limelight during U.S. President Richard Nixon's historic 1972 visit.

Public reaction to acupuncture ranged from wholehearted enthusiasm to extreme skepticism. By this time, Western medicine had advanced substantially in its understanding of the cellular pathophysiology of the human body and the molecular biochemical phenomena of regulatory and defense mechanism. Because of this knowledge, many medical professionals rejected the validity of acupuncture, deploring the mystic philosophy surrounding the practice. Others, however, chose to apply Western scientific knowledge and methods to the understanding of acupuncture, producing a number of interesting research works. One such work was a two-volume German manuscript titled *Deutsche Zeitschrift für Akupunktur*, published in 1974; this book documented the scientific foundation of acupuncture techniques, pushing its application into new territory.

Acupuncture has begun to receive more international acceptance. Upon the recommendation of the World Health Organization (WHO), training programs in acupuncture were established in the Chinese cities of Beijing, Shanghai, and Nanking, open to students from all nations. Recently, formal Departments of Acupuncture and Moxibustion were set up in all traditional Chinese medical colleges, to educate and train thousands of specialists in the uses of acupuncture as a healing tool. International conferences and symposia have been held in many different countries over the last decade for the presentation and discussion of experimental and clinical data on acupuncture.

These forums have advanced our current knowledge of acupuncture substantially. This ancient art of healing has marched into a new era of scientific accomplishment, helping to strip away prejudices and ignorance of the technique, both within China and in the rest of the world.

References

1. Chen, Sui-lou. The Renowned Medical Physicians and Scholars in China (in Chinese). Jiangsu: Jiangsu Science Technology Publisher, Jiangsu, 1987.
2. Cowen, R. Medicine on the Wild Side. Science News 138:288, 1990.
3. Needham, J., et al. Clerks and Craftmen in China and the World. London: Cambridge University Press, 1970, p. 263.
4. Shi, S. M., ed. The Miraculous Technique of Acupuncture and Moxibustion (in Chinese). Tianjin: Tianjin Science and Technology Publisher, 1992.
5. Tang, D. A. Practical Acupuncture. Tianjin: (in Chinese)Tianjin Science and Technology Publisher, 1985.
6. Wang, S. T. A Brief History of Chinese Acupuncture (in Chinese). Acupuncture Research 9(3):161, 1984.
7. Wei, L. Y., from Kao, F. F., and J. J. Kao,eds. Recent Advances in Acupuncture Research. Garden City, NY: Institute for Advanced Research in Asian Science and Medicine, 1979, p.49.

3

Doctrine of Meridians

Chinese folklore holds that the practice of acupuncture originated with Huang Ti, the famed Yellow Emperor, who was thought to have ruled in 2697 B.C. He was the direct heir of the emperor Shen Nung, the Divine Plowman, who was thought to have developed herbal medicine. Huang Ti is credited not only with the institution of extensive civil laws in China, but with the invention of the rickshaw and a system of musical notes and the creation of many classic Chinese music instruments. Most important, he and his chief minister are credited with formulating many principles of anatomy and medicine that continue to be the basis for much of traditional Chinese medical practice even today.

When Huang Ti discussed methods of diagnosis and treatment of ailments, he introduced the term *Chien-Loh,* or *channels of meridians and collaterals. Chien* can be translated as "a longitudinal line," while *Loh* represents a transverse line. These lines were thought to connect the external surface and the internal organs of the human body. In all, there are twelve Chien, or meridians, plus two extra meridians along the midline of the chest and vertebrae. Through these, communication and coordination of the functions between the internal organs are established.

These statements appeared in the book *Huang Ti Nei Chian,* or the *Yellow Emperor's Classic of Internal Medicine,* written more than two thousand years after Huang Ti by unknown authors, around 100 B. C. The *Nei Chian* contains 162 chapters in eighteen volumes. It is divided into two parts—a section on "questions and answers, and the "Ning Chiu," or the well-known "Needle Classic." The "Ning Chiu" includes eighty chapters, fifty five of which involve topics on needles and the basic principles and fundamental applications of acupuncture. Here the term *Chien-Loh* was used to describe a means of transporting both *blood and Qi*—the physical nourishment and the vital energy of life. It also functions as a means of regulating Yin and Yang in the body, moistening the sinuses and bones and benefiting the joints (8).

As early as 300–200 B.C., during the Qin Dynasty, the Chinese learned much about human anatomy through the autopsies on executed prisoners, and the "Ning Chiu" includes certain descriptions of human anatomy. The work does not in any way suggest, however that the Chien-Loh represents any specific anatomic structures, tissues, vessels, or nerves. The "Ning-Chiu" discusses the circulation of blood and Qi, but the physiology of circulation and the functions of the brain and nerves were not understood. The term *Chien-Loh,* or *channel of meridians,* was used only to explain how abnormalities of the inner organs can be treated from the outside through the meridians.

The Chien-Loh doctrine suggests that our bodies contain certain circulatory pathways, the Chien, which have their own direction of circulation. Through anastomoses of Loh, these Chien communicate with each other. This establishes a correlation between one meridian and another, allowing interaction between the functions of different organs. From these, a complementary relationship of the outside and the inside can be expressed through the circulation of Qi.

The concept of Chien-Loh is based on the ancient idea that all matter can be divided into Yin and Yang, which are complements. Yin and Yang can each be divided into three types, which are identified by their strength of Yin Qi and Yang Qi. The strongest Yin Qi is Tai Yin, or Greater Yin;

the next is Xiao Yin, or Lesser Yin; and the weakest is Jui Yin, meaning Final Yin, showing that Yin is at the final state of development, in transition to the Yang phase. The strongest Yang Qi is Yang Ming, or Radiant Yang, the next is Tai Yang, or Greater Yang, and the weakest is Xiao Yang, meaning "lesser Yang."

The six types of Yin and Yang are broadly used in Chinese traditional medicine, in herbal medicine as well as acupuncture. In the doctrine of meridians, the main channels distributed on the flexor side of the upper extremities are called Hand Three Yin, while those distributed on the extensor side are called Hand Three Yang. These are illustrated in figures 3-1 and 3-2. Following the same principle, the Foot Three Yin meridians are lined up on the inside of the lower extremities and the Foot Three Yang meridians are lined up on the extensor side, as illustrated in figures 3-3 and 3-4.

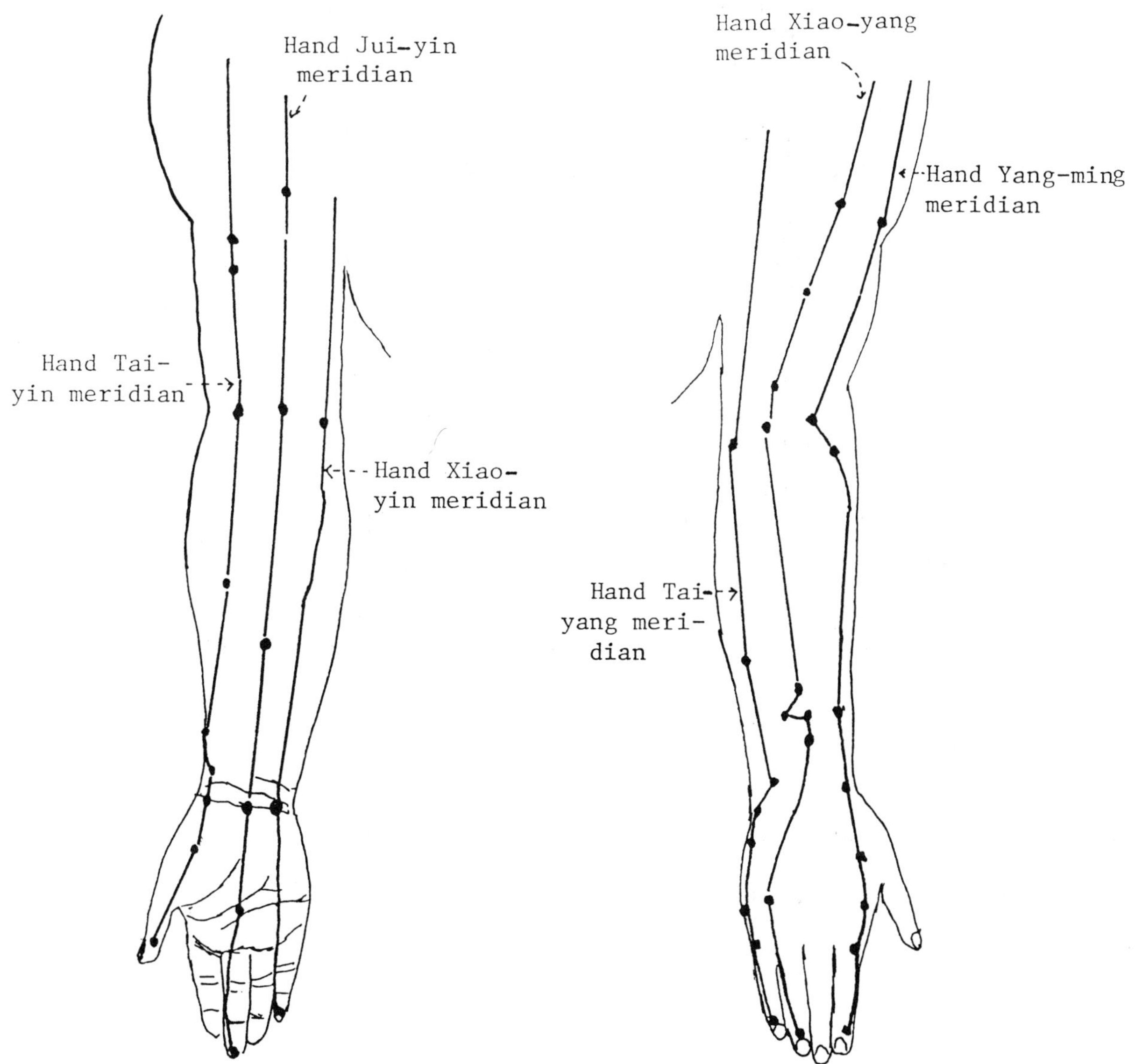

Figure 3-1. The Hand Three Yin Meridians

Figure 3-2. The Hand Three Yang Meridians

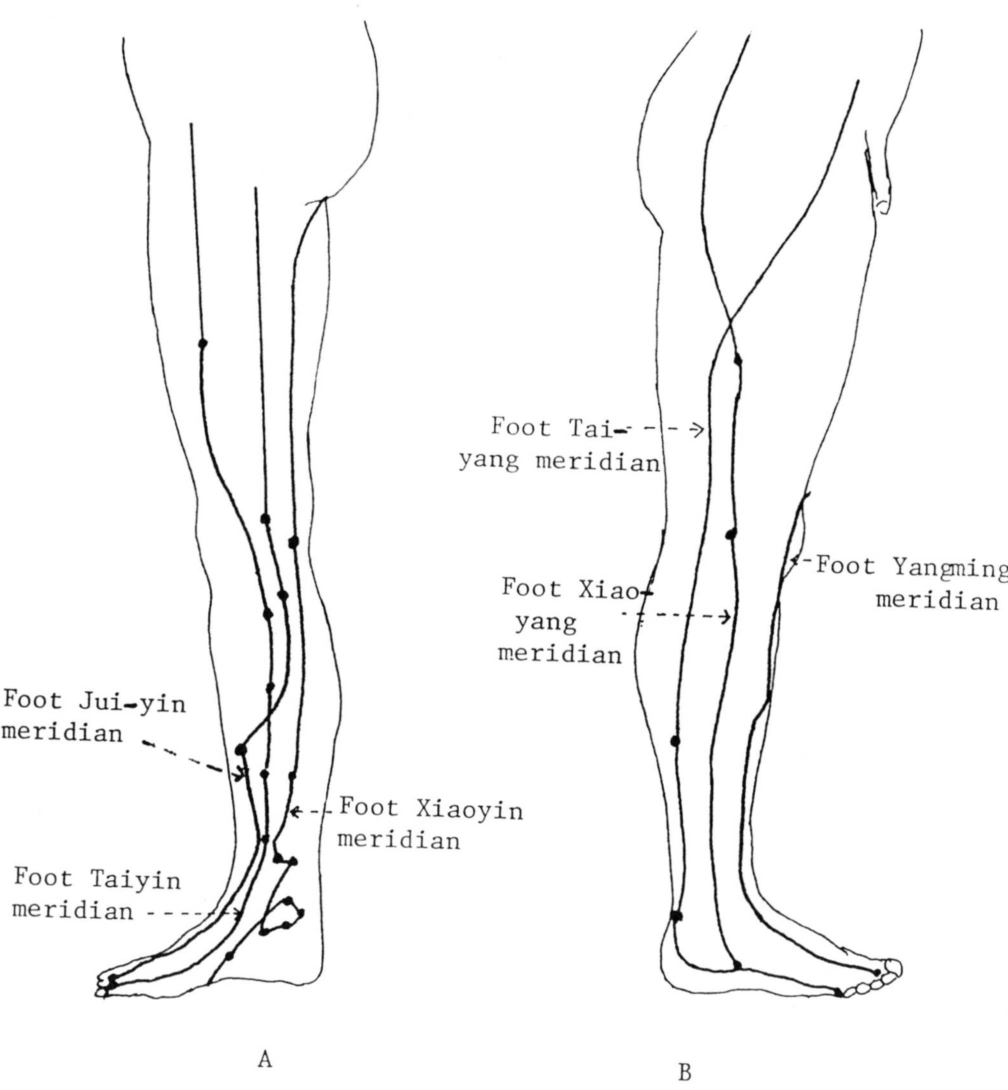

Figure 3-3. A: The Three Foot Yin Meridians

B: The Three Foot Yang Meridians

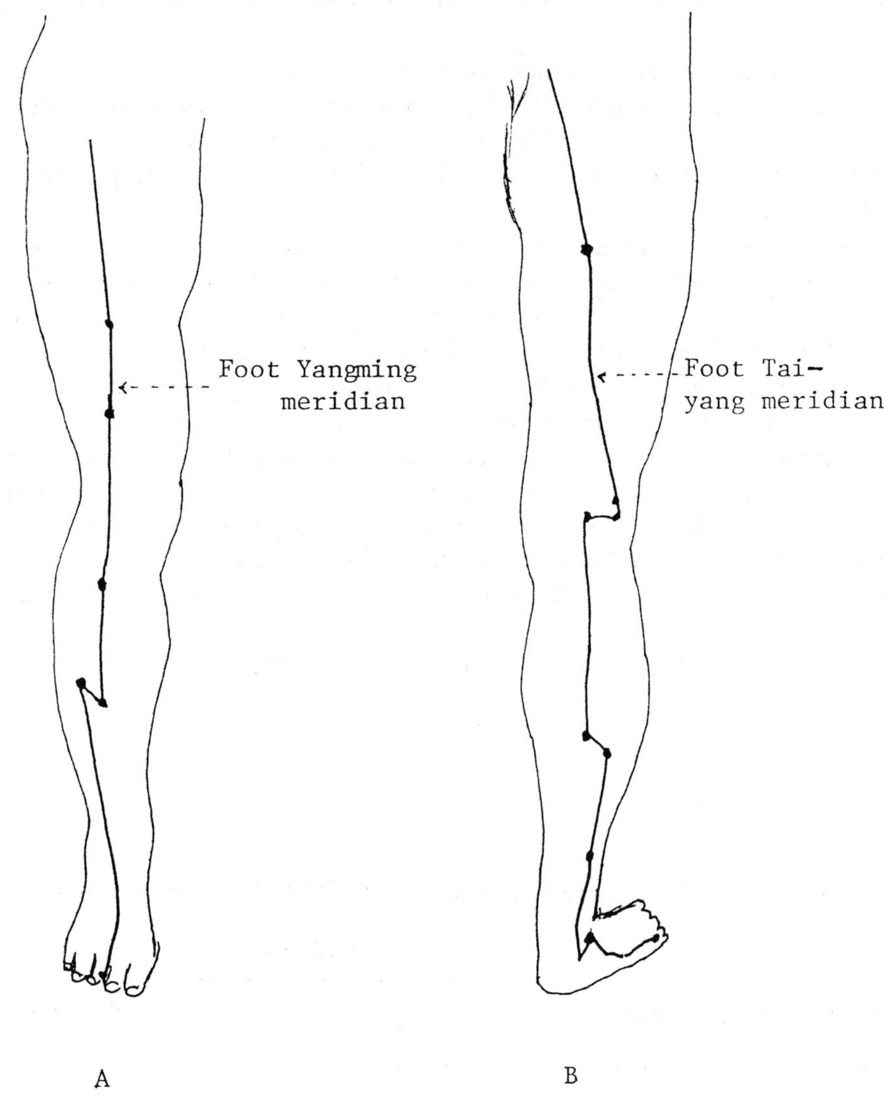

Figure 3-4. A: The Foot Yang-ming Meridians

B: The Foot Tai-Yang Meridian

Each of the main meridians can be divided into internal and external channels. The internal channels are associated with the organs and viscera or, as the Chinese call them, the *zhan and fu*. The external channels are connected to the bones and muscles, via the *yao* or loci. The *yao,* serve as stations on exact areas along the meridian line and send information from the surface to the deep internal structure when stimulated; methods of stimulation of *yao* can include application of a needle, heat, or electric current.

Ten of the twelve main meridians correspond directly with distinct organs within the body, such as the liver or heart. The eleventh, the Hand Jui Yin Chien, corresponds to the pericardium rather than to an organ. The twelfth, the Hand Xiao Yang Chien, is referred to in Chinese as the meridian of the "Triple Burner," corresponding to the viscera of the chest cavity, upper abdomen cavity, and lower abdomen cavity.

In addition to the twelve main meridians, the *Nei Chian* identifies two extra Chien, or meridians, which are alternatively thought to either supplement the primary meridians or control them. Classic acupuncture texts associated the extra Chien with a "governing vessel" or *du* and a "conception vessel" or *ren* in the body. The former was an unidentified organ thought to control bodily processes but was not associated by the Chinese with the brain; the latter may be construed as the reproductive organs. Nowadays, these extra Chien are referred to as the *du* and *ren* meridians.

Table 3-1 summarizes the twelve main meridian channels and their distribution and projection to the organs or viscera that they influence. It has been suggested that meridians affect not only their primary associated organs, but any organs which may be embryologically related (5A). For example, acupuncture treatment along the Foot Lesser Yin can be used for treatment not only of the kidney, but the ovary, testicle, uterus, and fallopian tube—all organs formed in the same region of the embryo.

Table 3-2 gives the detail of distribution area of each meridian and how they project.

Table 3-1. The Internal Association of Each of the Twelve Main Meridians

	Hand Meridian	Foot Meridian
Greater Yin (Tai-yin)	Lung	Spleen
Lesser Yin (Xiao-yin)	Heart	Kidney
Final Yin (Jui-yin)	Pericardium	Liver
Radiant Yang (Yang-ming)	Large intestine	Stomach
Greater Yang (Tai-yang)	Small intestine	Bladder
Lesser Yang (Xiao-yang)	Triple Burner	Gallbladder

Table 3-2. The Distribution and Projection of the Meridians

MERIDIAN		DISTRIBUTION AREA			PROJECTION to:		
		Extremity	Body	Neck	Head	Organ	Viscera
Extra:							
Du			Midline vertebra	middle post. neck	middle	nose, mouch, jaw and eye	brain, spinal cord scrotum
Ren			Midline sternum & abdomen	middle ant. neck	-	eye & mouth	scrotum
Hand Three Yin:							
Hand Taiyin	Upper Extremity	Flexor side, lateral	Chest lateral	-	-	lung	lung, larynx, and intestine
Hand Juiyin	Upper Extremity	Flexor middle	Breast lateral	-	-	-	pericardium, triple burner
Hand Xiaoyin	Upper Extremity	Flexor middle	Axilla	-	-	vision, cardiovascular, pharynx	heart. small intestine
Hand Three Yang:							
Hang Yangming	Upper Extremity	Extensor lateral	Shoulder front	neck front	face	nose & mouth	large intestine lung
Hand Xiaoyang	Upper Extremity	Extensor middle	Shoulder upper	neck, back side	ear back side	eye & ear	triple burner, pericardium
Hand Taiyang	Upper Extremity	Extensor medial	Shoulder lower	neck lateral	ear front	eye, ear, nose and throat	small intestine stomach and heart

Table 3-2. (continued)

Foot Three Yang: Foot Yangming	Lower Extremity	Extensor lateral	Chest abdomen lateral	neck front	face	eye, nose, mouth upper jaw, and breast	stomach, spleen large intestine, small intestine
Foot Xiaoyang		Extensor middle	Lumbar lateral	neck back and lateral	-	eye & ear	gall-bladder, liver
Foot Taiyang		Extensor medial	Lumbar back side	neck back side	head front	eye and nose	urinary bladder, kidney
Foot Three Yin: Foot Taiyin		Leg: inside & medial Thigh: inside & front	Chest, abdomen No. 1 & 2 lateral lines	-	-	triple burner, pharynx	spleen, stomach heart
Foot Hueyin	Lower Extrenutt	Leg: inside & front Thigh: inside & medial	Abdomen, central region	-	-	vision, nose, pharynx, mouth larynx and genital organ	liver, gall-bladder, lung, stomach
Foot Xiaoyin		Leg & thigh: inside & lateral	Chest, abdomen No.1 lateral	-	-	tongue, throat	kidney, urinary bladder, liver, lung, heart, spinal cord

Circulation of Qi and Blood

In the early centuries B.C., the Chinese theorized that blood and Qi are continuously circulated throughout the human body, acting in a state of homeostasis. The meridians serve as the avenues connecting the inner organs with the external surface. This was thought to keep Yin and Yang in balance, thus enabling the body to function in a harmonious state. If the blood and Qi do not circulate properly, the body will experience a tilt to excess or deficit in either Yin or Yang, resulting in sickness in an organ or tissue. Such an illness would either manifest itself on the surface or spread to other organs via connecting meridians. Thus the Chinese thought of the channel of meridians not only as analogous to a communicating system of highways and streets, but as a means for diagnosing illnesses. For centuries, both the Chinese and Japanese have devoted much time to investigating the exact nature of the channel of meridians, attempting to map out a total picture of the connections and anasthomoses between organs and tissues. Table 3-2 shows the ancient Chinese theory of the connections between the twelve pairs of meridians and the two extra *du* and *ren* meridians.

Although ancient Chinese literature frequently made use of the term *blood circulation,* the meridians were never considered to be structurally similar to the blood vessels of the circulatory system. They were described only by function, serving to circulate blood and Qi, nourish the body, regulate the activity of internal organs, and defend against "devilish" invasions. Qi was termed *the jury of life and death, handler of all ailments.* Only the channel of meridians allows the circulation of Qi and blood in the body.

Table 3-3 illustrates the interconnection between the meridians.

Table 3-3. The Interconnection between the Twelve Pairs of Meridians and the Two Extra Meridians

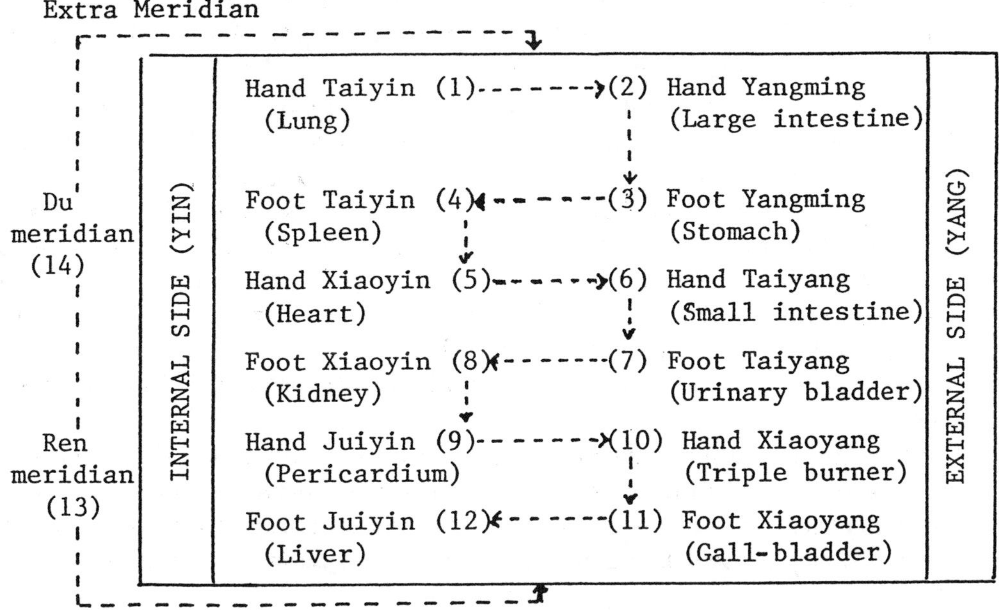

Electrophysiological Phenomenon

From our modern scientific viewpoint, we must consider what the meridian lines really are. There is no evidence that there is a special anatomical structure for each meridian line, although some researchers have proposed a special lymphatic system in the body that represents the meridians (14). From electrophysiological studies we understand that the cellular membrane of living cells exhibits an electrical potential between intracellular and extracellular fluid. A resting potential difference of 80 mV is recorded, with the inside negative. Nerve cells, nerve fibers, and muscle cells are examples of such electrical phenomena. When stimulation is applied—electrical, mechanical, or other, including laser, pressure, or magnetic fields—a change in potential occurs, and a current of a few mAmp in intensity is produced. A nerve fiber propagates this electrical potential change continuously from one end to the other, from one neuron to the next. The cells under the skin, however, act as a leaky membrane, and the change in electrical potential difference is dissipated rapidly after it is produced. An exception would be the electric eel: because the cells of the electric eel's organs are almost perfectly insulated, any electrical current produced from stimulation tends to accumulate, reaching levels of more than one hundred volts, since the cells are hooked up in series.

Let us visualize the meridian line as a similar type of structure. Suppose there is only slightly less leakage—between 1 and 5 percent—compared with other subcutaneous cells. When the meridian lines are stimulated, a slight but detectable electrical current would be produced, although no significant anatomical difference in structure would be apparent.

Rydoraku Channels

In the early 1950s, Y. Nakatani of Japan proposed an electroconductivity theory to explain certain pathological abnormalities of organs. He theorized that different areas of the body can have abnormally higher or lower conductivity and that there is a direct correlation between different illnesses and the abnormal conductivity that can be measured under the skin (10). He found that such abnormal conductivity is very closely related to the twelve meridian lines and called it *Rydoraku,* which in Japanese means "a good conductive line."

Nakatani also objectively pointed out certain points, which he called Reactive Electro-Permeable Points (REPP), which can be measured and assessed for higher or lower conductivity, thus indicating an abnormality or imbalance. According to this theory, the electrophysiological properties of each organ or tissue project onto a certain area on the surface of the body. Their resistance and conductivity correspond to their physiological or pathological condition and change accordingly. Furthermore, Nakatani theorized that stimulation of a REPP point in a certain area would induce an impulse via the sympathetic nervous system, thereby regulating the visceral organs. The Rydoraku theory thus generally follows the principles set out in the *Huang Ti Nei Chian:* treatment of a REPP point along the relevant channel or meridian line would tonify the weak (the Yin) and disperse the strong (the Yang).

To prove his hypothesis that abnormalities in conductivity can be measured in certain unhealthy states, Nakatani experimented with measuring electrical currents between two points on the upper arm. A decrease in electrical resistance was observed when a sympathomimetic or cholinergic agent was administered; similarly, the resistance increased when a sympatholytic or cholinergic blocking agent was used.

The electrophysiological phenomena expressed in the Ryodoraku theory do not, however, satisfactorily explain some emotional and psychological activities. When we are in a state of wakefulness—whether thinking, perspiring, excited, stressed, or in pain—the resistance of the skin falls abruptly. While we are at rest, however—during sleep, anesthesia, coma, or fatigue—the recorded resistance moves in the opposite direction, going up. These changes in resistance can be explained by the closing or opening of the pores in the skin. This leads to yet another question: does a meridian represent a line under the skin where the pores are more likely to be opened or closed than pores outside of the meridian lines?

Bidigital O-Ring Imaging

In 1986, Y. Omura developed a molecular identification and localization technique called bidigital O-ring imaging" (11). He performed extensive experiments using a device that was claimed to be able to investigate electrical fields within the body, graphing images of hitherto-unidentifiable structures. While Omura published many papers on his findings, no other investigators have made use of this technique. His findings thus have been neither proven nor refuted.

Using this technique, he outlined normal and abnormal organs. Even when working with human cadavers, Omura could demonstrate the meridian lines corresponding to the same specific organs and acupuncture points found in a living body. He therefore concluded that the descriptions in the ancient Chinese medical classics were essentially correct, with some variations and inaccuracies. The image outline shows that from the surface each internal organ line or network of lines extends to other parts of the body. Such a line resembles the classic meridian line described in the *Nei Chian.*

The width of the lines of a meridianlike network usually ranges between one and two millimeters. Areas as close as one millimeter to the lines exhibit distinctly different characteristics from the meridian lines. There appear to be specific channels that can propagate some types of information in an electrical or magnetic field, thereby regulating functions throughout the body.

Omura further theorized that each meridian line is connected to a specific organ and to a representative area within the cerebral cortex corresponding to that internal organ. He also speculated that each meridian line and its acupuncture point are associated with unique hormones. Upon stimulation of an acupoint or locus along the meridian, hormones in the organ-representative area of the brain will be rapidly released. For example, the Triple Burner meridian, Hand Xiao Yang, is associated with testosterone in males; in females, it is associated with estriol, estradiol, and progesterone, along with acetylcholine and prostaglandin (PGE_1). The stomach meridian, Foot Yang Ming, is associated with gastrin and PGE_1.

In other tests, it has been documented that stimulation of an acupoint along certain meridians results in an increased release of certain neurotransmitters and opiatelike peptides. (See chapter 6.) No such release could be detected when areas outside of the meridian line borders were stimulated.

Bidigital O-ring imaging is said to be able not only to outline internal organs, but also to outline malignant tumors (11). With this technique, it is postulated that a correct diagnosis of certain pathological abnormalities can be made without the risks associated with X-ray exposure. This technique can also identify which of the twelve pairs of meridian channels correspond to each internal organ. It is also suggested that this technique can give quick and reliable indication of a dysfunctioning meridian system, and this in turn can be used to determine the site of disturbance fields caused by pathogenic factors (6). It is also possible to apply this technique to search for the location of pathological conditions of organs and extend the use of acupuncture to treat these abnoralities (15). Omura and his coworkers also used this technique to detect the change of various neurotransmitters in the pineal gland under the influence of electromagnetic field (EMF) (12). They also claimed that the abnormal EMF or electric field (EF) can be detected by the bidigital O-ring test. EMF is a contributing factor to the genesis of cancer, Alzheimer's disease, stroke, and lead poisoning in the brain (13).

Additionally, the technique has been used as a guide to determine whether the performance of acupuncture on patients would be feasible if an abnormality in meridian lines has been observed (5). Cases of meridian line abnormality have been documented in a variety of situations. For instance, Ti Kobayashi reported observing certain abnormalities in the acupuncture meridians of cancer patients (9). Meridian abnormalities have also been observed in cases of stress and excessive tension in parasympathetic nerves.

Propagated Sensation Channels (PSCs)

In most Chinese acupuncture texts, it is suggested that a dull aching numbness or itching is felt by the person receiving acupuncture. Chinese acupuncturists call this *tai qi*,, or an indication of success in reaching the meridian line, predicting good results from acupuncture treatment in cases where this is observed.

Today acupuncturists have termed this a latent propagated sensation channel, or PSC. After at least ten minutes of stimulation with the needle, subjects report a sensation similar to that of a local anesthetic, which indicates the presence of PSC. It is a reversible phenomenon and can be blocked by mechanical compression—using pressure at approximately 800 gm/cm^2—or by local anesthetic, procaine, or by lowering the skin temperature with ice to twenty-one degrees Celsius (1, p. 268).

Studies on 170 individuals have shown when acupuncture was done at the acupoint Neiguan (P 6), seventy-six of them showed a marked change of their cardiac functions correlated with a significant PSC and ninety-four cases showed less degree of change and no PSC. It suggests that PSC is of importance for the improvement in cardiac function and has obvious regulative effect on the organs projected from the meridian where the needling was pierced (22).

In studies on 200 patients with various illnesses, investigators observed that 68. 5 percent of the subjects had a positive propagated sensation along the channel of meridians when acupuncture was performed (19). In clinical studies on fifty-one patients, the skin surface along the stomach meridian—the Foot Yang Ming—was tapped, together with electrical stimulation of the ear. These studies reported that fifty of the fifty-one patients (98 percent) exhibited a positive latent PSC, coincident to the stomach channel (20).

The Biophysics Institute Academica Sinica released a report based on the records of twenty-eight institutes of Chinese acupuncture. These studies showed that of the 63,228 people who were treated with acupuncture during a three-year period, only 12 percent to 24 percent expressed a feeling of positive propagated sensation along the meridian channels (PSC). No common factors were apparent among these patients—no statistical difference was found based on age, sex, or physical condition (1, p. 260).

Two other independent reports showed similar results. In one study, a total of 2,107 subjects received acupuncture, including 788 cases with normal health, 1,211 patients with varying illnesses, and 100 deaf mutes; among these, 495 cases exhibited PSC, or 23.5 percent (1, p. 263). A study in China's Anhui Province observed the acupuncture treatment of 11,853 peasants, with 3,437 cases exhibiting PSC (29 percent) (1, p. 265).

Other studies have shown a higher percentage of cases exhibiting PSC. In one study, 104 patients were treated with auricular acupuncture; 90 of these, or 86.5 percent, had PSC (1, p. 267). Zhang (2, p. 259) also reported a higher percentage of PSC in his clinical experiences in Guinea. He treated 123 Guineans with acupuncture, with 118 (95 percent) showing PSC running through the whole course of the meridian. A similarly high percentage of PSC has also been reported among other subjects living on the African continent. Zhang speculated that climate plays an important role in this phenomenon; race is also a possible factor, though no major studies have been published in this area.

Z. M. Chai and C. Zhang (4) discussed four different needling sensations, so called *tai qi,* which can be identified differently in different people at different acupoints, such as numb, swelling numb, aching and heavy (press) feeling. They tested the needling sensation at several acupoints, HoKu, Zusanli, and Sanyinjiao, of sixty-one patients with coronary disease and repeated it three or more times at the same acupoints. It was found that 91 percent of the patients express a consistent same kind of feeling.

Other Empirical Evidence

In experiments with dogs and studies of both healthy and unhealthy people, investigators have made quantitative measurements of the bioelectrical potential of the skin at different acupuncture points along the stomach and small intestinal line, using high- and low-frequency electrical stimulation. They detected a significant change in bioelectrical potential (BEP) affecting the organ-meridian line (24).

In experiments on dogs, electrical measurement of the acupoints along the meridian network have shown decreased electrical skin impedance compared with points outside the meridian border (18). In another study, electrical conductivity during acupuncture was measured in ten healthy volunteers and twenty-nine sick patients, leading to a possible correlation in the energy dynamics of the lung and heart meridian (7). Investigators found some variation in conductivity in patients suffering from cardiovascular disorders.

To support the existence of meridian channels in connection with internal organs, T. P. Feng (6) used a semiconductor effect to measure the difference in resistance between the left and right meridian, and between organs along the meridian line. Such differences can be used to diagnose diseases among the organs. Below are the differences in resistance he found among the meridians:

Based on his studies in twenty-five cases of acquired or congenital amputation, C. C. Xue observed an acupuncture-induced phantom limb and meridian phenomenon. To his surprise, he found that the phantom limb sensations elicited by acupuncture were complete, alive, and nearly the size of the actual limbs the patients should possess. He proposed that the nervous system contains a meridian center, accounting for this phenomenon (21). Reichmanis has confirmed the finding of lower electric resistance among some acupuncture points along meridians and postulates that the meridian system is likely to be the major pathway of electric current on the body's surface (16).

Meng postulated that the channel of meridians represents an additional system of equilibrium operating in the body, supplementing the somatic nervous system, the autonomic nervous system, and the endocrine system. Based on measurements of propagated sensation along the meridian channels, Meng noted that the speed of conduction along the meridians is approximately 0.1 m/sec, serving to maintain somatic visceral equilibrium. Rejecting the classic charts of the fourteen meridian channels, Meng and his colleagues have drawn a new set of charts for these channels, but do not have solid anatomical proof of these structures. (2, p. 244).

Meridian	Resistance (Ohmes)	
	Left Side	Right Side
Hand Yang-ming (large intestine)	78	70
Hand Tai-yang (small intestine)	25	21
Hand Tai-yin (lung)	25	38
Hand Xiao-yin (heart)	22	27
Hand Jui-yin (pericardium)	22	23
Foot Tai-yin (spleen)	38	38
Foot Jui-yin (liver)	48	54
Foot Yang-ming (stomach)	46	40
Foot Xiao-yin (kidney)	27	23
Hand Xiao-yang (triple burner)	17	90

Gong, et. al., injected ink into the acupoints along the three Foot Yin meridians of twelve postmortem fetuses. They observed that the ink appeared in the lymphatic vessels running along these meridians, converging and closing at the point referenced as Sanyinjiao (Sp 6) of the Foot Tai Yin (2, p. 247). When the Sanyinjiao acupoints of rabbits were stimulated by acupuncture, it was found that both T-lymphocytes and B-lymphocytes increased from 42.56±2.22 percent to 55.3±2.15 percent.

G. S. Sekhon, et al., believed that the channels and collaterals do exist in the body and play a role in the treatment of diseases deep inside the body and in analgesic induction. They further speculated that these meridians also function to moderate normal healthy perception (17).

A close correlation between the twelve primary meridians and the underlying nerves has been proposed by Xue (21). Table 3-4 outlines these correlations and their anastomoses.

Many texts written either in Chinese or in English have described the details of each meridian and collateral where it starts and ends in the body. They are more or less explaining what was in the old Chinese classics on acupuncture. Reader interested in this subject should refer to the books by J. Y. P. Chen (1A), X. N. Cheng (2A), and F. Mann (5A).

Books on Meridians

1A. Chen, J. Y. P. Acupuncture Anesthesia in PRC. U.S. Department of Health, Education and Welfare. DHEW 75–769, 1975.

2A. Chen, X. N., ed. Chinese Acupuncture and Moxibustion. Beijing: Foreign Languages Press, 1987.

3A. Chung, I. Y., ed. An Outline of Chinese Acupuncture. Oxford: Pergamon Press, 1975.

4A. Lan. Y. K. *Atlas of Meridians and Collaterals* (in Chinese). Fuchow, PRC: Fukian Technology & Science Publisher. 1991.

5A. Mann, F. Acupuncture, the Ancient Chinese Art of Healing. New York: Random House, 1971.

Table 3-4. The Meridian and Peripheral Nerves Correlation

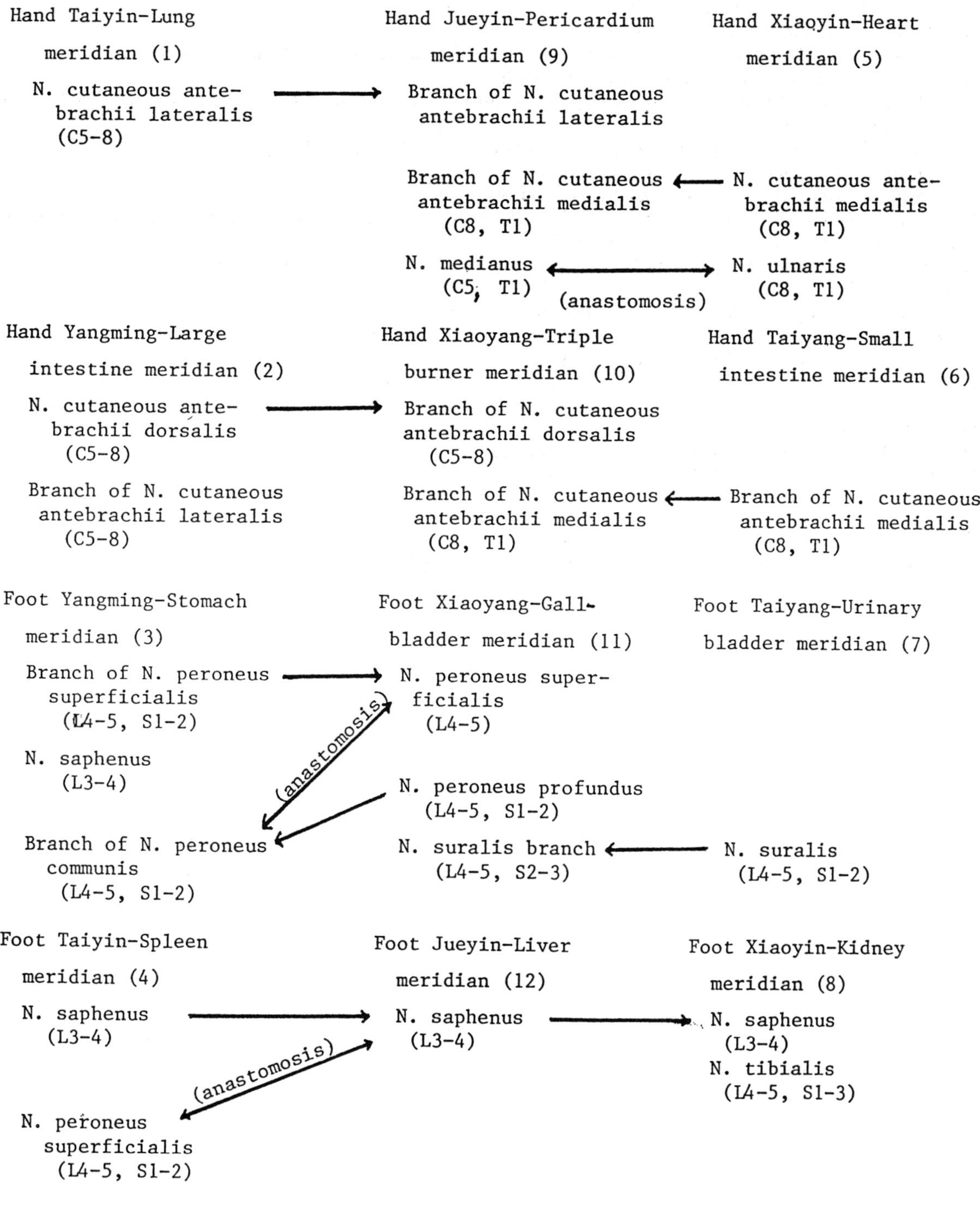

(Modified from Cai W. (3))

References

1. All China Society of Acupuncture and Moxibustion. First National Symposium on Acupuncture and Moxibustion and Acupuncture Anesthesia. Beijing: 1979.
2. All China Society of Acupuncture and Moxibustion. Second National Symposium on Acupuncture and Moxibustion and Acupuncture Anesthesia. Beijing: 1984.
3. Cai, W. American Journal of Chinese Medicine 20:331, 1993.
4. Chai, Z. M., and C. Zhang. Beijing Journal of Traditional Chinese Medicine. February 1994, p. 41.
5. Chan, J. C. Acupuncture Electro-Ther. Res. 13:44, 1988.
6. Feng, T. P., from Kao, F. F., and J. J. Kao, eds. Recent Advances in Acupuncture Research. Garden City, NY: Institute for Advanced Research in Asian Science and Medicine, 1979, p. 77.
7. Gheorghe, N., et al. Rev. Roum Morphol. Embryol Physiol. Physiol. 21:261, 1984.
8. Authors unknown, Huang Ti Nei Chian, written in 100 B.C.
9. Kobayashi, T. American Journal of Acupuncture 14:139, 1986.
10. Nakatani, Y. A Guide for Application of Ryodoraku Autonomic Nerve Regulatory Therapy. Tokyo: Japanese Society of Ryodoraku Autonomic Nervous Systems, 1972.
11. Omura, Y. Acupuncture Electro-Ther. Res. 13:153, 1988; 14:155, 1989; 12:53, 1987; 11:219, 1986.
12. Omura Y., et al. Acupuncture Electro-Ther. Res. 18:125, 1993.
13. Omura Y., et al. Acupuncture Electro-Ther. Res. 16:143, 1991.
14. Pinto, C. M. *Science of Charlatanry in Acupuncture. Why?* Guatemala: C.A., 1973.
15. Pontinen, P. J. Acupuncture Electro-Ther. Res. 11:217,1986.
16. Reichmanis, M. Modern Bioelectricity. New York: M. Dekker: 1988, p. 762.
17. Sekhon, G. S., et al. Chinese Medicine Journal 95:912, 1982.
18. Still, J. American Journal of Acupuncture 16:55, 1988.
19. Van Benschoten, M. M. American Journal of Acupuncture 16:119, 1988.
20. Xiang, Z. Z., et al. Acupuncture Electro-Ther. Res. 9:157, 1984.
21. Xue, C. C. Chinese Medicine Journal 99:247, 1986.
22. You, Z. Q., et al. Journal of Traditional Chinese Medicine. 7:195, 1987.
23. Yu, S. Z., et al. American Journal of Chinese Medicine 9:291, 1981.
24. Zukanskas, G., et al. Acupuncture Electro-Ther. Res. 13:119, 1988.

4

Acupuncture Points

The term *acupuncture point* refers to the site at which the acupuncture needle is applied. The term is also used interchangeably with the terms *acupuncture locus, acupoint,* and *meridian point.* According to Chinese theory, this is the point at which one of the internal meridian channels comes into proximity with the skin surface. This point can conduct external influences to the internal organs.

A total of 361 classical acupuncture points are listed in *Huang Ti Nei Chian.* The points lie along the meridians. The Chinese call them *shue yao,* meaning "circulation hole." They serve as transit stations along each meridian line, through which the *qi* and *blood* are transported. Qi, or the vital energy of life, is concentrated or accumulated on the surface of the skin; acupoints are therefore also called *Qi points.*

Chinese acupuncturists generally claim that when a true acupoint is correctly localized and needled, a sensation called *tai qi* is felt by the subject. This is a feeling of numbness or paresthesia, heaviness, and warmth at the site of acupoint; in some cases, the sensation may travel slowly up or down the body. It is not felt at nonacupoints.

Although there is no anatomical means of identifying a special locus for the acupoint, the literature claims that acupoints can be detected by palpitation or by electronic point finders. When stimulation is applied to a certain acupoint, it generates a functional activity that is propagated to the internal organs. Acupuncturists believe that this can regulate and strengthen body resistance, as well as prevent and treat diseases. Forms of stimulation can include finger twisting of a needle, electrical impulse, or moxibustion—a type of acupuncture performed not by needling, but by burning a Chinese herb or paper on a selected acupoint.

Y. Omura (31) described the acupoint as circular or slightly oval shape in a three-dimensional space, with a boundary three to thirty-seven millimeters in diameter. The majority of acupoints in the human adult normally have a diameter between six and twelve millimeters; those in the nailbeds of the fingers and toes are somewhat smaller. He also reported that most acupoints along the meridian lines have a high level of neurotransmitters and hormones, such as acetylcholine, enkephalin, ß-endorphin, ACTH, 5HT, cholecystokinin, norepinephrine, secretin, and GABA.

Classification

In addition to the 361 classical acupoints listed in *Nei Chian,* other points have been identified, but not all are commonly used. In clinical applications, according to the type and shape of the Shue Yao, acupoints can be classified either by "meridian" or by "body parts":

1. The acupoints of the fourteen meridians, or the Chien-Yao meridian loci. These are the major

acupoints located along the twelve pairs of hand and foot meridians, plus the extra *du* and *ren* meridian.

2. The extraordinary acupoints are certain loci identified as having specific effectiveness despite being located outside of the 14 meridian channels. These are considered to be supplemental acupoints to the regular Chien-Yao loci. The expanded use of auricular acupuncture in China since 1956 has led to the identification of numerous extraordinary acupoints used in this technique.
3. The *Ashi* points, which are commonly used in moxibustion. In cases of severe pain, it has been reported that when a moxa, or pressure, was applied to the painful area, the patient would suddenly yell loudly, and the pain would subside. This locus is called an *Ashi* point. The "Needle Classic" states that "the pain point is the Yao," while some call it an "indefinable point." It is located at the site of the pain.

Since the meridians are distributed from either the hand or the foot, centripetally toward the body or the center, they differ in length. Thus the number of acupoints along each meridian line is different. They are summarized in table 4-1.

Table 4-1. Number of Acupoints Listed in Nei Chian

Meridian	Acupoints	Meridian	Acupoints
Hand Tai-yin	11	Hand Yang-ming	20
Hand Xiao-yin	9	Hand Tai-yang	19
Hand Jui-yin	9	Hand Xiao-yang	23
Foot Tai-yin	21	Foot Yang-ming	45
Foot Xiao-yin	27	Foot Tai-yang	67
Foot Jui-yin	14	Foot Xiao-yang	44
Du	28	Ren	24
Total Acupoints	361		

The total number of acupoints has increased with the passage of time. Chinese scholars who considered themselves acupuncture specialists would invariably add a few more extraordinary acupoints to the list, as a means of demonstrating their authority on the subject. In the early Ming Dynasty, Wa Shou (A.D. 1304–1386), an expert acupuncturist, wrote a book titled *A Collection of Fourteen Meridians,* which was published in three volumes and mentioned 647 acupoints. He discussed each point in detail, including its correspondence to the meridians and internal organs. His writing was well respected, and the acupoints described in his book are still used.

Commonly Used Acupoints

In practical applications, only a few acupoints are commonly used by most acupuncturists. In a recent article, D. Evans suggested that not more than twenty loci be used for acupuncture analgesia, based upon various sizes of the body surface (13). In addition to his recommendations, we have added several other points and indicate the meridians and nerves to which they project. The name for each acupoint is a translation from the Chinese; each has been assigned a series number according to its meridian.

1. Head and Neck (figure 4-1)

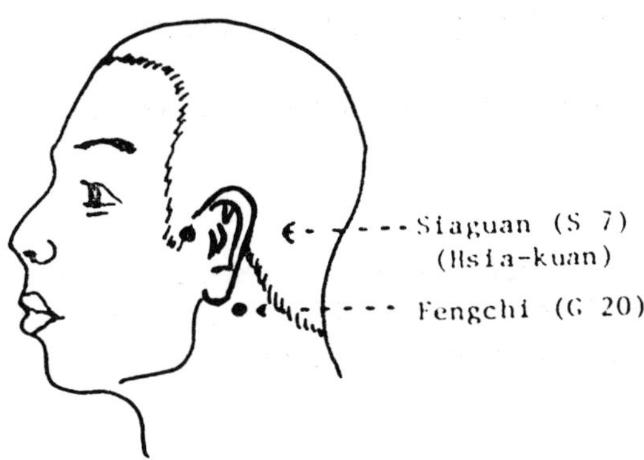

Figure 4-1. Acupoint Hsia Kuan or Siaguan (S 7) and Feng Chi (G 20)

HSIA KUAN or SIAGUAN (S 7), at the inferior border of the zygomatic branch of the N. facialis and the branches of N. auriculotemporalis. It is the point used in the treatment of trigeminal neuralgia and temporomandibular arthritis, deafness, tinnitus, toothache, and facial paralysis. Meridian: The Foot Yang Ming, or stomach meridian. This is the convergent point of this meridian and the Foot Xiao Yang (gallbladder) meridian.

FENG CHI (G 20), located between the upper portion of M. sternocleidomastoideus and M. trapezius. It is used in the treatment of occipital headache and neck pain, blurred vision, glaucoma, tinnitus, epilepsy, infantile and febrile convulsions, and the common cold. The nerve comes from N. occipitalis minor, which originates from the C2 to C5 vertebrae. Meridian: The Foot Xiao Yang, or gallbladder meridian.

SHANG HSING or SHANGXING (Du 23), on the midpoint of the forehead, close to the anterior hairline. It is used in the treatment of frontal headaches, ophthalmalgia, epistaxis, and mental disorders. It corresponds to the branches of the frontal nerve. (See figure 4-2A.) Meridian: The *du* meridian.

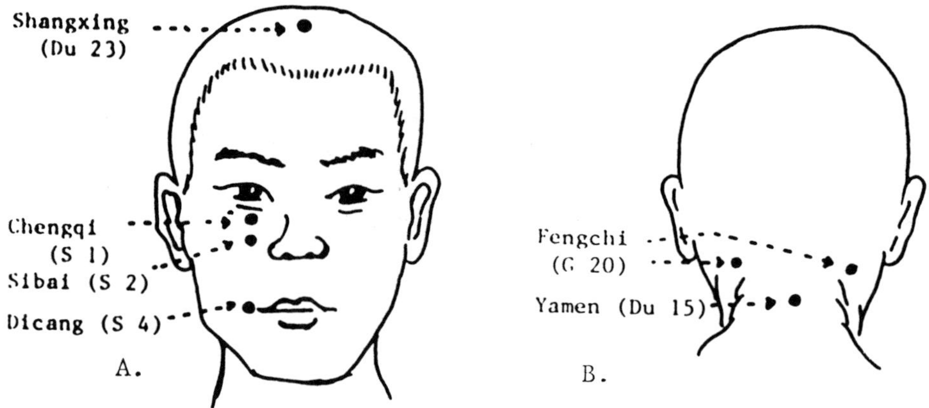

Figure 4-2. A: Acupoints Shangxing (Du 23), Cheng Qi (S 1), Sibai (S 2) and Dicang (S 4)

B: Acupoints Feng Chi (G 20) and Ya Men (Du 15)

YA MEN (Du 15), located slightly above the midpoint of the posterior hairline and below the spinous process of the C1 and C2 vertebrae. It is used in the treatment of occipital headache, epilepsy, deafness and muteness, sudden hoarseness, and aphasia. (See figure 4-2B.) Meridian: The *du* meridian.

CHENG QI (S 1), directly below the pupil of the eye. The nerve supply is the branch of N. infraorbitalis, the inferior branch of the N. occulomotoris. It is used in the treatment of eye disorders (pain, swelling, and blindness) and facial paralysis. (See figure 4-2A.) Meridian: The Foot Yang Ming, or stomach meridian.

2. The Back (figure 4-3)

DAZHUI (Du 14), between the C7 and T1 vertebral spinous processes and close to the dorsal branch of the eighth cervical nerve and first thoracic nerves. It is used in the treatment of neck pain and rigidity, epilepsy, and asthma. Meridian: The *du* meridian. This is the convergence point between the *du* and Foot Tai Yang (urinary bladder) meridians.

ZHIYANG (Du 9), on the midline of the T7 vertebra, close to the medial branch of the posterior ramus of the seventh thoracic nerve. It is used in the treatment of chest and back pains. Meridian: The *du* meridian.

MING MEN (Du 4), meaning "the Gate of Life," on the midline between the second and third lumbar spinous processes and close to the dorsal branch of the second lumbar nerve. It is used to treat lower back pain, lumbago, and impotence. Meridian: The *du* meridian.

CHIEN CHING or JIANJING (G 21), at the high point of the shoulder, in the upper part of the trapezius muscle. It is used in the treatment of neck pain, shoulder pain, insufficient lactation, mastitis, and difficult labor. Meridian: The Foot Xiao Yang, or gallbladder meridian.

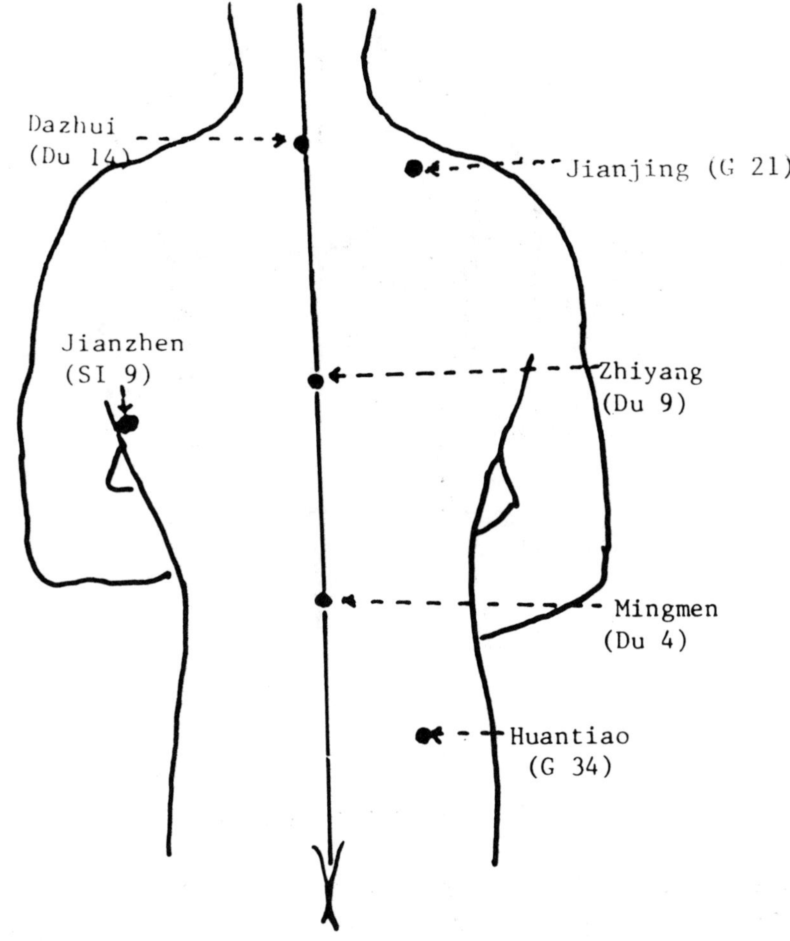

Figure 4-3. The Commonly Used Acupoints on the Back of the Body

3. Chest and Abdomen (figure 4-4)

YUAN YE (G 22), on the midaxillary line, below the axilla. It corresponds to the lateral cutaneous branch of the fifth N. intercostalis. This point is used in the treatment of fullness of the chest, swelling of the axillary region, and arm pains. Meridian: The Foot Xiao Yang or gallbladder meridian.

SHANG CHUNG or TANZHONG (Ren 17), located in the midline of the sternum, midway between the nipples. It is supplied by the branches of the fourth N. intercostalis and is used to treat chest pains, palpitation, and asthma. Meridian: The *ren* meridian. It is the selective point of the Hand Jui Yin, or pericardium meridian, and is the influential point of Qi.

CHUNG CHI or ZHONGJI (Ren 3), in the center line of the abdomen, four inches below the umbilicus. It is supplied by the branches of the N. iliohypogastricus from the L1 vertebra. It is used in the treatment of enuresis, noctural emission, impotence, hernia, and genitourinary disorders. Meridian: The *ren* meridian. It is the convergent point between the *ren* and three Foot Yin meridians. It is also the selective point for the Foot Tai Yang (urinary bladder) meridian.

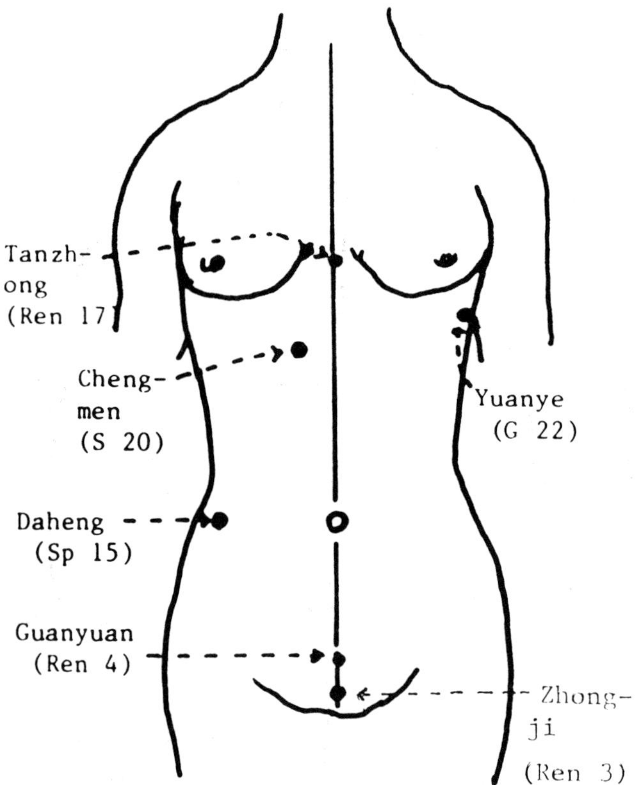

Figure 4-4. Acupoints on the Chest and Abdomen

TAI HENG or DAHENG (Sp 15), on the lateral side of M. rectus abdominus, at the level of the umbilicus. The nerve supply is from the tenth N. intercostalis. It is used to treat abdominal pains, diarrhea, dysentery, and constipation. Meridian: The Foot Tai Yin or spleen meridian.

CHENG MAN (S 20), at the front of eleventh rib. The nerve supply is from the branch of the tenth N. intercostalis. It is used in the treatment of gastric pain, vomiting, and anorexia. Meridian: The Foot Yang Ming or stomach meridian.

4. Upper Extremity (figures 4-5 and 4-6)

HOKU or HEGU (LI 4), on the back of the hand, between the first and second Os metacarpale, near the center point of the radial side of the second Os metacarpale. The nerve supplies are from the branches of the C5 to T1 nerves, the dorsal branches of N. radialis, and the N. medianus. This acupoint is very commonly used in the treatment of many neurological disorders and internal illnesses, including headache, neck pain, ophthalmological disorders (swelling and pain), toothache, rhinorrhea, deafness, abdominal pain and intestinal trouble (dysentery, constipation), amenorrhea and delayed labor, and weakness and paralysis of muscles (especially of the upper extremity). Meridian: The originating point of the Hand Yang Ming or large intestine meridian.

CH'IH TSE or CHIZE (L 5), in the striae transversae of the fossa cubitalis, in the radial depression of the biceps brachii. It is close to the branches of the C5 to T1 nerves, as well as the N. cutaneous antibrachiilateralis in the deep layer of the N. radialis. It is used in the treatment of elbow pains. Meridian: The uniting point of the Hand Tai Yin or lung meridian.

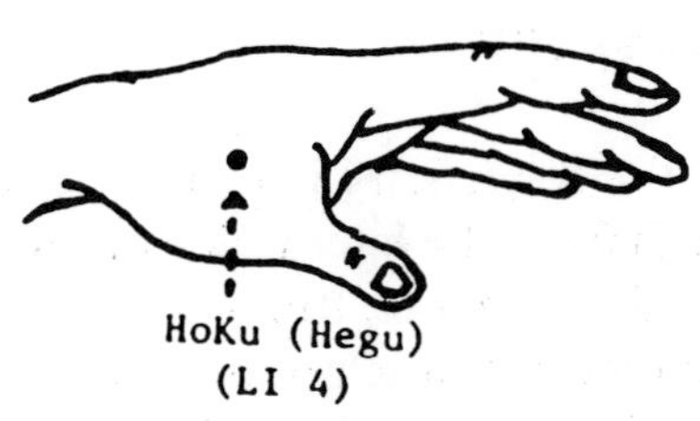

Figure 4-5. Acupoint HoKu or Hegu (LI 4)

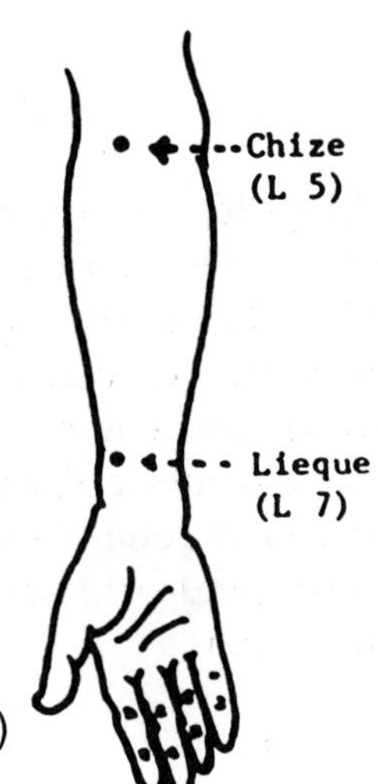

Figure 4-6. Acupoints Chize (L 5) and Lieque (L 7)

LIEH CHUEH or LIEQUE (L 7), a joint point between meridian and collateral. It lies slightly superior to the styloid process of the radius. In the first century A. D., some Chinese poets used the term *lieh chueh* to express lightning, suggesting that this point can conduct electric current as fast as lightning in transporting the message to internal organs. The underlying nerve supplies come from the lateral antebrachial cutaneous nerves and superficial ramus of the N. radialis. It is commonly used to treat headache, migraine, neck pain, asthma, sore throat, and toothache. Meridian: The main station along the Hand Tai Yin or lung meridian, branching to the Hand Yang Ming (large intestine) meridian. It is also linked to the *ren* meridian.

SHOU SAN LI (LI 10), *Shou* meaning "the hand," and *San Li* meaning "three Chinese miles." This is an exaggerated expression implying that the effects of this point could reach three miles. It is located one inch below the transverse line on the lateral side when the elbow is flexed. The nerve supplies come from the posterior antebrachial cutaneous nerves and the deep ramus of N. radialis. One of the classic acupuncture texts, the *Bronze Man's Illustration of Acupuncture,* states that "Shou San Li treats numbness of the arm, spastic contraction, toothache, and jaw swelling." It is commonly used in present times in the treatment of abdominal pain, diarrhea, and shoulder pain. (See figure 4-7.) Meridian: The main locus of the Hand Yang Ming or large intestine meridian.

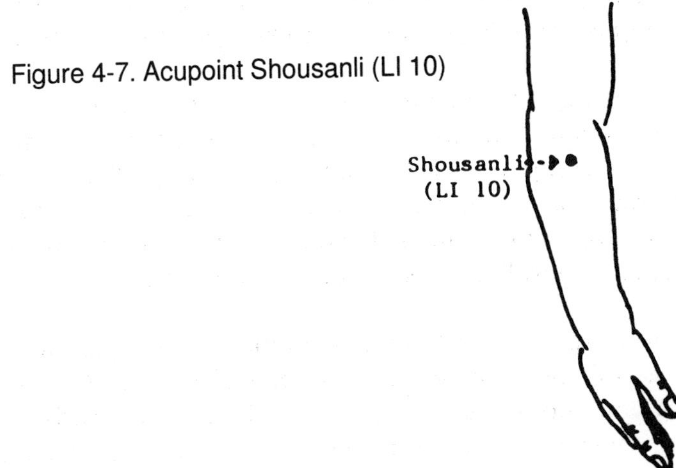

Figure 4-7. Acupoint Shousanli (LI 10)

5. Lower Extremity (figures 4-8 and 4-9)

ZUSANLI (S 36), meaning "foot–three miles," similar to the Shou San Li (LI 10). This point is three inches below the lateral knee depression, one finger width from the lateral side of the anterior crest of the tibia. The nerve supplies originate from the L4 to S1 vertebrae; those in the superficial layer come from the N. cutaneous surae lateralis and the cutaneous branch of N. saphenus, while those in the deep layer come from the N. peroneus profundus. In humans, this point is chiefly used for treating gastroenteric diseases, various chronic diseases, allergenic and urogenital diseases, insomnia, mania and general nervous disorders. In animals, usually used for treating pain, gastroenteral dysfunctions, and arthralgia syndrome (37). Meridian: The uniting point of the Foot Yang Ming or stomach meridian.

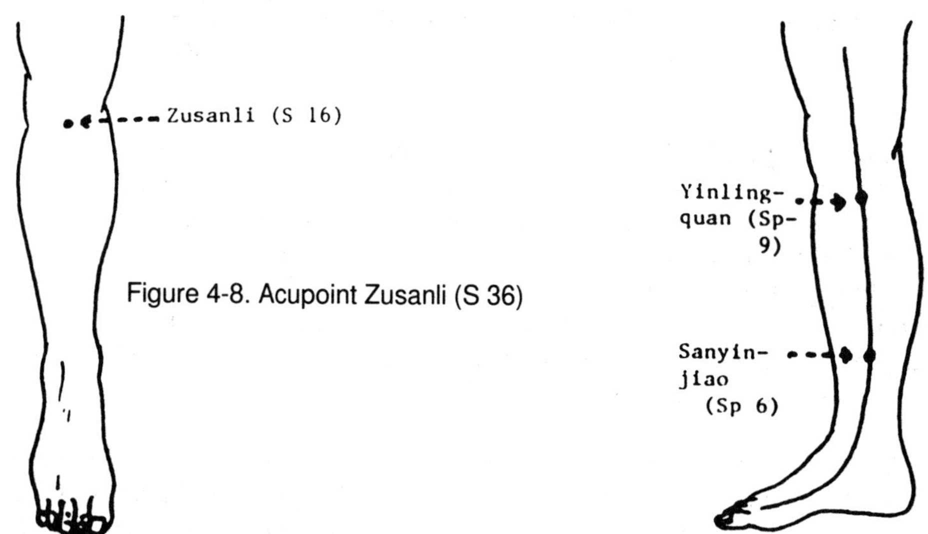

Figure 4-8. Acupoint Zusanli (S 36)

Figure 4-9. Acupoints Sanyinjiao (SP 6) and Yinlingquan (SP 9)

SANYINJIAO (Sp 6), located approximately three inches above the tip of the inner ankle, on the posterior margin of the metatarsal bone. In the superficial layer is the Nervus cutaneus medialis of the leg, which starts from the N. sapheus from the third to the fourth segments of the lumbar vertebra. In the deeper layer, there is the N. tibialis, which originates from the fifth lumbar vertebra to the second segment of the sacral. The supplied vessels include the great saphenus vein and the posterior tibial artery and vein.

Sanyinjiao is one of the commonly used acupoints in acupuncture therapy and acupuncture anesthesia beside Zusanli. It is used in the treatment of abdominal pain, borborygmus, abdominal distension, diarrhea, dysmenorrhea, uterine bleeding, morbid leukorrhea, prolapse of the uterus, sterility, delayed labor, nocturnal emission, impotence, enuresis, edema, hernia, muscular atrophy, motor impairment, paralysis and pain of the lower extremities, headache, dizziness and vertigo, insomnia. Meridian: The Foot Tai Yin or spleen meridian. It is the convergent point of the three Foot Yin meridians.

EAP at the Sanyinjiao acupoint of the ovariectomized rat can modulate and regulate the function of hypothalamo-pituitary-ovarian axis through the effect on certain Fos-labelled neurons in CNS, such as the arcuate nuclei (AR), lateral and medial preoptic nuclei (LPN and MPN), the suprachiasmatic nuclei (SCN), the periventricular and paraventricular nuclei of hypothalamus (PVNH and PANH) (19).

HUAN TIAO (G 30), located at the boundary of the lateral one-third and the medial two-thirds of the line connecting the highest point of the major trochanter of the femur and the hiatus sacralis. Nerve supplies come from the branch of the N. cutaneous gluteus inferior and N. gluteus inferior; in the deep layer, it comes from N. ischiadicus. It is used to treat sciatic and back pain, and hemiplegia. (See figure 4-10.) Meridian: The Foot Xiao Yang or gallbladder meridian. It is the anatomosis point between this meridian and the Foot Tai Yang (urinary bladder) meridian.

Li, et al., studied on anesthetized rats and recorded the nociceptive discharge of spinal dorsal horn. Acupuncture at the Huan Tiao point on the ipsilateral side gave a greater inhibitory effect than on the contralateral side. When acupuncture was done at the Renzhong (Du 26), it produced no significant inhibitory effect (24). In clinical practice Huan Tiao is an important point in relieving pain of the lower limb, probably transmitting the signal through the afferent fibers from the sciatic nerve.

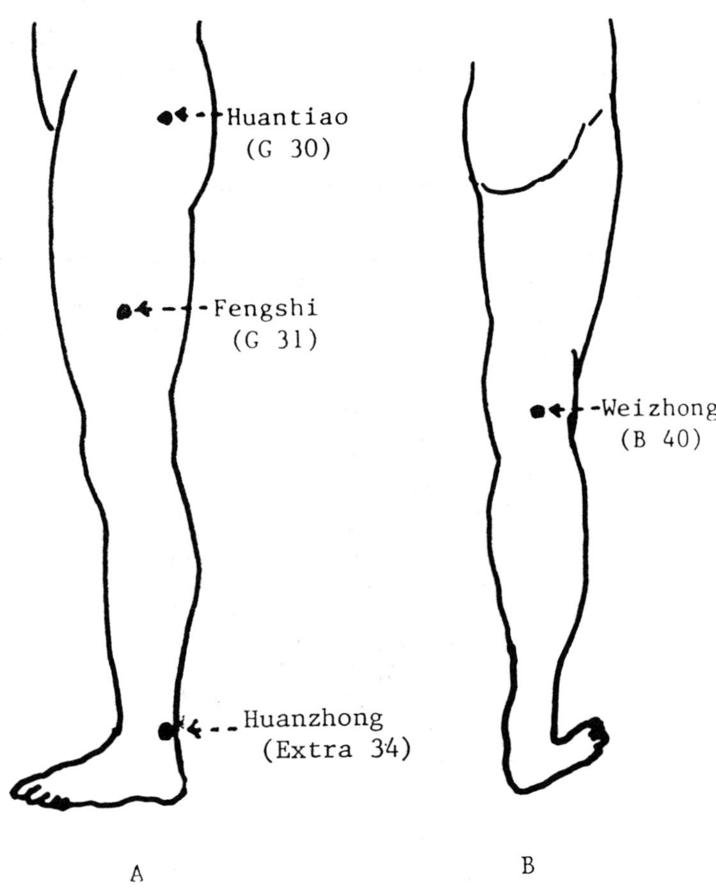

Figure 4-10. A: Acupoints Huantiao (G 30), Fengshi (G 31), and Huanzhong (Extra 34)

B: Acupoint Weizhong (B 40)

WEI ZHONG (B 40), at the center of the striae transversae of the popliteal fossa. The nerve supplies at the superficial layer come from the N. cutaneous femoris posterior from the S3 vertebra, and in the deep layer from N. tibialis from the L5 to S2 vertebrae. It is used in the treatment of sciatica, low back pain, knee pains, and abdominal pain. (See figure 4-10.) Meridian: The uniting point of the Foot Tai Yang or urinary bladder meridian.

FENG SHI (G 31), just under the middle finger of the hand when standing upright with the hand falling straight down. The nerve supplies come from the N. cutaneous femoralis lateralis from the T12 to L3 vertebrae. The deep layer is supplied from the muscular branch of the N. femoralis. It is used in the treatment of sciatica, back pain, and hip pain. Meridian: The Foot Xiao Yang or gallbladder meridian.

HSUAN CHUNG or XUANZHONG, also called **CHUEH KU** (G 39), approximately three inches above the tip of the external ankle, on the rear margin of the M. peroneus. The nerve supplies come from the superficial N. peroneus profundus. It is used in the treatment of apoplexy, hemiplegia, neck pain, abdominal pain, muscular atrophy of the lower extremity, and spastic pains. Meridian: The Foot Xiao Yang or gallbladder meridian. It is the convergent point of the three Foot Yang meridians and is considered to be the influential collateral point.

6. Auricular Acupoints

According to acupuncturists, the ear has a close relationship with the entire body. Points along the ear are said to represent specific points of the body. This relationship between the internal organs and channels was recorded in the *Huang Ti Nei Chian.* The "Needle Classic" states that "the ear is the place where all channels meet."

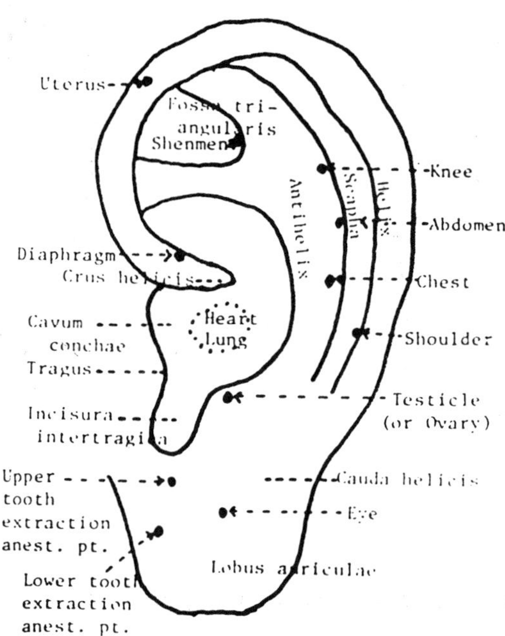

Figure 4-11. Diagram of Distribution of Auricular Acupoints

Since 1956, auricular acupuncture has become very popular in China. The many writings on the use and application of auricular acupuncture describe more than two hundred points that have been identified through repeated experimentation and clinical practice. These are points that exhibit low resistance and good conduction of electrical or mechanical stimulation. Only a few of these, however, are commonly used.

In the distribution of nerves to the ear, both the medial and lateral auricle receive innervation from the N. vagus, N. glossopharyngeus, and the combination branch of the N. facialis and N. occipitalis minor. The medial ear also receives branches from N. auriculotemporalis, N. auricularis magnus, and N. occipitalis major.

Generally, the lower part of the ear represents the hand and face, while the upper part of the ear represents the foot. The fossa of the antihelix and the cavum condae represent the internal organs. (See figure 4-11.) Studies of the skin of rabbits' ears have shown that after electro-acupuncture treatment, the biological active points (BAP) of the ear are more intensive vascularization and innervation and have more pronounced nerve fasciculi. In the nervous fasciculi, there are myelin and amyelin fibers, as well as an increase in acetylcholinesterase activity and a degranulation of mast cells in the BAP area (22).

Table 4-2. The Anatomical Position of Auricular Acupoints

Position of the Ear	Acupoints Propagated to:
Spina helicis	Diaphragm
Helix	Lower section of rectum; urethra; external genital
Scapha	Finger; wrist; elbow; shoulder; shoulder joint; and collar bone
Spina suprameatum of antihelix	Toe; ankle; knee; hip
Antihelix	Cervical vertebrae; thoracic and sacral vertebrae; neck; chest; abdomen
Triangular Fossa	Uterus; lowering of blood pressure; femoral joint
Tragus	Adrenal; pharynx-larynx; external and internal nose; parotid
Antitragus	Brain stem; brain; forehead; mouth
Periphery helix crus	Esophagus; cardiac orifice of stomach; duodenum; small and large intestine; liver
Cymba condae	Pancreas; kidney; ureter; bladder; heart
Cavum condae	Lung; trachea; spleen; triple burner; endocrine glands
Ear lobule	Eye; cheek; tongue; jaw; neurasthetic point; internal ear; tonsil; spinal cord
Back of the ear, Groove of inferior helix crus	Lowering the blood pressure; heart; spleen; liver; lung; kidney

Anatomical and Physiological Characteristics

Since there is no specific anatomical structure to the meridian channels, one has to ask how we can identify a specific acupoint that would respond differently from nonacupoints. N. L. Brown applied a pair of electrodes to the skin of the upper limb and found that some points of the skin demonstrate different electrical activity from others. He concluded that there is some evidence that these points correspond to points where the peripheral nervous system is especially accessible (7). Other investigators claim that natural quartz crystals or magnets can be used to read the vascular autonomic signals under the skin, thereby localizing acupuncture points and body field distortions (3).

H. C. Dung of Texas has contributed greatly to the study of meridians and acupoints (10). He states that the acupoints in the face and forehead region are located along the terminal or cutaneous branches of the trigeminal nerve and the motor points formed between the muscular branches of the facial nerve to the medial of facial exposure. The acupoints in the neck lie along the terminal branches of the cervical plexus, which have been divided into cutaneous and muscular components. Here the acupoints lie mainly along the route of their cutaneous nerve. Based on their clinical application, he classified the acupoints into four groups. The number of sensitive acupoints varied from individual to individual.

Recently Dung published six papers on acupoints, following anatomic nomenclature (11). He showed that typical spinal nerves have six cutaneous branches that reach the skin of the body wall in the thorax and abdomen. Each of these branches corresponds to an acupuncture point. He diagrammed the acupoints found in the thoracic and abdominal walls and their relation to the spinal cord.

For example, acupuncture points on the spleen and liver meridians are formed by the anterior branches of the lateral cutaneous nerves. He designated the acupoint Geshu (B 17), along the urinary bladder meridian, as a primary point; it is known to be the posterior cutaneous nerve point of T7. Additionally, he identified the Xinshu point (B 15) from the posterior cutaneous nerve of T5, and the Dushu point (B 16) from the posterior cutaneous nerve of T6.

Dung also illustrated the acupuncture points in the arm, forearm, and hand in comparison with the distribution of the axillary and radial nerves. The acupuncture points in the lower limb were correlated to the lumbar plexus. He further pointed out that while the sciatic nerve is the nerve with the greatest diameter in the body and lies deep beneath the layers of muscles, its distribution does not have a significant correlation with acupoints. Only one tertiary acupoint is derived from the sciatic nerve: the Fuxt point (B 38), which is also referred to as the sciatic point.

Wang, et al. (41) examined ten acupoints on the upper extremities of forty-eight patients. Nine were supplied by the N. medianus and one by the N. ulnaris. Fifty receptor units were observed under these ten acupoints and measured electrically. When the acupoints were stimulated, different sensations were felt by the patients. Five were rapidly adapting receptor units. Sensations from the needle lasted for a long time. Three of the tested acupoints are touch or pressure receptor units, two of which are located in deep tissues with abundant muscle spindles; one, the Da Lin point (P 7), is a Colgi tendon and/or pressure unit. The authors theorized that the receptors and the afferent fibers of acupoints take part in forming and maintaining needle sensations.

However, H. H. Dung in China (no relation to H. C. Dung) has suggested that the acupoints may be labile and related to pathological disease conditions (12). This was used to explain why there are so many acupuncture points, such as the extraordinary and *Ashi* points. Patients suffering from various diseases showed increased tenderness at different acupoints. The magnitude of tenderness increases as illnesses progress and decreases when pathological conditions subside. In healthy people, this tenderness was not observed. Thus he proposed that the acupoints exist in three states, according to whether the subject is healthy or asymptomatic (sick but without symptoms) or has a pathological condition. He terms these states as latent (normal or healthy), *passive* (asymptomatic), or *active* (symptomatic). If this hypothesis is correct, then the number of acupoints listed in both ancient and recent literature is vastly overstated.

Histological Properties

By studying the histology of acupuncture points, Croley (9) reported that human subjects consistently show twice as many papillae within the area of acupuncture points as nonacupuncture points. They observed a concentration of dermal papillae containing capillary loops with sympathetic wrappings, together with the contained nerve endings, within the loci of the acupuncture points. They further suggested that this is responsible for the increase in conductivity of the overlying skin.

C. C. Han reported that acupoints are endowed with more nerve fibers, including pressure and stretch receptors (17). His data show that acupoints have more myelinated fibers (approximately 2.7 times more), more Group II fibers (50 percent more), more large fibers (2.8 times more) in their afferent innervation, and more fast-velocity fibers (3.1 times more) than nonacupoints.

Histological investigation on micro- and macroscopic preparations has shown that some active acupuncture points contain a considerable amount of "specific" connective tissue in the form of meshwork (30). To determine whether acupuncture points are morphologically related to nerves and blood vessels, the radioactive isotope 99m Te (Technetium-99m) pertechnetate was injected directly into the Tai Xi (K 3) point along the kidney meridian, and Kun Lun (B-60) point along the urinary bladder meridian. The isotope rapidly appeared in the bloodstream with a higher peak activity and greater absorption rate, suggesting that the acupoints play a role in the drainage of soft tissue fluid into the vein (43).

A scintigraphic illustration of the meridians has been undertaken in twelve patients of unilateral nephroectomy and twelve normal subjects (served as control) (35). The radioactive isotope $^{99m}TeO_4$ was injected bilaterally into the Tai Xi (K 3) point of Foot Xiao Yin—kidney meridian. It was found that the migration of the isotope along the affected meridian of the nephroectomized side appeared more sluggish, dispersed, and broken, which was not seen in the contralateral side with a normal kidney, nor was it seen in the normal subjects served as control. Such altered scintigram of the affected meridian (the nephroectomized side) was characterized by a shorter laterency, a lower local clearance rate and a long disappearance of the radioactivity. As shown in figure 4-12, the time activity curve from the nephroectomized side is not only differerent from that shown in normal subject, but also different from the contralateral side (the normal kidney).

Using the radioactive technique, M. F. Chen, et al., (8) have found that subcutaneous injection of Tc-99m pertechnetate into the acupoint Xuehai (Sp 10) gives a significantly faster absorption pattern than those injected into the nonacupoint closed to Sp-10, evidenced by shorter phase 1, higher peak activity, and greater acceleration rate of phase 2.

The radioactive tracer technique with 99mTechnetium was also used to inject into certain acupoints to visualize the thyroid gland. After injection the radioactivity of the isotope is shown on the scintiscan and confirmed by venous blood counts. This indicates there is an anatomical connection between the injected acupoints and the thyroid gland via a lymphatic and venous system (36).

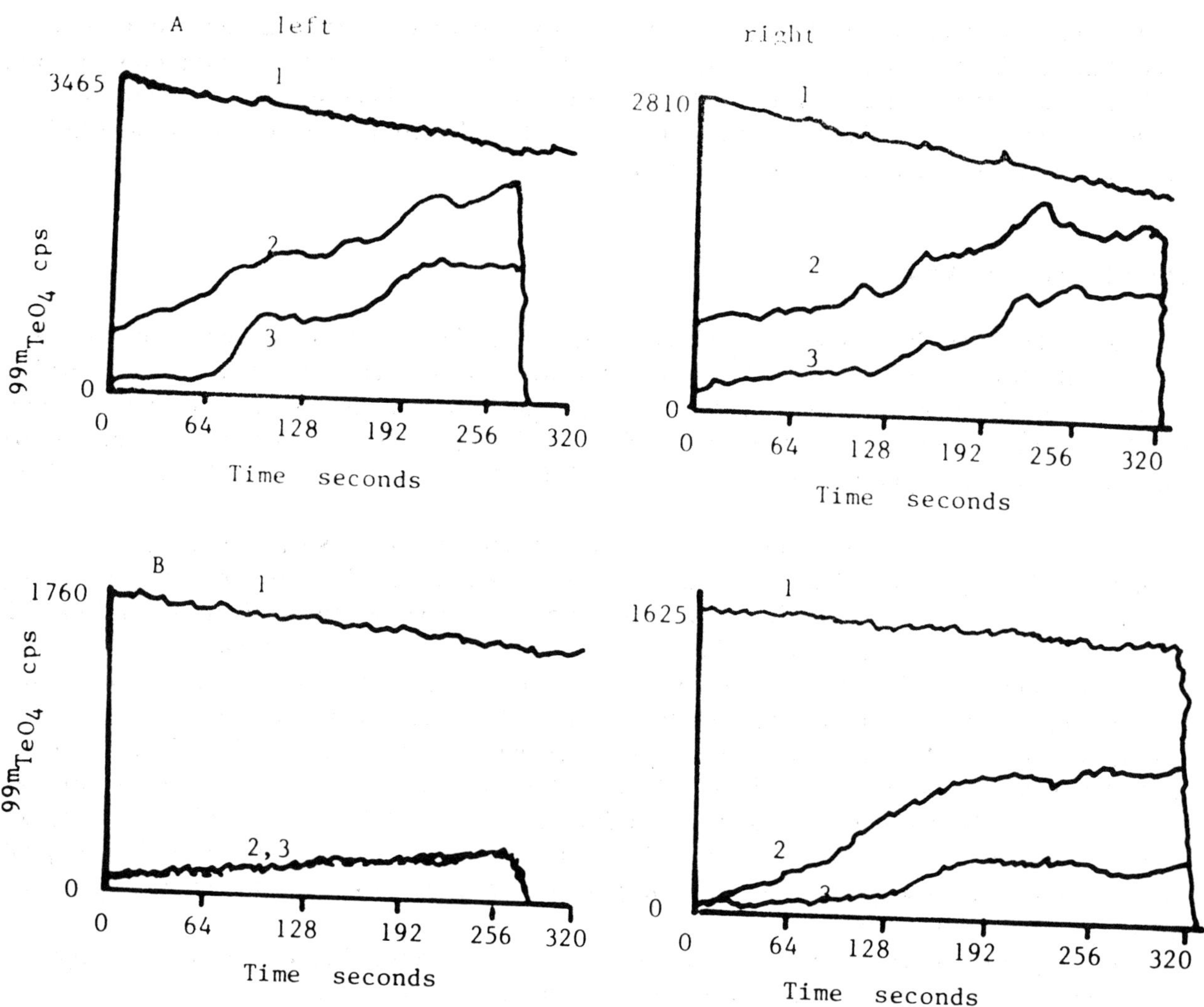

Figure 4-12. Scintigram from a Normal Subject (A) or a Unilateral Nephroectomized Patient (B) after Bilateral Injection of 99m-Te0_4 into the Acupoint Taixi (K 3).

Curve 1: radioactivity measurement at the injected acupoint vs. time;

Curve 2: measurement at the area closest to the injected acupoint;

Curve 3: measurement at the most remote area (3 inches away) from the injected acupoint.

left is the nephroectomized side

right is the normal kidney side

(From Shien (35))

Studies on sixteen anesthetized beagles have shown that the acupoints demonstrate a lower electric resistance than other skin area. When the radionucleides, 99m Tc pertechnetate, 201-Thallium chloride, 131-INa, or Rhenium sulfide was injected subcutaneously into some acupoints, only the 99m-Tc pertechnetate, not the other, gave rise to a rapid and longitudinal migration with a specific radioactive pathway, which is not the result of diffusion through nerve, vein, or lymphatic vessel, but its trajectory coincides with that described for one of the acupuncture meridian in the dog (23).However, by subcutaneous injection of three different radionucleides, 99m-Tc pertechnetate, Thallium-201 chloride (201-Tl) or Gallium-67 citrate (67-Ga), into the acupoint Tai Xi (K 3) of animals or human subjects, S. B. Jong, et al., (21) have shown that the absorption of these radionucleides is mainly through a passive pathway of diffusion process, depending upon the ionic radius of the agents. Administration of digitalis, a Na-K-ATPase inhibitor, does not block their absorption.

G. W. Lu (28) conducted studies with cats and rabbits, using EAP on the Zusanli point (S 36). This acupoint was chosen because it contains more myelinated large afferent nerve fibers. When electrical acupuncture was applied at the Zusanli point, a significant suppressive effect on jaw movement response and in the electromyogram of the digastric muscle induced by peroneal nerve stimulation was observed. This indicates that a longer-than-normal proportion of Class Aß fibers is involved. This predominance of large afferent fiber involvement was seen only when the needle was applied at the true acupoint, and not when it was outside the acupoint. Table 4-3 summarizes the histological findings of three different acupoints and their nerve innervations.

Table 4-3. Nerve Branches of Acupoints and Non-acupoints

Foci	Number of Foci	Number of fibers	Myelinated fibers %	Non-myelinated fibers %	Myelinated/ non-myelin.
High effective (Zusanli)	5	2,127	73	27	2.7*
Control					
non-effective	2	1,599	44	56	0.8
non-meridian	7	1,771	45	55	0.8

* $P < 0.01$ compared with the control

Following the monthly progress of seventeen human fetuses, Wang and his colleagues (42) studied the histology and embryonal development of two acupoints, Ho Ku (LI 4) and Ying Chuan (S 16). They found that before the fourth fetal month there are only small nerve bundles and nerve fibers under the skin in the area of these acupoints; no special encapsulated nervous receptors were observed. In the fifth fetal month, however, a primary type of Pacinian corpuscle was seen in the subcutaneous tissue. Rufini's corpuscle, muscles, and tendon spindle appeared in the sixth month. Before the sixth month, the muscle spindle was still in its primordial form. Capsule-differentiated nuclear bag and chain fibers and various nerve endings could only be identified after this period. In the eighth fetal month there were long fusiform receptors, and in the thirty-eight-week fetus tactile corpuscles were seen but were still immature.

Bioelectrical Properties

It has been postulated that at the acupuncture points the skin plays an important role in generating the pattern of bioelectric fields (34). Using an electric device, an electroacupointogram (EAG) of the acupoint can be recorded. This has been claimed to be useful in the differential diagnosis of the acupoint potential between healthy and pathological conditions (20).

Some acupoints represent an organizing center in the body (33,34). They contain a high density of gap junctions and a high level of electrical coupling. Such areas containing a high density of gap junctions mediate the rapid propagation of electric signals and optimization of metabolic activity. This is also a possible explanation of the phenomenon of distribution of radioactive substances through the acupoints.

Evidence indicates that acupoints are distinguishable from nonacupoints by means of their electrical properties. Applying two electrode probes on the skin, M. Reichmanis, et al., found some acupoints to be genuine local resistance minima (32). The resistance of the acupoints along the meridians tended to be lower than that of nonacupoints. These points, when connected by lines, resemble the acupuncture system of points and meridians.

Experimentation on animals has revealed that some acupuncture points vary in skin conductance. The epidermis at low resistance points is characterized by a high incidence of gap junctions (45).

T. E. Croley (9) measured the acupoint conductance in living and dead human subjects. He found that the electrical potential at the acupoints is higher than that of nonacupoints. In the cadaver, the electrical potential of the right-hand acupoints is significantly different from that of the left-hand acupoints. The reason for this difference is still unknown. The average range of electrical potenial for the HoKu acupoint of both living and dead subjects was 9.65 µA to 11.16 µA.

A group of researchers in Beijing measured the impedance of certain acupoints along the meridian channels (2, p. 280; and p. 284). In twenty-four young volunteer subjects, the acupoints along nine meridians showed lower impedance than nonacupoints. The average impedant of acupoints was measured at 16.33± 2.8 K ohm, whereas that of nonacupoints was reported at 18.55±3.74 K ohm. This phenomenon was also observed in cancer patients and in patients whose cancerous limbs had been amputated. Similar results were observed in rats, rabbits, and sheep.

Analgesic Effects and Pain Tolerance

E. M. Tsirulnikow, et al., applied acupuncture on the hands of nine healthy subjects, using ultrasonic stimulation. When the acupoint was stimulated, subjects reported feeling a particular sensation and a higher pain threshold than when stimuli were applied to nonacupoints (40).

The Zusanli point is one of the commonly used major acupoints, occasionally used as well as an adjuvant acupount. X. Liu, et al., (27) reported that the Zusanli acupoint is innervated by N. peroneus communis. In experiments with rats, Zusanli was stimulated electrically, an antidromic C wave was recorded, and it propagated to the Nucleus raphe magnus (NRM), a kind of feedback mechanism to modulate pain. T. P. Teng, et al., (38) recorded a pressure effect of tibialis anterior muscle and contraction after electrical stimulation of Zusanli. In experiment with cats and rabbits K. W. Lue, et al., (29) showed that a significant analgesic effect can be obtained by acupuncture on the Zusanli point, but not on nonacupoints. The effective Zusanli region contains 1,550 myelinated nerve fibers, much more than in the region of nonacupoints. The ratio of Aα , Aβ and Aτ to Aδ was 3.10 in the Zusanli region and 1.17 in the noneffective regions.

Han and his associates (1, p. 486–487) acupunctured rats at the Zusanli and Sanyinjiao points and found that 70 percent of the animals demonstrated an excellent analgesic effect. The pain thresholds of those animals increased, and there was also an elevation of the neurotransmitters, 5HT, and opioidlike substances in the brain. Z. Bing, et al., (5) performed acupuncture on rats at the Zusanli point of the right hind limb and found that acupuncture can trigger the neuronal mechanism involved in diffuse noxious inhibitory controls. Analgesia induced by either acupuncture or noxious thermal stimulation can be reduced significantly by administration of naloxone.

Another acupoint frequently used by acupuncturists is the HoKu locus. Wang, et al., (1 p. 424) studied the hands of two patients prior to amputation surgery and the morphology of the nerve endings of the HoKu acupoint. The patients were placed under acupointure anesthesia at the HoKu point. Once the propagation sensation or *tai qi* phenomenon was reported by the patients, the hand was immediately removed and studied. Wang reported that:

1. The sensory point is situated in the muscular layer. Around the neighborhood of the layer were many kinds of nerve endings, muscle spindle, motor end plates, and small nerve bundles.
2. In the superficial part of the corium, other morphological forms were observed. One of these manifests itself as a group of epithelial cells in which the nerve fibers were divided into it repeatedly and distributed into their intercellular space. Another specific form showed nerve endings distributed in and on the surface of a long spindle-shaped bundle of collagenous fiber.
3. In the deeper part of the corium, a noncapsulated receptor similar to a Raffini corpuscle was seen, measuring approximately 280 micrometers in length and 125 micrometers in diameter. The capsule contains about ten layers; under the capsule is subcapsular space, containing a cylindrical body. Another encapsulated receptor was also observed, resembling a round spindle approximately thirty micrometers in length and thirty micrometers in diameter.
4. Along the hair follicle of the HoKu point are many complex nerve endings, formed in a loose network. Some of these run parallel to the longitudinal axis of the hair.
5. The subcutaneous layer contains many comparatively large nerve bundles. Pacinian corpuscles may also be seen in this layer.

Z. L. Hou, (18) recorded the muscle action potential of the HoKu point of dogs and found that even after the nerve innervation was blocked by flaxedil, the muscle action potential of the HoKu point continued to be discharged for a certain period of time. (See figure 4-13.) Studies on awake, alert monkeys (*Macaca cyclopsis*) by Ha and Tan (16) showed that acupuncture would produce a significant analgesic effect and increase the pain threshold. The application of acupuncture at the acupoint HoKu (LI 4) or Zusanli (S 36) would induce a much more prominent effect and longer duration than when acupuncture was applied at other acupoints.

A. Brockhaus and C. E. Elger (6) tested on forty patients with acupuncture therapy at the acupoint HoKu and thirty-nine patients with laser acupuncture at the same point. They have found that acupuncture needling elicits an increase of pain threshold, but not on the patients treated with laser acupuncture.

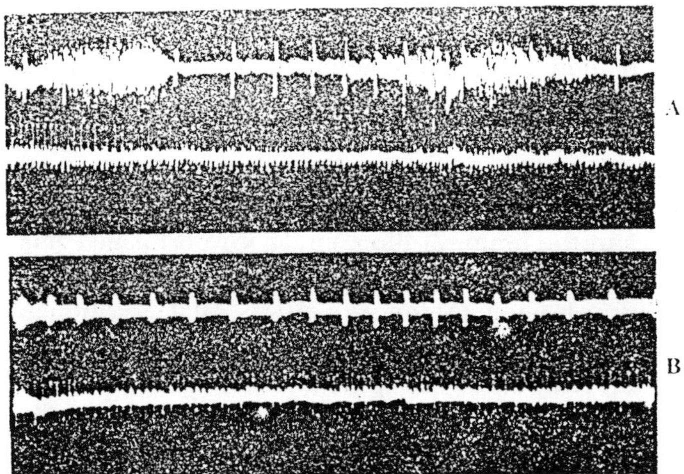

Figure 4-13. The Recorded Muscle Action Potential of a Dog before (A) and after (B) the Intravenous Injection of Flaxedil (2 mg/Kg)

Upper curve recorded at the pectoralis major, standard voltage 300 mV; time base 1.6 sec.

Lower curve recorded at the Acupoint HoKu (LI 4), standard voltage 50 mV; time base 1.6 sec.

(From Hou, (18))

Other Empirical Evidence

Reports have indicated that acupuncture along certain acupoints can cause an increase or decrease in skin temperature at distant sites. In nineteen healthy subjects who received acupuncture, either by manual stimulation or by electrical stimulation at the HoKu point (LI 4), a nonsegmental, long-lasting warming effect of the skin of the face and hand was observed. Manual stimulation was particularly effective in inducing elevation of skin temperature. When acupuncture was applied on the Zusanli point (S 36), both manual and electrical stimulation induced a long-lasting increase in skin temperature of the face and hands, but not the feet (24).

In other studies with eight normal human subjects, the Sanyinjiao (Sp 6) acupoint on the medial side of right leg was needled and stimulated. A vasoconstriction in the right leg and a decrease in skin temperature were observed, but there was no change in either the arm or the left leg. When the Neiguan (P 6) acupoint of the right arm was needled, vasoconstriction of both arms was observed, together with a decrease in skin temperature; neither leg was affected. When acupuncture was applied on the Qu Chi (LI 11) point of the left arm, vasodilation of both arms and an increase in skin temperature were observed, without affecting either leg (26).

Using a thermographic technique, M. Ernst and M. H. M. Lee measured the skin temperature of the face, hand, and foot during acupuncture procedures on healthy volunteers at the HoKu point. Both manual and electric stimulation produced a generalized long-lasting warming effect indicating a sympatholytic effect (14,15). In another experiment they measured the skin temperature during the acupuncture at the Zusanli locus and found that the electro-acupuncture produced a cooling effect in the foot by increasing the sympathetic activity; on the contrary, the manual acupuncture still produced a warming effect, as shown in the hand.

Figure 4-14 presents some of their data, which illustrate the change of temperature by manual or electrical acupuncture.

Figure 4-14. The Skin Temperature Change during Manual and Electrical Acupuncture at Acupoint Zusanli (S 36)

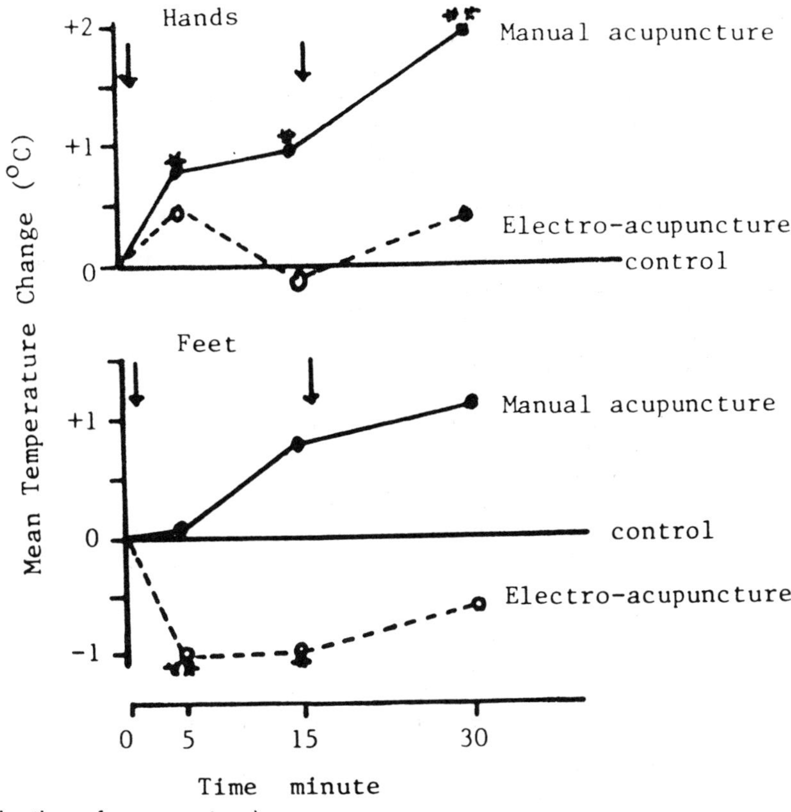

(arrow indicates the application of acupuncture)

* p .05; ** p .01

(From Ernst & Lee (15))

T. Yano, et al., (44) studied five healthy male volunteers using an ultrasonic diagnostic apparatus (Toshiba SSA-90A) to measure the cross-sectional area of the gallbladder. They performed an image analysis before, during, and after electro-acupuncture of certain acupoints along the Foot Xiao Yang (gallbladder) meridian. They did not detect any change in the gallbladder image. However, when the needle was applied on the extra point, Dan Nang Xue (Extra-390), about one to two inches below the G-34 point, the gallbladder contracted.

Z. Bing, et al., (4) have reported a lack of topographical specificity of the acupoints. In their experiments with animals, they found no difference between the capacity to activate subnucleus reticularis dorsalis neurons, whether EAP was applied directly on the Zusanli locus or on nonacupoints in the surrounding area.

References

1. All China Society of Acupuncture and Moxibustion. First National Symposium on Acupunture and Acupuncture Anesthesia. Beijing, 1979.
2. All China Society of Acupuncture and Moxibustion. Second National Symposium on Acupuncture and Moxibustion and Acupuncture Anesthesia. Beijing, 1984.
3. Badgley, L. American Journal of Acupuncture 12:219, 1984.
4. Bing, Z., et al. Neuroscience 44:693, 1991.
5. Bing, Z., et al. Neuroscience 37:809, 1990.
6. Brockhaus, A. and C. E. Elger. Pain 43:181, 1990.
7. Brown, N. L. American Journal of Chinese Medicine 2:67, 1974.
8. Chen, M. F., et al. American Journal of Chinese Medicine 21:221, 1993; Clinical Nuclear Medicine 19:426, 1994.
9. Croley, T. E. American Journal of Acupuncture 14:57, 1986.
10. Dung, H. C. American Journal of Chinese Medicine 12:80, 1984; 12:94, 1984.
11. Dung, H. C. American Journal of Chinese Medicine 13:39, 1985; 13:49, 1985; 13:133, 1985; 13:145, 1985.
12. Dung, H. H. Chinese Medical Journal 97:751, 1984.
13. Evans, D., from Raj, P. P., ed. Practical Management of Pain. 2nd ed. New York: Mosby, 1992, p. 934.
14. Ernst, M., and M. H. M. Lee. Pain 21:25, 1985
15. Ernst, M., and M. H. M. Lee. Exp. Neurol. 94:1, 1986.
16. Ha, H. C., and E. C. Tan. American Journal of Chinese Medicine 10:92, 1982.
17. Han, C. C. Chinese Medical Journal 97:223, 1984.
18. Hou, Z. L. Chinese Medical Journal 92(4):223, 1979.
19. Huk, Z., et al., Acupuncture Electro-Therp. Res. 18:117, 1993.
20. Ionescu-Tirgovistec, S., and S. Pruna. Rev. Roum. Medicine Interne 25:67,1987.
21. Jong, S. B., et al. Radioisotope 41:431, 1992.
22. Kiselveva, R. E., et al. Arkh. Anat. Gistol Embriol. 90:36, 1986.
23. Kovacs, F. M., et al. Journal of Nuclear Medicine 33:403, 1992.
24. Lee, M. H. M., and M. Ernst from Pomeranz, B., and G. Stux, eds. Scientific Bases of Acupuncture. Berlin: Springer Verlag, Berlin, 1989. p. 157.
25. Li, C. Y., et al. Journal of Traditional Chinese Medicine (in English) 7:29, 1987.
26. Lin, M. T., et al. American Journal of Chinese Medicine 9:305, 1981.
27. Liu, X., et al. Acta Physiology Sin. 42:523, 1990.
28. Lu, G. W. American Journal of Physiology 245:R606, 1983.
29. Lue, K. W., et al., in Chang, C. T., et al., eds. Research in Acupuncture and Moxibustion. Beijing: Science Publisher, 1986, p. 331.
30. Novikov, I. I., et al. ZH Nevropatol. Psikhiatr. I M S S Korsalova 87:58 1987.
31. Omura, Y. Acupuncture Electro-Ther. Res. 14:155, 1989.
32. Reichmenis, M. Modern Bioelectricity. 1988, p. 762.
33. Shang, C. American Journal of Chinese Medicine 17:119, 1989.
34. Shang, C. American Journal of Chinese Medicine 21:91, 1993.

35. Shien, P. Y. Journal of Chinese Acupuncture and Moxibustion 11(3):147, 1991.
36. Simon, J., et al. Presse Medicine 17:1341, 1988.
37. Sun, B. L., et al. J. Chin. Soc. Veterinary Sci. 20:118, 1994.
38. Teng, T. P., et al., in Chang, C. T., eds. Research in Acupuncture and Moxibustion. Beijing: Science Publisher, 1986, p. 319.
39. Thomas, O. L. American Journal of Acupuncture 14:205, 1986.
40. Tsirulnikow, E. M., et al. Fiziol. Chel. 12:414, 1986.
41. Wang, K., et al. American Journal of Chinese Medicine 17:145, 1989.
42. Wang, Z. T., et al. Jeipou Xuebao 17:203, 1986; 17:207, 1986.
43. Wu, C. C., et al. Radioisotopes 36:261, 1990; American Journal of Chinese Medicine 22:114, 1993.
44. Yano, T.,et al. J. Jpn. Asso. Phys. Medicine Balmed. Climatol. 53:207, 1990.
45. Zhang, D., et al. Journal of Traditional Chinese Medicine (in English) 10:36, 1990.

5

The Physiology of Pain

We generally consider the body to have five primary senses, each of which conveys impulses to a specific area of the brain: *touch, taste, smell, hearing,* and *vision.* An additional sense is that of *pain,* which the body perceives from skin or deep tissues (viscerals, muscle, and bone). Physiologists still debate about how the sensation of pain occurs and whether there are specific nerves conducting the sensation analogous to those involved in the five primary senses.

In the Chinese language, the word *pain* is usually associated with a sensation of bitterness, a feeling from the heart. While acupuncture and other medical techniques were developed to relieve symptoms of pain, the Chinese had no direct theories about the sensation of pain itself. Instead, they believed that pain resulted from an imbalance of Yin and Yang or an obstruction of the circulation of blood and Qi in the body.

Buddha attributed pain to the frustration of desires. Theologists from all religions have advanced the idea that pain is a penalty from a *divine being,* and a means for the purification and redemption of men. Even Hippocrates, the father of Western medicine, believed that the Divine works to subdue pain.

It was in ancient Greece that physiological origins of pain were first proposed. Anaxagoras (500–428 B.C.) proposed that the brain is the organ that perceives pain and sensation. Later Herophilus (335–250 B.C.) and Erasistratus (310–250 B.C.) of Alexandria provided anatomical evidence that the brain was part of the nervous system and that the nerves are the basis for movement and for feeling.

Today we know that the sensation of pain originates from a cutaneous nociceptor, stimulated by an impending or actual tissue damage with no emotional or perceptual connotation. Pain is a complex sensation, which includes an unpleasant feeling and an emotional reaction. Sometimes pain can be so extreme, unbearable, and consistent over a long duration that it is the most severe suffering in human experience. As Trush summarized in his thesis (18), "without sensitivity to pain, one must live a miserable life. "

Pain is also a defense mechanism of the body to prevent or to escape from injury or stimulation. In some rare individuals who lack perception of pain, or when pain perception is lost during disease, such as in leprosy or tabes, this defense mechanism no longer functions. This frequently results in repeated severe insults to the body, leading to major tissue destruction.

Peripheral Nociceptors

There are free nerve endings under the dermis of the skin, as well as specific receptors. When cellular or tissue injury occurs for any reason, the noxious stimuli, as described by Sherrington, activate those specific pain receptors by either direct damage, nociception, or release of a certain chemical substance—for example, bradykinin, histamine, serotonin, prostaglandins, or acetylcholine in a process of chemoreception. The noxious stimulus, which is generally considered to be the cause of tissue damage, varies in intensity. In addition, other receptors, such as mechanoreceptors and thermoreceptors, have been identified under the skin.

The message or impulse created by stimulation of these receptors is transmitted by nonspecific afferent nerve fibers from the receptors to the spinal cord and then carried by specific pain pathways in the neuraxis into the pain center. The primary afferent spinal nerve fibers terminate at the dorsal root ganglia first and then project to the spinal cord. The transmitted impulse is modified at the first sy̆napsis within the dorsal horn, but also at multiple levels of the neuraxis. The impulse ascends to the thalamus and the brain stem and ultimately to the cortex. As pain per se, it is neither transmitted nor conducted: only the impulse is propagated through the nerve fibers. Figure 5-1 illustrates diagrammatically the cutaneous receptors.

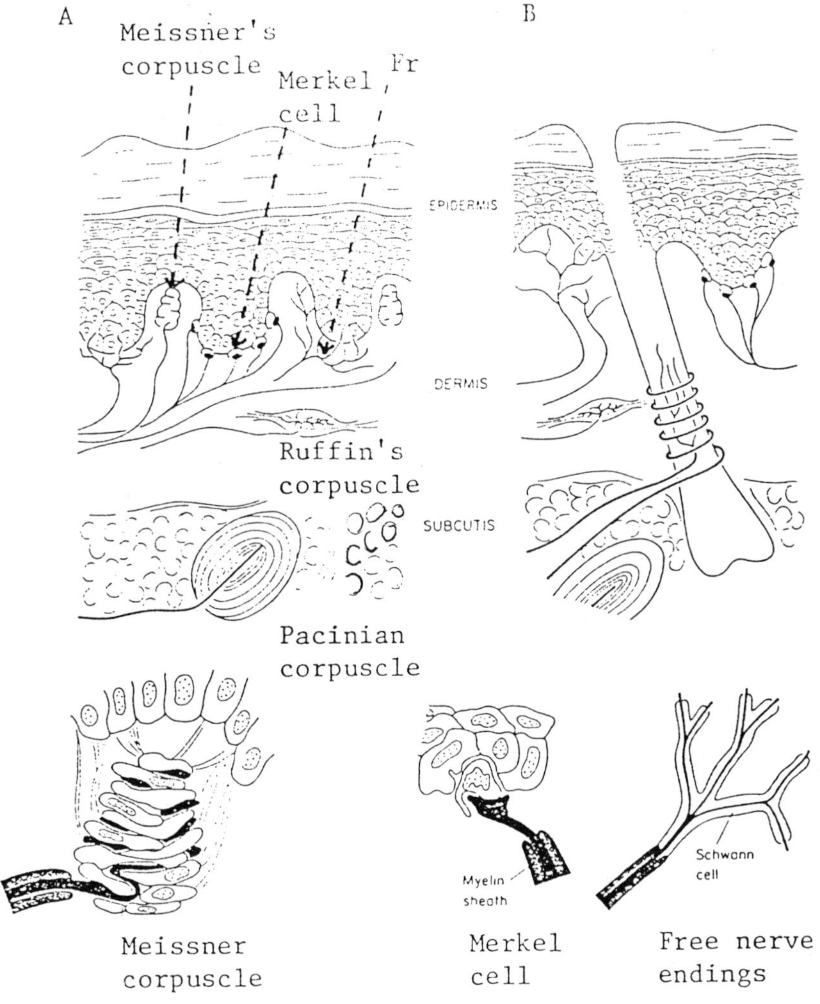

Figure 5-1. Cutaneous Receptors

(From Brodal: *The Central Nerve System*, p. 114)

Table 5-1. Classification of Afferent Nerve Fibers

Class	Diameter μ	Myelination	Morphologic Receptor	Conduction velocity m/sec	Functional type	Sensation evoked	Stimulation
A α (I)	large (6–17)	heavy	unmyelinated neurite-Schwann cell complex in basal epidermis, muscle spindle, Golgi, tendon, mechanoreceptor (applies to A α and A β)	70–120	somatic afferent	sharp stinging pain	noxious skin deformate (11–15 g/mm^2)
A β (II)		heavy		30–70			
A δ (III)	small (1–5)	thin	nociceptor (25%) (free nerve ending) mechanoreceptor (75%) thermoreceptor	6–30	somatic afferent		
C fibers (IV)	small (0.3–1)	none	free nerve ending nociceptor (25%) mechanoreceptor (50%)	0.4–1.5	visceral & somatic afferent	dull, burning pain, aching?	noxious skin deformate (6–26 g/mm^2), heat, chemicals

It is now well established that two types of afferent nerve fibers carry pain impulses, although not exclusively. They are Class A fibers and Class C fibers. Class A fibers are further differentiated as Aα , Aβ and Aδ , fibers. They are all myelinated but differ in their diameter and conduction velocity. Class C fibers are nonmyelinated and are very slow in conduction speed. There are, however, about four times more Class C fibers than myelinated Class A fibers in a somatic nerve trunk. The sympathetic trunk contains up to 20 percent Class C fibers. Table 5-1 illustrates the differences among the afferent nerve fibers.

In the early 1960s, some neurophysiologists believed that the speed of conduction plays a role in the intensity of the pain sensation, and a double pain system was proposed. But later, G. H. Bishop obtained evidence that the diameter or size of the nerve fiber is more important than conduction velocity for effectively transmitting the "essential metabolites from cell body to synaptic transmitting terminal" (2).

A pain message or impulse is conducted from the receptors in the periphery to the spinal cord via the dorsal root ganglia; then in the spinal cord or the medulla oblongata, conduction of the impulse is delayed and the conducting fiber synapses with a second neuron. In the spinal cord, the afferent fiber ends in the interneuronal substantia gelantinosa, which contains a large number of Golgi Type II neurons. The delay in impulse transmission at this site allows an important modification of pain sensation. The Gate Control theory proposed by R. Melzack and P. P. Wall (14) is based on this interneuronal regulation. Melzack and Wall also claim that the substantia gelantinosa functions as a storehouse for memories of pain. Figure 5-2 diagramatically illustrates the pathways for pain impulse transmission.

Figure 5-2. Primary Neural Pathways for Transmission of Nociceptive Information From Peripheral to the Brain, via the Spinal Cord, Medulla, Pons and Mesencephalon.

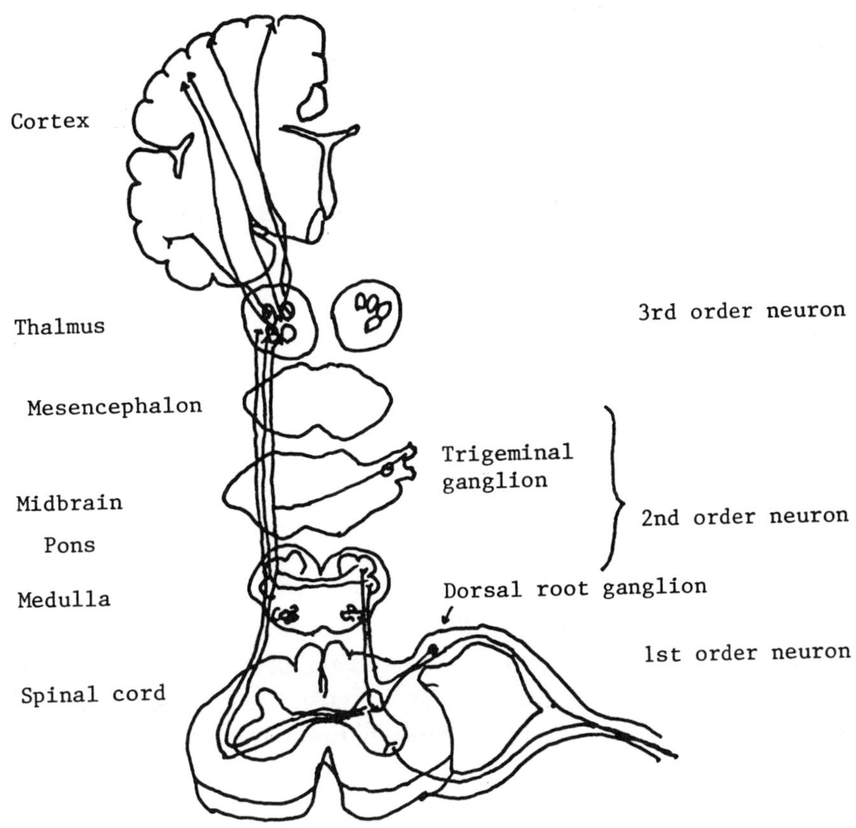

Gate Control Theory

In 1965, Melzack and Wall proposed a very attractive hypothesis to explain how the sensation of pain is modulated in the body. They submitted a model of sensory, motivational, and central control in the determination of pain. The modulating mechanism is located mainly in the spinal cord dorsal horn and the caudal trigeminal complex, which serve as a gate to control or filter and abstract the flow of impulses entering the central nervous system. An impulse may be either blocked or allowed to go through. In this theory, the substantia gelatinosa of the spinal dorsal horn functions as "a gate control mechanism that modulates the afferent pattern before the impulse influences the transmission cells (T cells); and the T cells activate neural mechanisms that comprise the action system responsible for perception and response" (13).

Melzack and Wall's model is presented diagrammatically in figure 5-3.

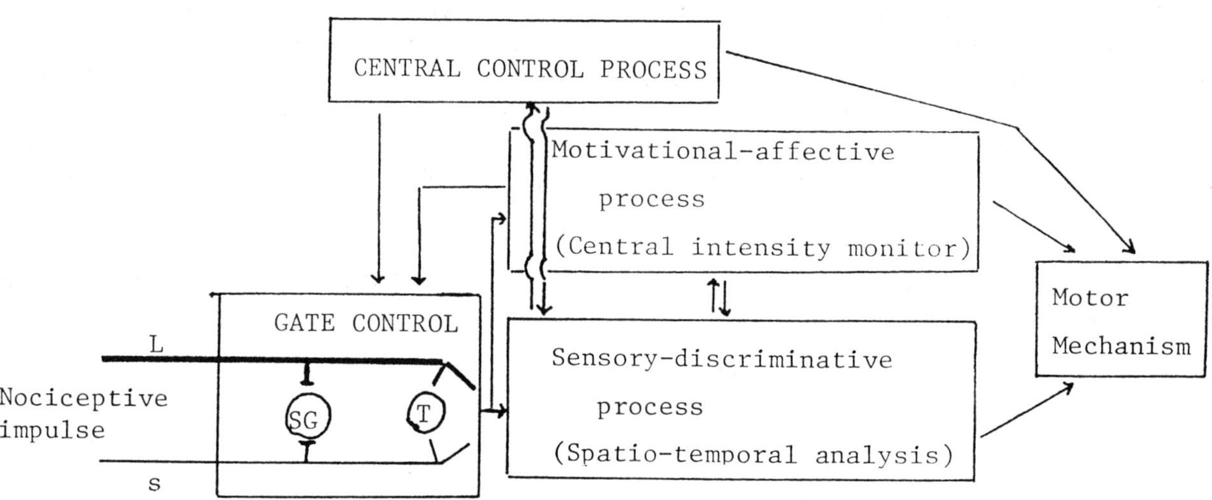

Figure 5-3. Conceptual Model of the Sensory, Motivational, and Central Determinants of Pain

L: large diameter afferent fibers;

S: small diameter afferent fibers;

SG: Substantia gelatinosa

T: Central transmission cells

(From Melzack and Wall (14))

When the pain impulse is initiated at the nociceptors, it is transmitted from the peripheral afferent fibers into the spinal dorsal horn. Transmission of the impulse is delayed in the interneuronal neurons in the substantia gelatinosa and a central transmission cell (T cell). The level of activation of the T cell is determined by a balance between the input from large-diameter fibers (Aß) and small-diameter fibers (Aδ and C). It is believed that impulses coming from the small fibers stimulate T cells or increase their effectiveness and that impulses from large fibers inhibit or decrease the effectiveness of the T cell.

Through the inhibitory activity of the substantia gelatinosa, the "gate" is closed and prevents the impulse from being conducted through the T cell. The thin myelinated Aδ fibers and nonmyelinated C fibers primarily conduct noxious stimuli, but the large-diameter fibers (Aß) influence the output of the second-order neurons in the brain stem, which affect discharges from the pain pathway neurons.

The output of the dorsal horn T cell is transmitted to the brain by two pathways: the anterolateral spinal tract via the neospinothalamic fibers into the thalmus and somatosensory center, and the paramedial ascending fibers into the reticular formation and medial intralaminar thalamus and the limbic system. A further assumption suggests that descending impulses from the brain also play a role in a presynaptic control mechanism. The conduction of pain impulses in the spinal cord is thus influenced both by the afferent activity and by central control processes in the brain.

Ascending Systems

The primary afferent fibers that transmit pain messages are first interrupted in the dorsal root ganglia. The impulses are then transmitted centropetally along two pathways. The first runs along the dorsal columns, which are composed of the ascending branches of large-diameter myelinated primary afferent axons whose bodies are in the dorsal root ganglia and terminate in the cuneate and gracile nuclei of the medulla oblongata; the other runs along the anterolateral ascending pathways, which are composed of axons of secondary-order neurons whose bodies are in the dorsal horn. The nociceptive impulses transmitted from the dorsal root ganglia are primarily modulated here, by the substantia gelatinosa and T cells.

The majority of the ascending neurons then cross the midline in the spinal cord and continue their ascent in the contralateral anterolateral funiculus, which projects to the lateral spinothalamic tract (neospinothalamic) fibers and the ventral spinothalamic tract (paleospinothalamic) fibers. Neurophysiologists identify these as the pain pathways. However, small numbers of axons have been identified ascending ipsilaterally to the brain stem, as the spinoreticular tracts. It has been shown that the spinoreticular tracts also play a part in pain mechanisms, and there are synaptic connections between the thalamic neurons receiving the spinothalamic axons and the brain stem reticular formation. This indicates that the reticular formation also serves as a relay station for nociceptive impulse transmission.

The lateral spinothalamic tract fibers project to and synapse in the ventrolateral and posterolateral thalamic nuclei, which then project to the primary somatosensory cortex. They are responsible for spatial and temporal discrimination of pain and touch sensations. The axons of ventral spinothalamic tract fibers terminate directly in the medial thalamic nuclei or terminate indirectly through the spinoreticular formation. It is believed that these fibers participate in suprasegmental reflex responses and are responsible for transmission of nondiscriminative pain. The spinoreticulothalamic pathway is believed to be responsible for transmission of diffuse slow pain.

Thalamus

The thalamus is divided into a ventral nuclear complex, posterior nuclear complex, and medial and intralaminar thalamic nuclei. The major portion of the ascending axons from the medial lemniscus and the lateral spinothalamic tracts terminate in both the ventral and posterior nuclear complex. Information is then relayed to the somatosensory area in the ipsilateral postcentral gyrus of the parietal lobe. The posterior nuclear complex contains more neurons than the other two complexes. This complex is responsive to nociceptive stimuli, which tend to be bilateral. It is more effective than the other complexes in functioning as a relay to the cortex.

Cortex

The somatosensory area receives the propagation of nociceptive impulses from the thalamus. It is still not completely understood whether this area is essential for pain recognition. It is, however, known that this somatosensory cortical area plays a role in modulating the cognitive and noncognitive features of pain. The evaluation of the pain sensation occurs through association with other neurons in the central nervous system and prior experiences. This somatosensory area is probably important for the production of effective responses to stimuli and the initiation of avoidance and escape behavior.

Studies of unanesthetized rabbits or cats have shown that when an animal is given a microinjection of opioid peptides (EK and endorphins), morphine, or EAP, there is a unidirectional change in both spontaneous and nociceptive-stimulated neuronal activity of the sensorimotor cortex, mesencephalic reticular formation, and giant cell reticular nucleus of medulla oblongata being observed. Such changes can be abolished by administration of naloxone (19).

Descending Systems

When the afferent fibers transmit their input to the CNS, many terminate or send collateral branches to the brain stem reticular formation. Here a negative feedback system is established to send a descending impulse back to the spinal cord, resulting in modulation of the pain sensation.

Using the antidromic activation technique Z. Q. Chen, et al., (4) demonstrated that the cortical neurons in somatosensory area II (S II) projecting directly to the centromedian nucleus (CM) were identified intracellularly. EAP could activate these cortical neurons, which in turn inhibited the nociceptive response to induce analgesia, confirmed that the cerebral cortex plays a role in descending modulation of the acupuncture-analgesia.

It has been shown that the mesodiencephalic periventricular and periaqueductral gray (PVG and PAG) and the rostral ventromedial medullar (RVM) area play a role in such descending systems. PAG is chemically heterogeneous, receiving its afferent fibers mainly from the hypothalamus and frontal granular and insular cortex, and also from the amygdala. The input from the PAG, which is predominently excitatory, is not directly transmitted to the spinal cord. Instead, it goes to the RVM, which includes both the medullary nucleus raphe magnus (NRM) and reticulus magnocellularis (RMC). The RVM is the major source of axons from the brain stem to the spinal cord. These axons are densely concentrated in the superficial layer of the dorsal horn, where the small-diameter primary afferent fibers (Aδ and C) terminate. Electrical stimulation of fibers in this descending system results in suppression of nociceptive spinal dorsal horn neurons and the phenomenon of stimulation-produced analgesia (SPA). Figure 5-4 illustrates diagrammatically the descending system.

Figure 5-4. Diagrammatic Illustration of the Descending System in Modulating the Pain Sensation

PAG: Periagueductral gray

PGL: Paragiantocellularis nucleus

rm: raphe magnus nucleus

mc: reticularis magnocellularis

DLF: Dorsolateral funiculus

NE: Norepinephrine

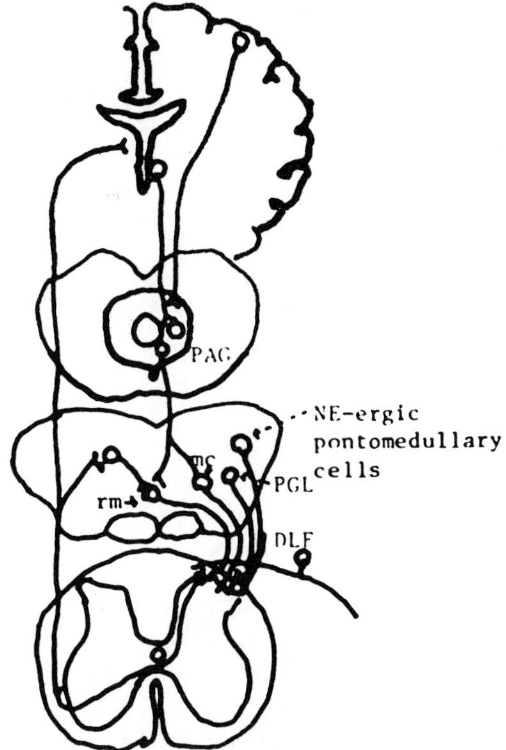

In this descending system, it is believed that some type of chemical transmitter mediates the modulation of the pain sensation. Cells in these nuclei can release 5HT, catecholamines, and opioid peptides, which can influence the sensation of pain. In particular, the opioid peptides, including the enkephalins, ß-endorphins, and dynorphin, are found in these nuclei. Table 5-2 summarizes the chemical characteristics of these six nuclei.

It was shown in an experiment with rats that acupuncture stimulation of the muscle beneath the acupoint, e. g., Zusanli, is effective in producing an analgesic effect that can be abolished by hypophysectomy or by intracerebral-ventricular (icv) injection of anti-ß-endorphin serum (17). The acupuncture analgesic pathway is conducted to be from D-PAG converged to the hypothalamo-pituitary and then projected to the anterior hypothalamus. Injection of L-glutamate sodium into the hypothalamic paraventricular nuclei (PVNH) or electric stimulation could enhance the acupuncture-induced analgesia, while electrical cauterization of PVNH would abolish it, but removal of pituitary would not influence the L-glutamate effect (20). Experiments in conscious rats also showed that EAP at the acupoint Zusanli can increase the pain threshold, there is a positive involvement of specific C-fos protein-labeled neuron through the neuroaxis including the PVNH (5).

Table 5-2. The Opioid Peptides and Analgesic Effect in Various Neurons

SITE	OPIOID PEPTIDE*	OPIATE RECEPTOR	OPIATE MICRO-INJECTION	SPA#	NALOXONE BLOCKAGE
Amygdala	+	+	+	+	?
Periventricular Diencephalon	+	+	+	+	?
PAG	+	+	+	+	+
NRM	+	0	+	+	+
Nuclei reticularis paragigantocellaris	+	0	+	+	+
Dorsal horn	+	+	+	0	+

* ß-Endorphin, enkephalin or dynorphin;

\# SPA = stimulation-produced analgesia

\+ = yes; 0 = no; ?= not sure

Empirical Evidence

Experiments have shown that electrical stimulation of rats can cause an excitatory effect on the nucleus arcuatus hypothalamus (ARH) and NRM, which is abolished by decerebration of the animal, section of ß-endorphinergic tract, or administration of naloxone (8). Further, the activation of NRM neurons can be elicited by stimulation of dorsal PAG. Leucine-enkephalin (LEK) can mimic the activation and the opiate antagonist, while naloxone can reverse such activation (22). Experiments with rats and rabbits have also demonstrated that an analgesia can be effectively induced by microinjection of morphine into the PAG area or by direct electrical stimulation. Such analgesic effect can be reversed by naloxone (1,10,11). It has been shown that EAP applied to rats can provoke a descending slow potential recorded at the C6 vertebra; lesion of PAG by electrolytes markedly reduces such potential (21).

X. D. Cao (3) reported that the stimulation of the lateral preoptic area (LPO) of a rabbit by a microelectrode could cause an inhibitory effect on the PAG activity, which can be reversed by administration of naloxone. This suggests that either LPO stimulation or EAP can integrate in the PAG neuron and activate the interaction of endorphins and other opiate receptors and bring forth a stimulation of the nociceptive responses.

J. S. Han (9) implanted a cannula into the lateral ventricle of a rat or into the PAG region of a rabbit and performed the following experiments:

1. Intrathecal injection of dynorphin (DYN) into the neuron, it raised the pain threshold and produced an analgesic effect that lasted for three or four hours, such effect being dose-dependent;
2. Nalopxone or anti-DYN-IgG serum can abolish the analgesic effect induced by DYN;

3. Injection of DYN into the subarachnoid space of an acute morphine-tolerated rat can elicit a marked analgesic effect.

It has been shown in the rat that the analgesic effect induced by either morphine, EAP, or stress can be abolished by a lesion of the locus coeruleus at the floor of the fourth ventricle by electrolyte or by kainic acid. Injection of dexamethason only blocks the stress-induced analgesia, but not the other two. This suggests that these three analgesic effects involved some different endogenous analgesic system (6).

T. Sato, et al., (15) reported that application of low-frequency electrical stimulation at the Zusanli point in rats could produce an equivalent analgesic effect to an intrathecal application of 0.05 μg of morphine or intraperitoneal injection of 0.5 mg/kg of morphine. Naloxone can completely block such analgesic effect, whether induced via acupuncture or morphine. The morphine-induced analgesia can be abolished by bilateral lesion of the anterolateral tract (ALT) of the spinal cord, while the acupuncture-induced analgesia can be abolished by contralateral lesion. However, analgesia induced by large doses of intrathecal morphine (0.1–0. 2 ug) was not abolished, but persisted after ALT lesion, unilateral lesion of dorsal PAG, or hypophysectomy. Furthermore, it was found that the analgesia induced by dorsal PAG stimulation was not affected by ALT lesion, nor by intrathecal injection of nalaxone, but was abolished by lesion of dorso-lateral funicule.

The authors then concluded that there are probably two types of morphine action in the spinal cord that work to produce analgesia—one activating the ascending acupuncture analgesic pathway and the other via a direct inhibition of pain messengers in the spinal cord. The acupuncture analgesic pathway ascends contralaterally in the ALT and then bilaterally in the dorsal PAG.

It has been reported that the posterior hypothalamic arcuate nucleus (P-HARN) is the origin of the descending pain inhibitory system, which is enhanced by acupuncture. In studies with rats, C. Takeshige, et al., showed that lesions of the P-HARN or medial HARN (hypothalamic arcuate nucleus) can abolish such acupuncture analgesia effect, but lesion in anterior HARN does not. Microinjection of ß-endorphin, morphine, or dopamine into the P-HARN can produce an analgesia that is dose-dependent. Such analgesia is antagonized by naloxone or haloperidol, a dopaminergic blocking agent. Hypophysectomy can abolish the acupuncture analgesic effect, which can be restored when acupuncture and ß-endorphin or morphine are administered together, but not with the drug alone (16). Figure 5-5 illustrates such acupuncture analgesic effects in normal and hypophysectomized rats. It can be seen here that hypophysectomy abolishs the acupuncture analgesia. The microinjection of either ß-endorphin or morphine into the P-HARN would restore the abolishes acupuncture-induced analgesic effect but has no influence on normal acupuncture action.

Electrical stimulation of a rat's arcuate nucleus of hypothalamus (HARN) has been shown to induce analgesia that is attenuated by intrathecal injection of ICI-174864, an opiate δ-receptor antagonist, or ß-FNA, an opiate μ-receptor antagonist (12). However, injection of BNI, a kappa receptor antagonist, does not modify the descending inhibitory effect of HARN on spinal cord mociceptive reflexes or the basal pain threshold. Data suggest that the spinal δ and μ, but not kappa, opiate receptors, are involved in mediation of pain-relieving effects induced through HARN stimulation.

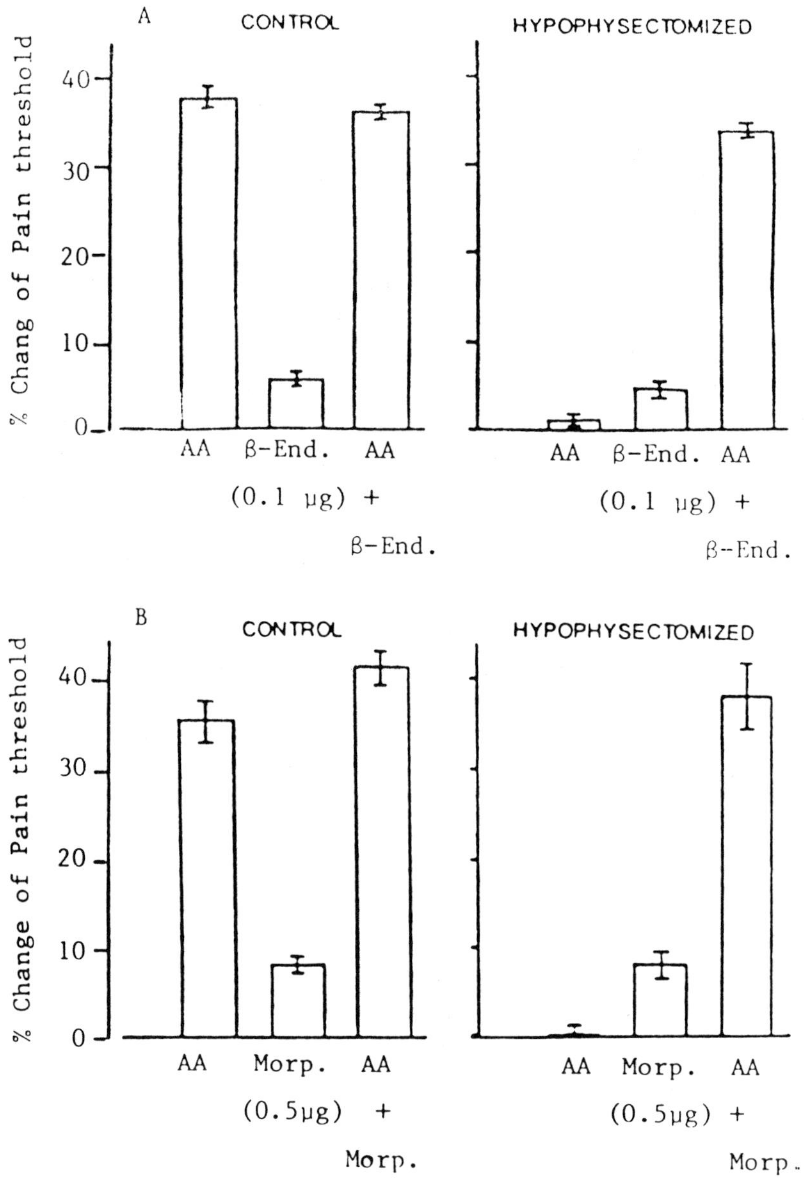

Figure 5-5. Acupuncture-Induced Analgesia (AA) in Control and Hypophysectomized Rats

(A) microinjection of β-endorphin or

(B) of morphine into the P-HARN nuclei

(From Takeshige et al. (17))

References

1. Akil H., et al. Science 191:961, 1976.
2. Bishop, G. H., in Knighton, R. S., and P. R. Dumbol, eds. Pain. Boston: Little and Brown, 1964, p. 83.
3. Cao, X. D. The Second National Symposium on Acupuncture and Moxibustion and Acupuncture Anesthesia. All China Soc. on Acupuncture and Moxibustion. Beijing: 1984, p. 360
4. Chen, Z. Q., et al. Journal of Traditional Chinese Medicine 6:195, 1986.
5. Dai, J. L., et al. Acupuncture Electro-Therap. Res. 17:165, 1992.
6. Di, S., et al. Acta Pharmacol. Sinica 4:153, 1983.
7. Fields, H., and A. I. Basbaum, from Wall, P. D., and R. Melzack. Textbook of Pain. 2nd ed. New York: Churchill A. Livingstone, 1989, p, 206.
8. Gao, Y. S., and Y. H. Ku. Acta Physiol. Sinica 35:409, 1983.
9. All China Society of Acupuncture and Moxibustion. Second National Symposium on Acupuncture and Moxibustion and Acupuncture Anesthesia. Beijing: People Health Publisher, 1984 p. 397.
10. Jacquet, Y. F., and A. Lajtha. Brain Res. 103:501, 1976.
11. Lianfang, H., and W. Q. Dong. Acup. Electro-ther. Res. 8:257, kd1983.
12. Mao, L. H., and J. S. Han. Chinese Journal Pharmacol. and Toxicol. 5:81, 1991.
13. Melzack, R., and P. P. Wall. Science 150:971, 1965.
14. Melzack, R., and P. P. Wall. in A. K. Jacox, ed. Pain. Boston: Little Brown 1977, p. 16.
15. Sato, T., et al. Acupuncture Electro-Ther. Res. 16:13, 1991.
16. Takeshige, C., et al. Brain Res. Bull. 26:113, 1991.
17. Takeshige, C., et al. Brain Res. Bull. 30:53, 1993.
18. Trush, D. C. Brain 96:369, 1973.
19. Yang, J., and B. C. Lin. Acupuncture Electro-Therap. Res. 17:209, 1992.
20. Yasnetsov, V. V., and V. A. Prevdivtsev. Byull Eksp. Biol. Medicine 94:53, 1982.
21. Zhang, Q. Y., and Z. F. Cheng. Acta Physiol. Sinica 45:142, 1993.
22. Zhu, L. X., and Q. Y. Shi. Journal of Traditional Chinese Medicine 4:111, 1984.

6
Opioid Peptides

As described in the previous chapter, the sensation of pain is a response to a nociceptive stimulus, whether chemical, mechanical, or thermal. In normal daily life, many things can result in pain—hunger, childbirth, and physical and emotional pressure. Even in primitive times, men searched not only for food, but for painkillers to relieve their suffering.

An early Chinese medical pharmacopeia, the *Herbal Classic of the Divine Plowman,* was written in approximately 101 B.C., about one hundred years earlier than the *Huang Ti Nei Chian* (17). This book recorded the methods of Sheng Nung, the Divine Plowman, born in 2900 B.C., who taught the people to use herbs in treating their illnesses. Among the 365 plants, minerals, and animal products listed in the classic were certain herbs considered to be painkillers.

In ancient Greece, Theoplastus (third century B.C.) was the first to mention the use of opium as a pain reliever. Later, Celus and Dioscordes wrote extensively on the use of opium and hemp to relieve pain. Opium, the unripe juice obtained from *Papaverum somniferum,* was not originally grown in China and was unavailable in early Chinese society. The Chinese people have mainly depended upon herbs and other remedies, such as acupuncture and moxibustion, for relief of pain.

Before 1975, most Western investigators considered acupuncture to be some sort of mystic art, with little basis in science. No one understood how acupuncture produced analgesia. It should be remembered, however, that the same question was originally asked of opium, before its active principle, morphine, was understood.

In 1975, however, researchers found that the central nervous tissue can synthesize and release endogenous peptides, which exert their antinociceptive effect by binding to specific receptors, sometimes called opiate receptors, in the central nervous system. J. Hughes first reported that he and his colleagues had isolated two closely related pentapeptides from the brain tissue (18,31). These were methionine-enkephalin (MEK) and LEK, which exhibit very similar chromatographic behavior and the same sequence of the first four amino acids: Tyr-Gly-Gly-Phe. Hughes' work led to extensive investigation of the chemical structure of several fragments from a prohormone isolated from the brain tissue, ß-lipotropin. Table 6-1 gives a generic relationship between the ß-lipotropin and its fragments, as well as other opioid peptides.

The two pentapeptides, LEK and MEK, have been found to be present over a large area of the brain. Their distribution is closely similar to that of opiate receptors. The striatum of a guinea pig brain contains MEK at approximately 750 pmol/g and LEK 180 pmol/g at a ratio of 4:2. The hypothalamus contains MEK 453 and LEK 54 pmol/g at a ratio of 8:4. However, only a minute amount of these pentapeptides is found in the cerebellum or in the pituitary gland. Using radio-immunoassay, Han and his coworkers in Beijing (31) analyzed the content of MEK and LEK in the rat's brain and reported that the ratio of these two neuropeptides is close to 3:1. Their results are presented in table 6-2.

Zhou, et al., of Shanghai applied manual acupuncture to rabbits and EAP to rats and found

Table 6-1. The Amino Acids Sequence of Opioid Peptides

Name	Amino Acid Sequence
	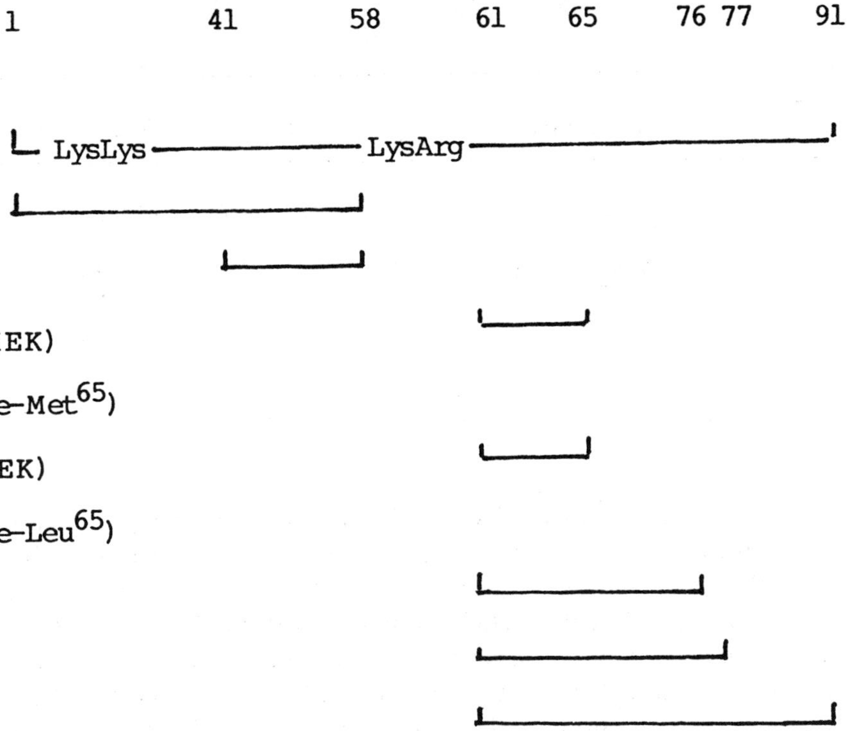 1 41 58 61 65 76 77 91
β-Lipotropin (β-LPH)	LysLys —— LysArg ——
γ-LPH	
β -MSH	
Met-Enkephalin (MEK) (Try-Gly-Gly-Phe-Met[65])	
Leu-Enkephalin (LEK) (Try-Gly-Gly-Phe-Leu[65])	
α-Endorphin	
γ-Endorphin	
β -Endorphin (β-Lipotropin[61-91])	

The other non-lipotropin fragments:

Dynorphin

(13 amino acids peptide): Tyr——Leu[5]——Pro[10]-lysleu-lys)

The first 5 amino acids sequence is similar to that of LEK

Naga:

(a tetrapeptide): Asn-Ala-Gly-Ala

that the enkephalin level in the striatum and hypothalamus was greatly increased (1, p. 34). Han, et al., (1, p. 486) studied twenty-one volunteers given EAP and reported that their plasma levels of endorphin increased significantly. LEK has also been found to be present in the dorsal horn of the spinal cord of rabbits; acupuncture could raise the LEK level more than 60 percent (34).

Table 6-2. Concentration of Immunoreactive MEK and LEK in Rat's Brain

Neuropeptide	Brain Area			
	Striatum	Hypothalamus	Thalamus	Pons-Medulla
	(µg/mg of tissue)			
MEK	371 ±29 (22)*	284 ±21	151 ±10	144 ±18
LEK	129 ±11	95 ±6	46 ±15	39 ±5

* Mean ± S.D. (number of animals)

Q. L. Jian, et al., (21) reported that LEK in the trictum and hypothalamus in a rat was increased markedly when the animal was exposed to hyperbaric oxygen condition. When the rat was acupunctured electrically at the acupoints Sanyinjiao and Zusanli, a marked acceleration of the release of EK at the ipsilateral side of the dorsal horn of spinal cord and the contralateral ventromedial medulla (especially in the lateral paragiantocellular reticular nucleus) occurred (20). S. X. Yuan, et al., found that injection of vitamin K_3 (63 mg/Kg) to rats could cause an increase of the content of LEK in the caudate putamen nucleus and hypothalamus, but not in the hippocampus and thalamus (38).

Experiments carried out in rats have shown that acupuncture or focal stimulation of the dorsolateral part of PAG could cause an activation of most neurons of NRM, which was reversed by iontophoretic naloxone. Microinjection of leucine-enkalephalin near the NRM area could mimic the activated action of acupuncture (46). It is suggested that the activation of NRM neuron by acupuncture is at least in part mediated by opioid peptides released from the enkephalin-containing neurons in PAG.

In rats acupuncture at the Zusanli point would significantly increase the release of MEK-like material from the perfusate of the cervicotrigeminal zone, but not of the lumbar area. (3).

Opioid peptides are not only found in the CNS, but also in the peripheral. Adrenal medulla is a neural tissue in nature. A MEK-like peptide has been isolated from this tissue; it is a Met-enkephalin-Arg-Phe (MEAP). When MEAP was injected intra-PAGly into a rabbit, analgesia was observed. Captopril, an inhibitor of MEAP degradation enzyme, injected intra-PAGly could produce a marked analgesic effect, which can be antagonized by anti-MEAP serum, but not by anti-MEK serum. EAP-induced analgesia would be potentiated by captopril injection and abolished by the intra-PAG injection of anti-MEAP serum (13).

The region of HARN has been shown to be the main site where ß-endorphin and ACTH are synthesized. Physiologically, this region has a close connection to the nucleus raphe dorsalis (NRD) and locus coeruleus (48). Rats treated neonatally with monosodium glutamine (MSG) showed HARN size decreasing by 72 percent and brain ß-endorphin of just 67 percent of the control value; the effectiveness of EAP applications on these animals was significantly reduced. If the MSG-treated rats were hypophysectomized, acupuncture-induced analgesia completely disappeared and the level of norepinephrine (NE) in the brain postacupuncturally was significantly higher than that of prior to acupuncture.

Studies on conscious curarized rats showed that the excitatory effect of stimulation of HARN on unit discharge of NRM were abolished by section of ß-endorphinergic tract and by microinjection of naloxone or anti-ß-endorphin serum into PAG, suggesting that the excitatory effect of HARN on NRM conducted through a direct connection between axons of ß-endorphinergic HARN neurons and the PAG-NRM system (14). It was also shown that the activation of NRM neurons by EAP was abolished after decerebration at the superior colliculus level, indicating that EAP depends mainly on the supramidbrain structure. The ß-endorphinergic pathways between AR and the PAG-NRM system is mediating the major excitatory effect of EAP on NRM neurons.

Analysis by radio-immunoassay has demonstrated that endorphins are predominately located in the pituitary gland. The gland contains 34 nmol/g of endorphins (assayed as ß-endorphin) and only negligible amounts of enkephalin. The striatum contains both EK and ß-endorphin, but in a relative smaller quantity (19). Among the endorphins isolated, it was found that the longer the peptide chain, the higher its potency in analgesic effect and the longer its duration of action. This indicates that ß-endorphin is far superior to either the α - or γ-endorphin. It was also found that ß-endorphin, the C fragment of ß-lipotropin 61-91, produces an analgesic and hyperglycemic effect 100 times greater than that of morphine. However, the analgesic effect of enkephalin is much less potent than that of ß-endorphin. Analysis of human patients' CSF (cerebro-spinal fluid) ß-endorphin levels during thirty-minute acupuncture sessions shows that the ß-endorphin level rises from 59.3 ±15.7 fmol/ml to 186 ±32.5fmol/ml, and both pain thresholds and pain tolerance are elevated (2, p. 403).

Studies on ten volunteer individuals have shown that EAP would increase the pain threshold and the ß-endorphin like immunoreactive substance (ß-EPIS) in the CSF. There is a direct relationship between the percentage increase of ß-EPIS in CSF and the pain threshold or pain tolerance (6).

There is also a circadian effect on the release or secretion of ß-endorphin in the rat's brain. It is higher at the nighttime and lower in the daytime (36).

Enkephalins are rapidly inactivated in vitro and in vivo by both nonspecific and specific peptidase. Their half life, $t_{1/2}$, is on the order of one minute or less, whereas the endorphins retain their activity for several hours. It was reported that both trypsin and chymotrypsin can degradate the endorphins rapidly. Bacitracin, an inhibitor of peptidase, has no analgesic effect by itself, but when it is injected IVC into mice, LEK content in the brain tissue greatly increased and the analgesic effect induced by EAP was potentiated. It was also found that intraperitoneal injection of Ca^{++} ions would anatagonize such analgesic effects, whether induced by acupuncture or by morphine. Such antagonist action would be altered by pretreatment with apomorphine, a dopamine (DA) agonist, or droperidol, a dopamine antagonist (42). D-Phenylalanine (DPA), a nonspecific peptidase inhibitor, can slow down EK degradation. Xu, et al., (2, p. 345) injected DPA directly into the nucleus amygaloid and found that analgesic effect induced by either acupuncture or morphine increased by 135 to 216 percent. Analgesia induced by acupuncture in rats can be abolished by intrathecal injection of anti-MEK serum, but not antidynorphin serum. Additionally, the antagonistic effect of anti-LEK serum is much inferior to that of anti-MEK serum.

Thiorphan is a potent enkephalinase inhibitor, and bestatin is a potent aminopeptidase inhibitor. When either one of these is injected icv into mice, rats, or rabbits, the content of both EKs in the brain was elevated and greater analgesia was observed (37). Such effects can be abolished by naloxone or administration of the anti-MEK-IgG serum and the less effective anti-LEK IgG serum. Figure 6-1 and figure 6-2 illustrate these effects.

Z. F. Zhou, et al., (44) injected either thiorphan or bestatin into a rabbit through the preimplanted microcannulae and the pain threshold was increased, which is dose-dependent and is potentiated by morphine and can be reversed by administration of naloxone. The authors also found that thiorphan or bestatin can potentiate the EAP-induced analgesic effect by 126 percent and 52 percent, respectively. Data do suggest that EAP or morphine analgesia is mediating at least partially by enkephalin relased in the CNS.

Han and his coworker (15) applied EAP to rats for thirty minutes and found that both MEK and LEK content in the striatum and hypothalamus were 40 percent higher than prior to acupuncture. If the animal was pretreated with Thiorphan, Bestatin, or D-Phenylalanine, the EAP analgesic effect was greatly enhanced and the MEK and LEK content was raised to 120 percent above the original level, indicating that EAP stimulation accelerated the biogenesis as well as release of EKs from neurons located in the striatum and hypothalamus. The rate of inactivation of the opioid pentapeptides under normal physiological conditions plays an important role in the nociceptive sensation of human subjects.

In order to facilitate studies on the role of opioid peptides in the regulation of physiological functions, hundreds of enkephalin analogues have been synthesized. Some are resistant to peptidase degradation. The replacement of glycine with a D-amino acid at the [2] position and the replacment

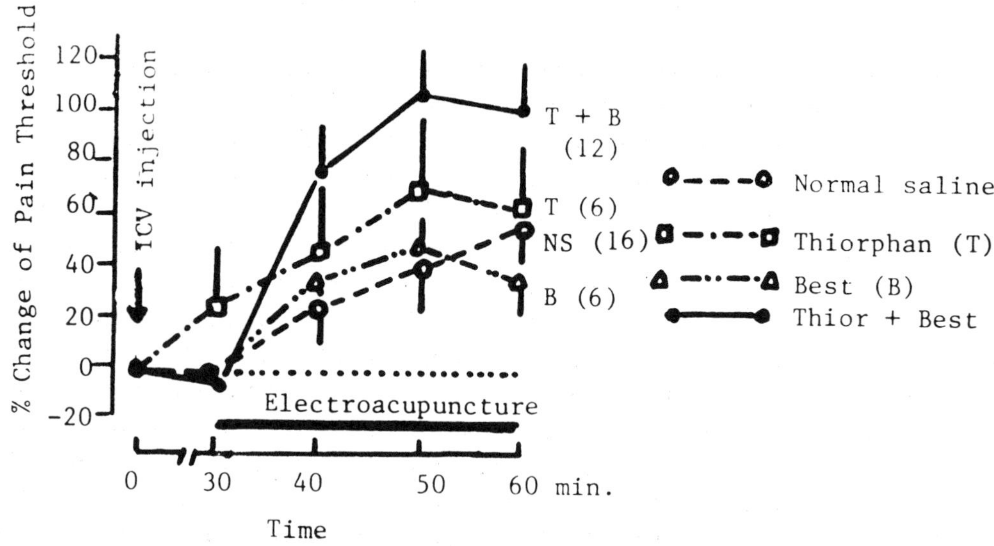

Figure 6-1. Effect of Intracerebroventricular (ICV) Injection of Bestatin (B) and/or Thiorphan (T), 50 µg each, on Electroacupuncture-Induced Analgesia

Mean ± SEM (number of rats)

(From Yuan & Han (37))

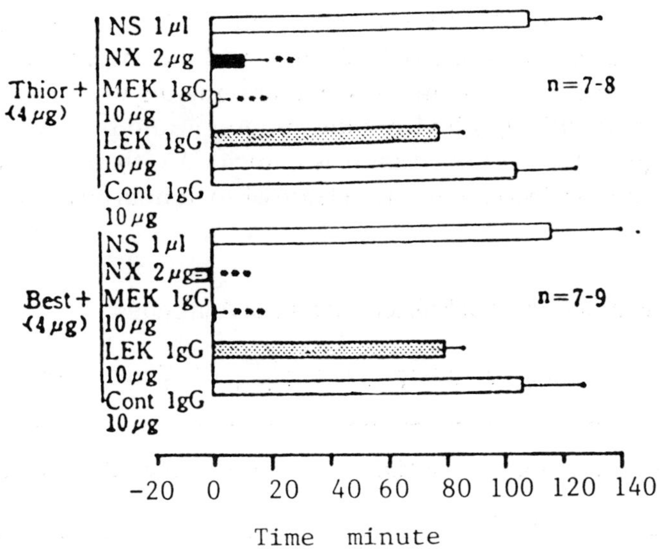

Figure 6-2. Analgesic Effect Elicited by Thiophan or Bestatin Injected into the N. Accumbenz of Rats.

NS: Normal saline

NX: Naloxone

MEK IgG: anti-MEK serum IgG

LEK IgG: anti-LEK serum IgG

Cont IgG: control serum IgG

** $p<0.01$; *** $p<0.001$

(From Jin et al. (22))

of leucine or methionine at the [5] position by another D-amino acid gives an analogue such as Tyr-D-Ala2-Gly-Phe-D-Leu or Tyr-D-Ala2-Gly-Phen-D-Met, both of which are highly resistant to metabolism. These were used to compare the action of natural opioid neuropeptides and opiate agonists in binding with specific opiate receptors. Table 6-3 summarizes research on structural activity on receptor binding, or contraction of vas deferens and guinea-pig ileum(25).

In experiments with mice, administration of the D-amino acid analogues of EK has been shown to exert a greater analgesic effect than the l–amino acid analogues, especially analogues with -NH_2 terminal.

Rabbits equipped with bilateral preimplanted cannulae directed to habenula or PAG were given microinjection of $CaCl_2$ solution. The EAP-induced or morphine-induced analgesia was significantly reduced, more than 50 percent as compared with the $CaCl_2$ injected into the vicinity of the nuclei. The $CaCl_2$ itself does not change the pain threshold at all. Furthermore, the intra-PAG injection of $CaCl_2$ gives a greater reduction effect on EAP-induced analgesia (84 percent) than on morphine-induced analgesia (only 54 percent). Data suggest that the ability of morphine and endogenous opioid peptides in blocking neuronal Ca^{2+} influx in certain CNS structure, including PAG and habenula, may constitute the basic mechanism of EAP and morphine analgesic action (45). T. Kunno (23) explained that the cytosolic free Ca^{2+} is an intracellular signaling for release of the neurotransmitters such as 5HT, NE, and opioid peptides from the aminergic and peptidergnic neurons in the brain. An oscillatory change in Ca^{2+} concentration is coincided with the burst potentials in the neuron resulting in an increase or decrease of the release of such neurotransmitters.

Table 6-3. The Inhibitory Effect of Enkaphalin and its Analogues

Peptide	IC_{50} of Morphine/ IC_{50} of Test Compound		
	Receptor Binding (Na^+-free)	Vas deferens	Guinea-pig Ileum
Leu5-EK	0.318	38	0.13
Met5-EK	0.175	32	0.36
(D-Ala2-Leu5)-EK	1.094	267	0.66
(D-Ala1-Met5)-EK	0.921	227	0.41
(D-Ala2-D-Leu5)-EK	1.346	1227	1.95
(D-Ala2-D-Met5)-EK	0.435	228	0.92

(From Miller et al. (26))

Physiological Importance

Antinociceptive Mechanism

In many respects, opioid peptides could be considered neurotransmitters that serve as a homeostasis mechanism of the central nervous system, balancing the activity of other neurotransmitters. In the early 1960s, some investigators proposed that an endogenous antinociceptive mechanism exists in the nervous system. After Hughes's successful isolation of pentapeptides from the brain, this proposition was strongly supported by most neurophysiologists and by psychiatrists. The opioid peptides are named because they possess similar functional and biochemical characteristics to opiate agonists in suppressing the sensation of pain. They are synthesized and released in the brain and play a role in antinociceptive function. The opiate antagonist, naloxone or naltrexone, can reverse all actions of these opioid peptides while providing practically no action of its own.

Although the first two pentapeptides isolated from brain tissues are only slightly different in their amino acid sequence, their specific function is quite different. Laboratory assays have shown that MEK is about twenty times more potent than LEK in analgesic effect. Both MEK and LEK can enhance the immunoactivity of B-lymphocytes, but have no effect on T-lymphocytes. LEK and ß-endorphin can enhance the activity of macrophage, with action reversible by naloxone (8). Injection of an anti-MEK or anti-ß-endorphin serum in the PAG area of a rabbit's brain can cause a decrease of EAP-induced analgesia. The anti-MEK serum is more potent than anti-ß-endorphin serum and is also active in the spinal cord. This suggests that MEK plays a more important role in the descending modulating mechanism than does ß-endorphin.

The isolation of the opioid neuropeptides from human tissues began in the late 1970s. A. Z. Zhang, et al., isolated a relatively pure substance from human brain tissue by use of a chromatographic technique. This substance is analytically identical to endorphin and exerts a remarkable analgesic effect when administered ICV into rabbits (39, 40). Figure 6-3 illustrates the analgesic effect of this endorphinlike substance on rabbits.

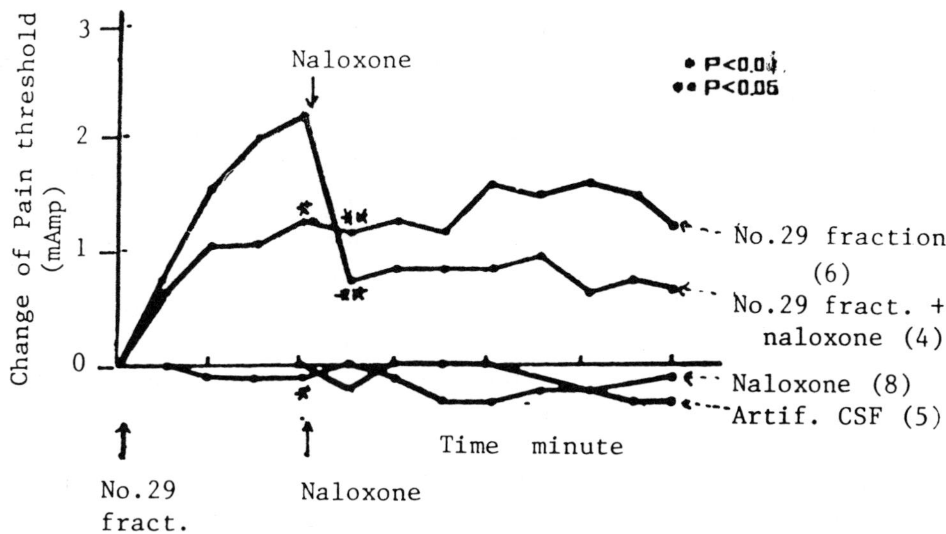

Figure 6-3. Analgesic Effect of a Substance, No. 29 Fraction, Isolated from Human Brain Tissue on Rabbits. Number of animals is shown in the parentheses

(From Zhang, A. Z. (39))

It has been reported that patients suffering chronic pains have lower endorphin levels in their CSF than normal persons. When EAP was performed on those patients, the level of endorphins in the CSF was elevated (31), as was the CSF ß-endorphin concentration (9). A similar phenomenon was observed in patients who suffered other malignant diseases, such as cancer (1, p. 30). Intrathecal administration of ß-endorphin produces a long-lasting analgesic effect in cancer patients (28).

Studies on healthy human subjects have shown that the CSF level of ß-endorphin significantly increases during EAP (10, 32). When acupuncture was performed on rats, the CSF level of LEK and dynorphin was elevated, but there was no change in plasma levels.

In patients who have had operations on their neck area or abdomen, under auricular acupuncture anesthesia and electrical stimulation it was found that levels of ß-endorphin and ACTH in the CSF were significantly elevated. Such elevation was suppressed if the patients were pretreated with cortisol medication (25). Figure 6-4 illustrates the effect of acupuncture on ß-endorphin and ACTH concentration and the suppressive effect of cortisol.

The correlation between acupuncture analgesia and elevated levels of opioid peptides in the brain has been demonstrated repeatedly via animal experimentation. In one study, anesthetized rabbits with a cannula implanted into the preoptic area and perfused with normal saline were subjected to EAP for twenty minutes. It was found that the ß-endorphin-like substance in the collected perfusate was elevated from 57.66 ±8.06 pg/100 µl to 92.43±7.95 pg/100 µl (47). Conscious rabbits with chronically implanted cannula in the PAG area of the brain also showed similar results when stimulated by EAP at the HoKu point (16): an increased content of opioid peptides coincided with an increase of the pain threshold.

In their recent studies, Han's team gave morphine to a rabbit by microinjection into the nucleus accumbens and collected the perfusates from their PAG or amygdala nuclei and found that the ir-ENK and ir-ß-endorphin content was markedly increased; naloxane can block such increase (24). The result is illustrated in figure 6-5.

Studies in rats have shown there is increased release of ß-endorphin and Dynorphin A_{1-13} from nucleus reticularis gigantocellularis lateralis (RPGL) nucleus of the brain during EAP, and a direct correlation between the change in Dyn A_{1-13} and ß-endorphin concentration and the pain threshold (43). Figure 6-6 illustrates such effect. Acupuncture also induces an elevation of LEK content in the plasma, caudate nucleus, hypothalamus, and thalamus and a decrease in the adrenal medulla (8). Studies also report that the MEK and LEK content in the hypothalamus and caudate nucleus increases significantly during acupuncture, with a positive correlation to the time of stimulation. There is, however, no significant change in the MEK level in the thalamus, other brain tissue, and spinal cord. This suggests that only MEK in the caudate nucleus and hypothalamus plays a role in mediating the analgesic effect induced by EAP (32).

When a small dose of ß-endorphin (100 to 250 µg/ml) was microinjected into the nucleus amygdaloideus centralis of the anesthetic rats, a falling of the blood presssure and heart rate was observed. Such effect was antagonized by injection of naloxone or by ß-endorphin antiserum, or by phentolamine and propranolol, indicating that such effect is mediated by the adrenergic neuron (33). Figure 6-7 illustrates such effect to lower the blood pressure by ß-endorphin and reversed by phentolamine.

ICV injection of anti-ß-endorphin serum (AEPS) can attenuate the EAP-induced analgesic effect in rats, but not the enhancement of EAP analgesia by oxytocin. The icv injection of anti-Dynorphin A_{1-13} (ADYNS) serum also would reduce the EAP analgesia, but if the injection of ADYNS was prior to the injection of oxytocin, the ADYNS could potentiate the enhancement of EAP analgesia by oxytocin. Such potentiation of the enhancement effect was exerted by the injection of neither anti-MEK serum nor anti-LEK serum. This suggests that ß-endorphin and enkephalin do not affect the role of oxytocin in analgesia. The enhancement of EAP-induced analgesia by oxytocin is not dependent upon the endogenous opioid peptides in the brain (30).

It was also found that in rats icv injection of a small dose of pancreatic polysaccharide could cause a fall of ß-endorphin and prolactin level in the plasma, but a larger dose would increase the ß-endorphin level and significantly lower the prolactin concentration (35).

Stress-induced analgesia is most commonly observed in repeated or prolonged electric shock and can be abolished by the administration of naloxone or by immersion in cold water or foot shock.

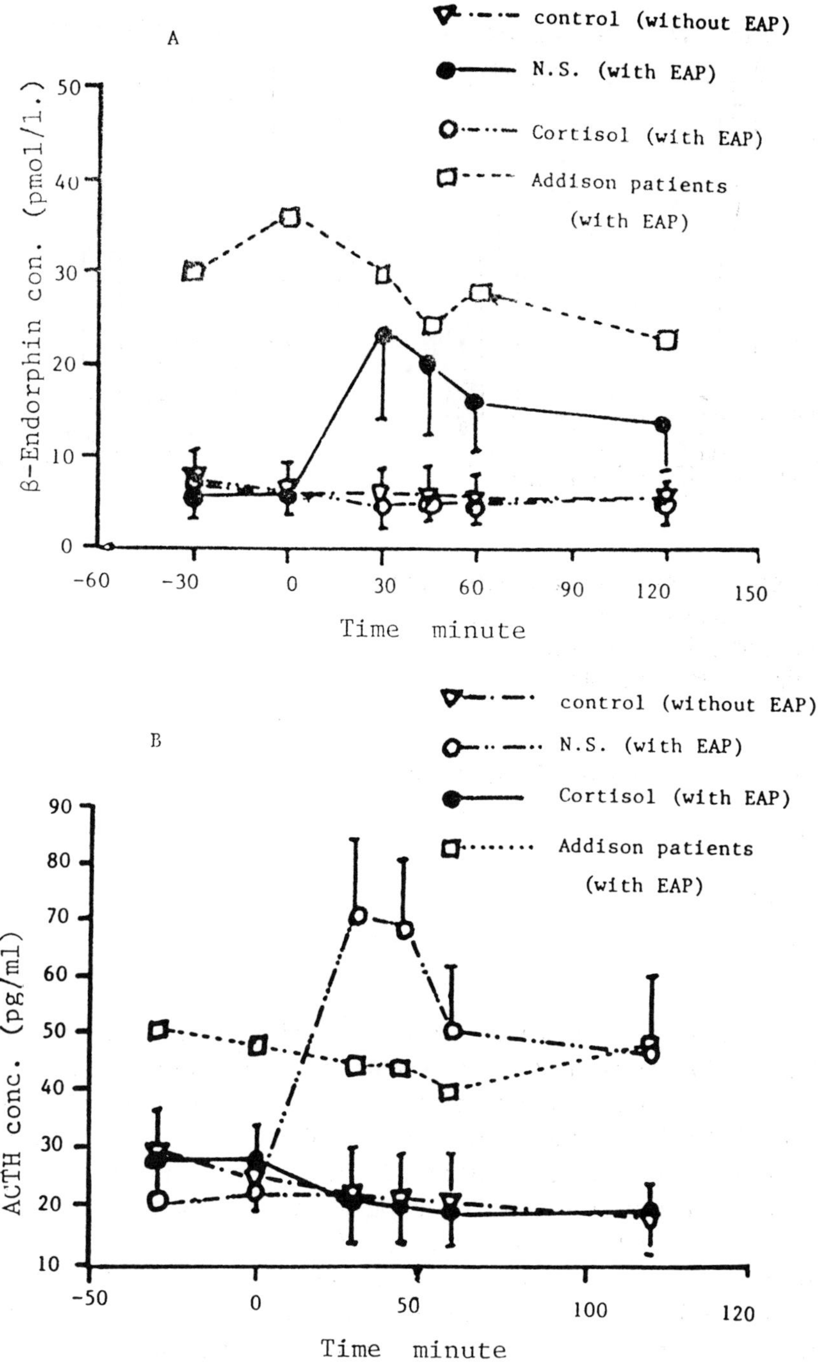

Figure 6-4. Effect of Electro-acupuncture (EAP) on β -Endorphin (A) and ACTH (B) Concentration in CSF of Normal Individuals or of Addison Patients

(Drawn from Masula et al.'s data (25))

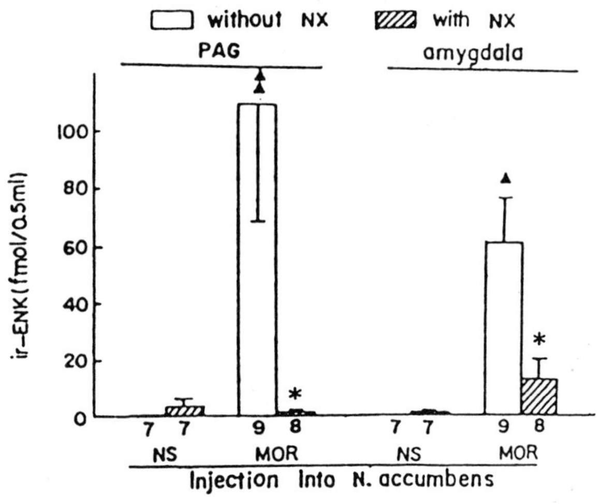

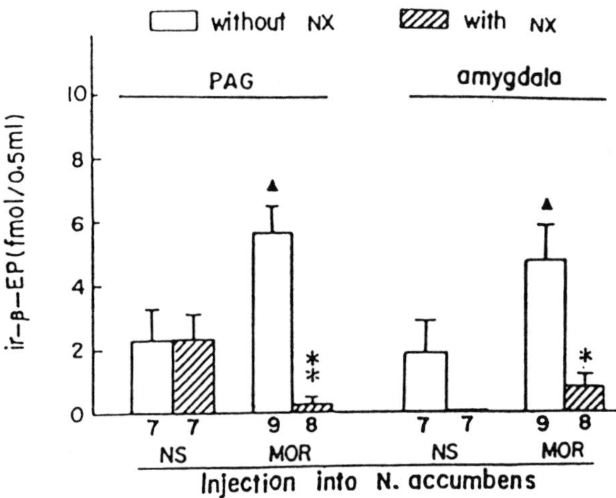

Figure 6-5. Concentration of Enkephalin (ENK) and β-Endorphin (EP) in the Perfusates Collected from PAG or Amygadla Nuclei of Rabbits after Microinjection of Morphine into the N. accumbenz.

NS: normal saline; MOR: morphine; NX: naloxone

* p<0.05; **p<0.01

(From MA & Han (24))

It has been shown that stress can cause a release of pituitary opioid peptides and ACTH. The ß-endorphin level in the plasma and pituitary gland is elevated after shock therapy. Lesions of the ventromedial hypothalamus (VMH) would attenuate such stress analgesia. It has been suggested that such lesions of VMH causes a reduced level of ß-endorphin and enkephalin. However, the administration of Dexamethasone, a synthetic corticosterone, can block stress analgesia, but not acupuncture-induced or morphine-induced analgesia; this indicates that the mechanisms of these three analgesic phenomena differ from each other (11).

During childbirth, the ß-endorphin level has been seen to rise but was reduced by epidural anesthesia. It was found that newborn babies have a high ß-endorphin immuno-reactivity level, suggesting a protective action of the infant against stress during labor (27).

Recently L. Cao, et al., (4) analysed the plasma and CSF level of 3 opioid peptides (LEK, ß-endorphin, and Dyn-A_{1-13}) on 44 asphyxia neonatal cases as compared with the normal nonasphysia neonatals. They have found that all three opioid peptides were markedly increased in asphyxia cases, especially in the severe cases (fourteen of forty-four neonatals) they were three- to four-fold higher than the normal. Such higher opioid peptides level was much greater in those with fetal distress or with cerebral injury than those suffering asphyxia without fetal distress or without cerebral injury.

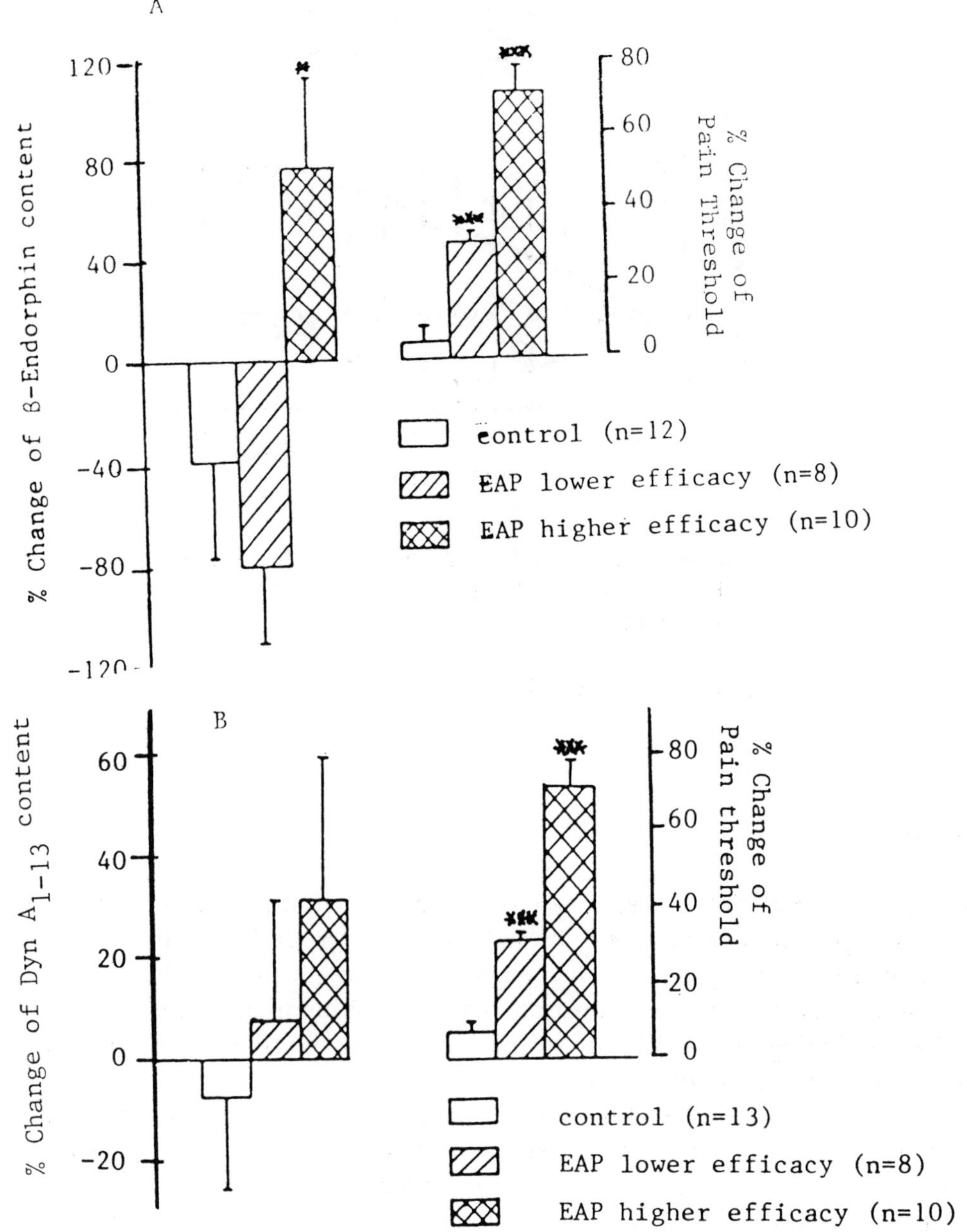

Figure 6-6. Effect of Electro-acupuncture (EAP) on β -Endorphin content (A) and Dynorphin A_{1-13} Content (B) in the Perfusate Collected from N. reticularis gigantocellularis laterailis

* p<0.05; ***p<0.0001 compared with the control

(From Zhou et al. (43))

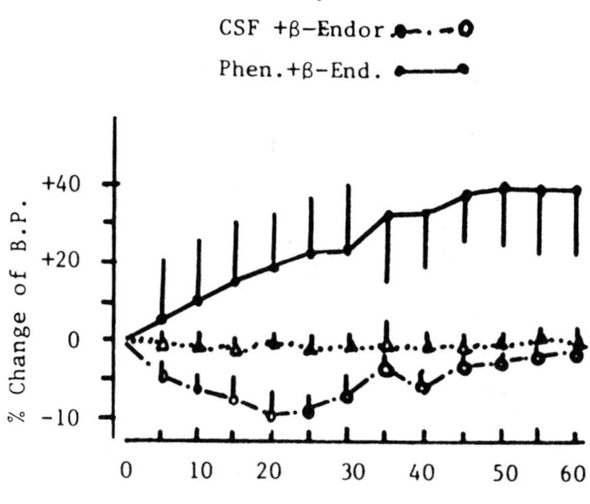

Figure 6-7. Effect of β -Endorphin in the Absence (o) or Presence (•) of Phentolamine on Blood Pressure of Rats

(From Xiao et al. (33))

Dynorphin

Dynorphin is one of the three major opioid neuropeptides that have been identified in the central and peripheral nervous system. It was first isolated from the pituitary gland; now it is known to be widespread in every area of the CNS, excluding the cerebellum and dorsal thalamus. Immuno-cytochemical findings demonstrate that dynorphins are present in the nociception-related area of CNS, including the dorsal horn of the spinal cord, the trigeminal complex, Nucleus raphe, PAG, cuneiform nuclei, and pretectal.

Dynorphin is a 13-amino acid peptide. Physiologically, it is quite different from either LEK or MEK. It has a broad spectrum of neural and somatic functions. It involves the antinociceptive mechanism of the brain; the cardiovascular, respiratory, and thermoregulatory function; ingestion and mobility of the alimentary tract; hormonal modulation;control of water balance, reproduction, and immuno-modulation. This opioid peptide is also involved in the body's reactions to seizure, trauma, and stroke. It also plays a role in circadian rhythms.

Dynorphin has little effect when injected into the brain but can produce a potent analgesic effect when injected into the spinal cord. It can decrease the analgesic potency of other opiate analogues.

J. S. Han and G. X. Xie (15) administered DYN to rabbits via intrathecal injection and observed an analgesic effect twenty times more potent than that of morphine. It requires a 50 percent larger dose of naloxone to reverse it. Intrathecal injection of antidynorphin antibodies in animals can block EAP effects by 77 percent; this antagonistic effect lasts a very long time. However, in contrast to endorphins, injection of DYN directly into the PAG area of the brain may produce no analgesic effect. Data suggest that dynorphin reduces the nocifensive response in the spinal cord and plays a role in mediating acupuncture analgesia. Figure 6-8 illustrates the effect of DYN on the pain threshold of a rabbit.

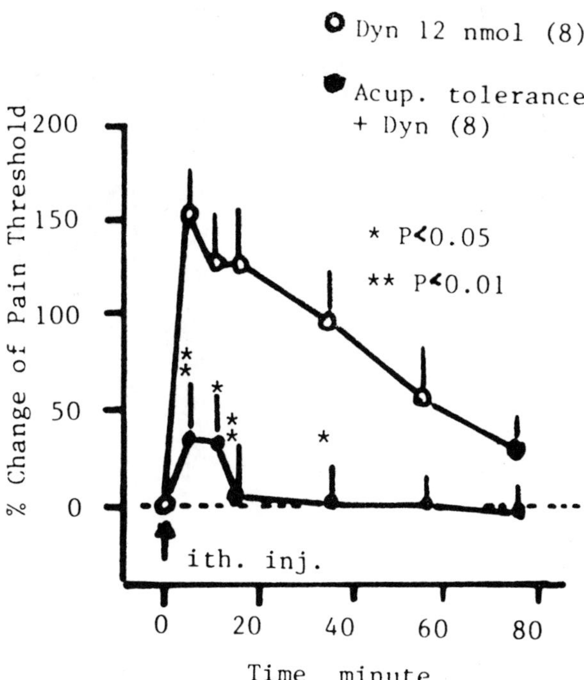

Figure 6-8. Analgesic Effect of Dynorphin on Acupuncture-tolerant Rabbits
(Arrow indicates the time of intrathecal injection)

* p<0.05; **p<0.01 compared with the non-acupuncture tolerant group

(From Han & Xue (15))

Studies on rabbits undergoing continuous EAP for six hours showed development of a tolerance to acupuncture analgesia. When DYN was intrathecally injected into the same animal, the analgesic effect was greatly reduced. This suggests there is a cross tolerance between acupuncture and DYN analgesia. There is no cross tolerance between morphine analgesia and DYN analgesia, however, indicating that the opioid activity of DYN in the spinal cord is mediated via the kappa, rather than the μ, opiate receptor. The DYN in the spinal cord, but not the brain, exhibits a potent antinociceptive effect and plays an important part in mediating acupuncture analgesia.

When Dyn. $A_{1\text{-}13}$ was injected icv into rats, it would increase the diuretic effect with insignificant action on the mean arterial pressure and heart rate. Such diuretic effect was started 20 minutes after injection and lasted to 120 minutes and can be blocked completely by nalaxone (41). Figure 6-9 illustrates such diuretic effect by dynorphin.

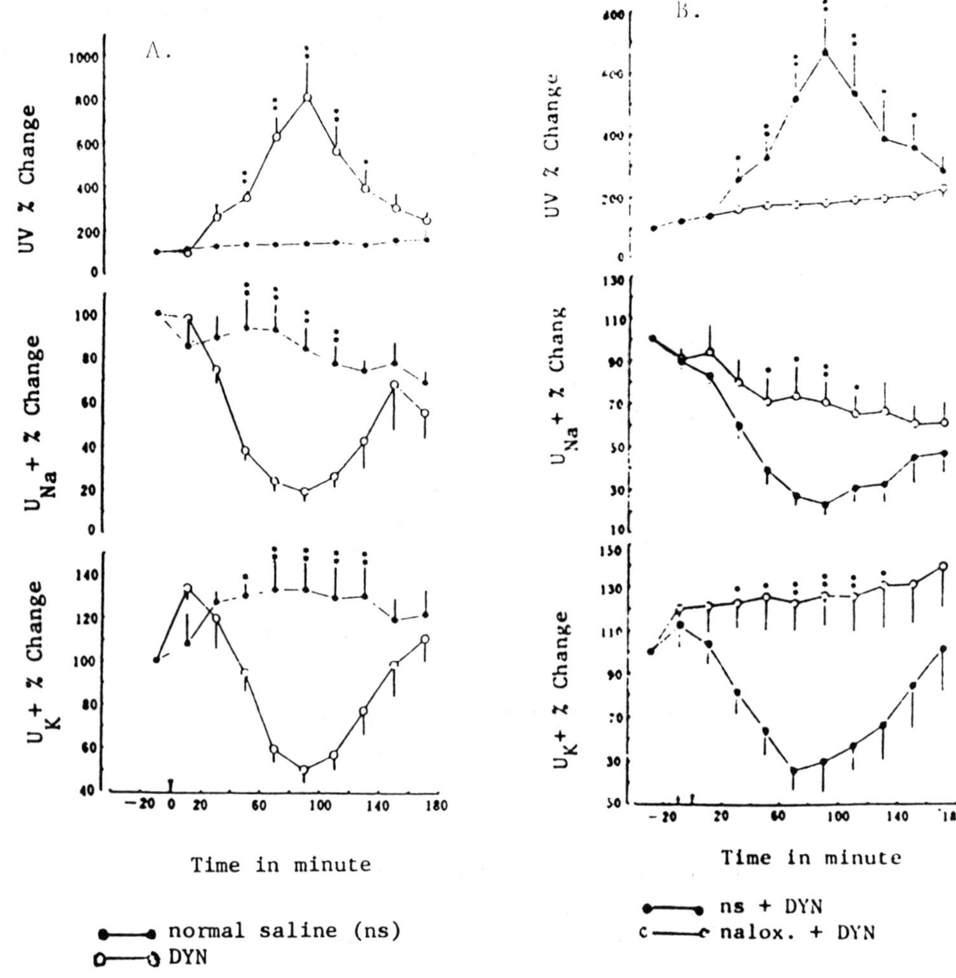

Figure 6-9. Effect of Dynorphin A_{1-13} on Urinary Volume, U_{Na} and U_k in Rats, in the Absence (A) or Presence (B) of Naloxone

Naga

Naga is a tetrapeptide isolated from human brain tissue by Chinese investigators (29). The amino acid sequence of naga differs from that of other opioid neuropeptides. It was found that naga can produce a potent analgesic effect after administration to mice and is resistant to enzyme degradation. The duration of action is long, lasting more than sixty minutes, and can be blocked by naloxone. Acupuncture can increase the naga content in the central gray neuron of the animal, and also in the CSF of human patients. This increase paralleled the increase in ß-endorphin content and the pain threshold. Table 6-4 illustrates such effects of acupuncture on naga and ß-endorphin concentration.

It was also found that the injection of naga into rabbits' PAG area would raise the LEK level in the CSF, as well as the pain threshold. This is illustrated in table 6-5.

Cranial surgery was performed in tumor patients under EAP, the opioid peptides concentration in CSF of lateral ventricle was determined, it was found that the content of ß-endorphin, naga, peptide and acetylcholine was significally increased during the EAP period and graduatedly subsides to normal level after the operation (7). The result is summarized in table 6-6. Figure 6-10 presents a dose-dependent analgesic effect of naga, its amide, and LEK on mice.

Opioid peptides also play a role in the modulation of eating and drinking. One of the areas of the brain known to influence eating is the VMH. A surgical lesion of the medial hypothalamus neighboring the VMH area produces hyperphagia and weight gain. Such effects can be reversed by administration of naloxone, suggesting that the medial hypothalamus serves as an inhibitory mechanism of the opioid system (mainly VMH). However, plasma ß-endorphin level analysis supplies little evidence to support the suggestion that opioid peptides are involved in human obesity. Despite this, Chinese clinicians claim to obtain a high success rate in treating obesity with acupuncture (27).

Recently J. Erchegyi, et al., (12) have isolated a tetrapeptide with an opiate and antiopiate activity from human brain cortex. It is not yet understood what role this tetrapeptide plays in the CNS. The author gives the structure of its peptide as follows: Tyr-Pro-Trp-Gly-NH2.

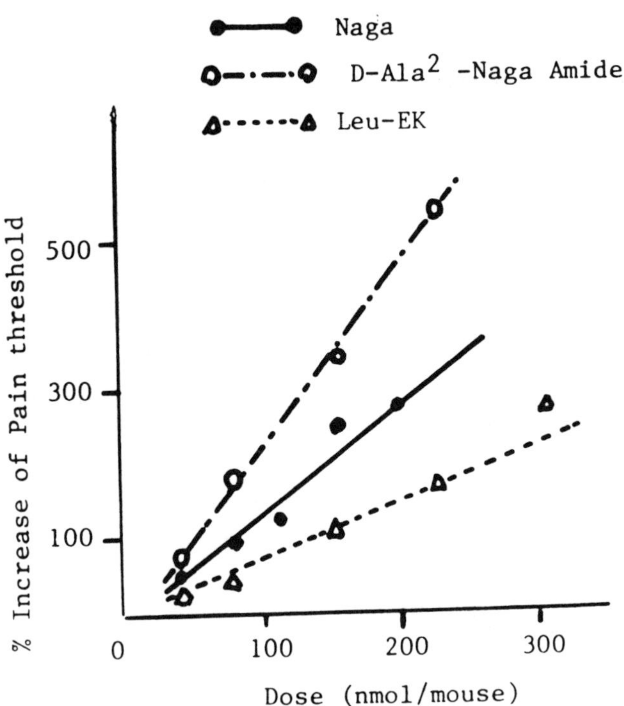

Figure 6-10. Dose-Dependent Analgesic Effect of NAGA, Its Analog and LEK in Mice

(From Pan et al. (29))

Table 6-4. Effect of Acupuncture on CSF Concentration of Naga, β-Endorphine and Pain Threshold in Human Individuals

	Time after Acupuncture				
	0	20 min.	30 min.	50 min.	110 min.
Naga (pmol/μl)	288.8± 11.2 (10)*	741.1±32.5	780 ±96.5	578 ±55.3	568.3 ±79.9
β-Endorphine# (fmol/μl)	59.3± 19.7 (10)	110 ± 18.8	186 ±32.5	110±14.7	84.4±15.3
Pain threshold (gm)	375± 35.9 (10)	-	553 ±27.9	-	333 ± 45.9

* mean ± SD (number of patients)

\# determined by radio-immunoassay

(From Pan et al (29))

Table 6-5. Change of CSF Concentration of LEK and Pain Threshold after Microinjection of Naga into Rabbit's PAG Region

Group	Time After the Injection			
	0	20 min.	50 min.	80 min.
Control (n.s.)				
LEK (pg/100 μl)	79.43± 11.06 (7)*	72.43±14.58	62.0±12.78	70.71±11.5
Pain threshold (mA)	0.43±0.03	0.47±0.04	0.44±0.03	0.43±0.03
Naga				
LEK (pg/100 μl)	81.0±16.2 (12)	184.4±44.4	185.0±41.9	161.4±30.3
Pain Threshold (mA)	0.39±0.03	1.04±0.06	0.62±0.09	0.45±0.05

* mean ± SD (number of rabbits)

(From Pan et al. (29))

Table 6-6. Effect of Electro-acupuncture on CSF content of β-Endorphine, Naga and Acetylchlorine in Patients during Cranial Surgery

	Concentration in Lateral Ventricle CSF		
	Before EAP	During EAP	After EAP
β-Endorphin (fmol/ml.)	44 ± 12.3 (10)*	159.8 ± 32.2	79.9 ± 11.1
NAGA (nmol/ml.)	144.4	176.4	
Acetylcholine (ng/ml.)	2.23	4.01	3.31

* Mean ± S.D. (number of patients)

(From Chen et al. (7))

References

1. All China Society of Acupuncture and Moxibustion. First National Symposium on Acupuncture and Acupuncture Anesthsia. Beijing: 1979
2. All China Society of Acupuncture and Moxibustion. Second National Symposium on Acupuncture and Moxibustion and Acupuncture Anesthesia. Beijing: 1984.
3. Bing, Z., et al. Pain 47:71, 1991.
4. Cao, L., et al. Chinese Medical Journal 106(10):783, 1993.
5. Chen, B. Y., et al. Acta Physiol. Sinica 34:385, 1982.
6. Chen, B. Y., et al. Acta Physiol. Sinica 36:183, 1984.
7. Chen, G. B., et al. Journal of Traditional Chinese Medicine 4:189, 1984.
8. Chin, P. H. Journal of Chinese Acupuncture and Moxibustion (in Chinese) 11(5):31, 1991.
9. Clement-Jones V., et al. Lancet 2:946, 1980.
10. Demura H. Journal of Tokyo Women's Medical Coll. 58:1146, 1988.
11. Di, S., et al. Acta Pharmacol. Sinica 4:153, 1983.
12. Erchegyi, J., et al. Peptides 13(4):623, 1992.
13. Fei, H., and J. S. Hang, et al. Acta Physiol. Sinica 37:10,85.
14. Gao, Y. S., and Y. H. Ku. Acta Physiol. Sinica 35:409, 1983.
15. Han, J. S., and G. X. Xie. Pain 18:367, 1984.
16. He, L. F., et al. Pain 23:83, 1985.
17. Huang, K. C. Pharmacology of Chinese Herbs. Boca Raton C. R. C. Press, 1993.
18. Hughes, J. Brain Res. 85:295, 1975.
19. Hughes, J., et al., in Hughes, ed., Centrally Acting Peptides. Baltimore, MD: University Park Press, 1978, p. 179.
20. Ji, R. R., and J. S. Han, et al. Acta Physiol. Sinica 45:395, 1993.
21. Jian, Q. L., et al. Acta Physiol. Sinica 45:182, 1993.
22. Jin, W. Q., et al. Acta Physiol. Sin. 37:377, 1985.
23. Kunno, T. Biomedical Res. 11:7, 1990.
24. Ma, Q. P., and J. S. Han. Peptides 13:261, 1992.
25. Masula, A., et al. Acta Endocrin. 103:469, 1983.
26. Miller, R. J., et al., in Hughes, J. ed., Centrally Acting Peptides. Baltimore, MD, Univ. Park Press, 1978, p. 195.
27. Olson, G. A., et al. Peptides 6:769, 1985.
28. Oymama, T., et al. Lancet l:122, 1980.

29. Pan, X. P., et al. Journal of Traditional Chinese Medicine 4:273, 1984.
30. Song, C. Y., et al. Acta Physiol. Sinica 45:231, 1993.
31. Terenius, L., and A. Wahlstroem, in Hughes, ed., Centrally Acting Peptides. Baltimore, MD: Univ. Park Press, 1978, p. 161.
32. Xie, C. W., et al. Acta Physiol. Sinica 36:192, 1984.
33. Xiao, Q., et al. Acta Physiol. Sinica 46:77, 1994.
34. Xu, C. F., et al. Acta Physiol. Sinica 36:220, 1984.
35. Xu, R. K., et al. Acta Physiol. Sinica 45:215, 1993.
36. Yehuda, S., and D. I. Mostofsky. Peptides 14:203, 1993.
37. Yuan, H., and J. S. Han. Acta Physiol. Sinica 37:365, 1985.
38. Yuan, S. X., et al., Chinese Pharmacol. Bulletin 10(1):18, 1994.
39. Zhang, A. Z., and C. T. Chang, et al., in Research on Acupuncture and Moxibustion Anesthesia. Beijing: 1986, p. 189.
40. Zhang, A. Z. Chinese Medical Journal 93:673, 1980.
41. Zhang, Y. C., and L. Huang. Acta Physiol. Sinica 45:462, 1993.
42. Zhang, Z. X., et al. Acta Physiol. Sinica 35:172, 1983.
43. Zhou, L., et al. Acta Physiol. Sinica 45:36, 1993.
44. Zhou, Z. F., et al. Acta Physiol. Sinica 36:175, 1984.
45. Zhou, Z. F., et al. Acta Physiol. Sinica 37:463, 1985.
46. Zhu, L. X., and Q. Y. Shi. Journal of Traditional Chinese Medicine 4:111, 1984.
47. Zhu, J. M., et al. Acta Physiol. Sinica 42:188, 1990.
48. Zhu, M. Y., et al. Acta Physiol. Sinica 36:42, 1984.

7

The Role of Other Neurotransmitters and Endocrines

The complex role of brain neurotransmitters in producing analgesia has raised more questions than can be answered currently. It is well recognized that opioid peptides are distributed in almost all brain tissues, but in various quantities. Some areas of the brain also synthesize and liberate other neurotransmitters to modulate certain brain functions. Do these neurotransmitters play any role in the sensation of pain or in the antinociceptive process? Additionally, do the opioid peptides interact with any of these neurotransmitters, or do they interfere with or influence the biosynthesis and release of the opioid peptides in the brain tissue?

5-Hydroxytrytamine (5HT)

Han and his coworkers (10) have demonstrated from their studies in human subjects and animals that 5HT and acetylcholine, similar to the opioid peptides, can enhance the acupuncture analgesic effect; DA and NE can decrease it. When EAP is applied to rats, the 5HT concentration in the brain is elevated (42). Intraperitoneal injection of 5-hydroxytryptophane (5HTP), a precursor of 5HT, can augment the acupuncture-induced analgesic effect. Intracerebroventricular injection of p-chlorophenylalanine (pCPA), an inhibitor of 5HT synthesis, can partially lower the 5HT content in the brain and decrease the acupuncture analgesic effect. When animals were given a dose of just pCPA alone and dissected three to five days days later, the opioid peptides activity of the brain tissues was seen to be significantly higher. When acupuncture was administered to these pCPA-pretreated animals, a much greater increase of the opioid peptides in the brain tissue was observed than that of animals without acupuncture. Data also show an inverse relationship between the concentration of 5HT and opioid peptides in the brain. Figure 7-1 illustrates this relationship.

It is possible that 5HT is a prerequisite for the interaction of opioid peptides with the opiate receptors in order to exert an analgesic effect. It has also been postulated that acupuncture acts first by triggering the release of 5HT from the seratoninergic neurons; through the 5HT, the opioid peptides can then exert their antinociceptive effect. Without the presence of 5HT, no analgesic effect would be produced even if opioid peptides are present, and the peptides would be accumulated at the synaptic junctions. Microinjection of kainic acid into the NRD of a rat can provoke a marked reduction of 5HT and its metabolic product, 5HIAA, in the brain, significantly attenuating the acupuncture analgesic effect (36).

EAP was applied to rats at the acupoints Shousanli (LI-10) and Huantiao (G-30), and there was an increase of the pain threshold and a marked increase of 5HT content in the medulla, pons, and midbrain. If atropine was injected to the animal before the EAP application, such effect can be blocked. This further suggests that EAP-induced analgesia is mediated through the serotoninergic system in the brain. (32).

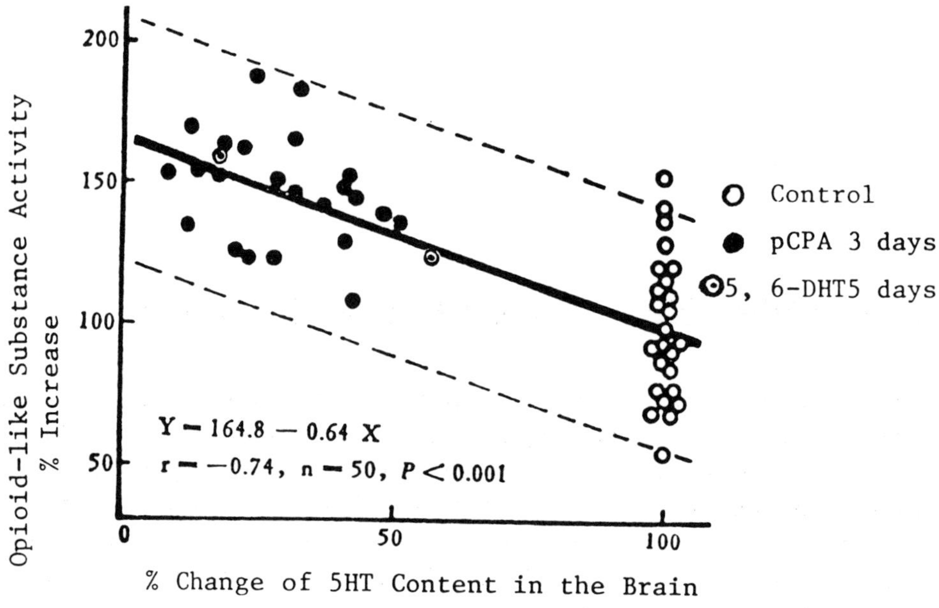

Figure 7-1. Inverse Relationship between the Brain Opioid Peptides Activity and Brain Tissue 5HT Concentraton in Rats

Solid Line is the Regression Line from 50 Rat's Experiment; Dotted Lines Are within 95% Range

(From Han (10))

In other studies, rabbits preimplanted with a cannula in the PAG and NRM or in the spinal cord were given acupuncture. During the acupuncture procedure, saline was perfused into the cannula and the perfusate was collected. It was found that acupuncture can raise the pain threshold of the animal, increase levels of 5HT and 5HIAA (the metabolic product of 5HT) in the PAG, NRM, and spinal cord perfusate, and also increase the release of LEK in the dorsal horn of spinal cord. However, the norepinephrine concentration in the PAG and NRM perfusate was markedly lower (29).

Figure 7-2 illustrates the increase of LEK concentration in the perfusate of dorsal horn of spinal cord after acupuncture application.

When dihydroxytryptamine (DHT) is injected directly into the locus coeruleus of the pons in rats, the acupuncture-induced analgesic effect is substantially reduced. Seven days after injection, a 76 percent to 82 percent reduction of the 5HT content in the locus coeruleus and pons was found (7).

Animal experimentation has shown that the icv injection of naloxone in rats at a dose of 20 μg will only slightly reduce acupuncture-induced analgesia. If the animal is pretreated with pCPA, however, the same dose of naloxone can completely abolish the acupuncture effect. This suggests a close correlation between 5HT and opioid peptides on the antinociceptive mechanism.

Similarly, 5HT also shows a correlation to morphine-induced analgesia. J. S. Han and G. X. Xie (8), demonstrated that analgesia can be produced by intra-PAG injection of morphine into a rabbit, which can be blocked by intraaccumbens injection of Cinanserin, a 5HT antagonist, and augmented by intraaccumbens injection of 5HTP. This suggests that morphine or endogenous opinoid peptides

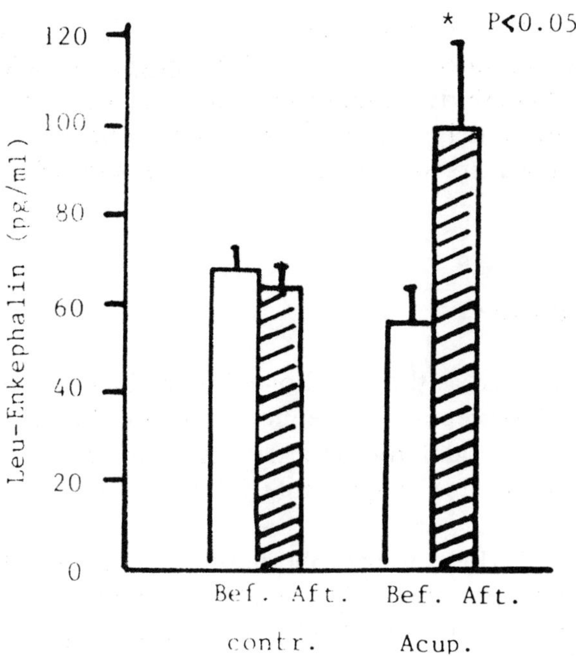

Figure 7-2. Leu-enkephalin Concentration in the Perfusate of Dorsal Horn of Spinal Cord

contr.: control (sham acupuncture)

Acup.: acupuncture

(From Xu (29))

in PAG may activate the ascending serotoninergic neurons that release 5HT in Nucleus accumbens to synergize such analgesic effect. It has also been shown that bilateral intraaccumbens injection of an anti-EK-IgG serum will attenuate the intra-PAG injected morphine effect and intraaccumbens injection of d-phenylalanine will potentiate the intra-PAG injected morphine effect. His team also studied the rabbits with preimplanted cannula that received a dose of 100 µg of 5HT either by icv or by intrathecal (iTH) injection (17). There was only a slight fall of blood pressure in the animals by ICV injection, but a marked decrease by 29.5+3.4 mmHg by iTH injection. Such hypotensive effect can be reversed by iTH administration of 100 µg of Cinanserin, a 5HT receptor blocker. They also reported that in hypovolumic-shock rabbits the iTH injection of Cinanserin can produce a significant increase of blood pressure without change of the heart beat.

By using the bidigital O-ring test method Omura and his coworkers (20) can localize the electromagnetic resonance phenomena from the pineal gland representative (rep) area on the surface of the head. They have found that the concentration of several neurotransmitters such as 5HT, melatonin, NE, DA, GABA and Ach was changed greatly, either increased or decreased, depending upon whether the eyes were closed or opened, or whether the skin was exposed with a weak light beam, or an (+) or (-) electrical field, or a magnetic field from the South pole to a small permanent magnet, or from the North pole. Data indicate that our human skin is not only able to detect an electromagnetic field (EMF) that can influence a change of the concentration of 5HT, melatonin, NE, DA, GABA and Ach in the pineal gland. Also, the pineal gland rep area is the most sensitive to the EMF effect. They therefore speculate that such EMF effect would influence our physiological and pathological function in our daily life. An electric field coming from a 110 –115 volt electric cord placed less than thirty centimeters (about one foot) from the head may contribute to some insomnia, hypertension, ischemic heart, arrhythmia, and the growth or spread of cancer cells in some cancer patients by markedly reducing melatonin and Ach in the human pineal gland and other organs.

Dopamine and Norepinephrine

Other neurotransmitters such as the catecholamine analogues, DA and NE, have also been found to play a role in antinociceptive conception. Apomorphine, a DA agonist, can reduce acupuncture analgesia, and droperidol, the DA antagonist, can enhance acupuncture analgesia in animals and in human subjects. This suggests that DA exerts a negative effect on the analgesic mechanism (10).

l-Tetrahydropalmatine (l-THP), tetrahydroberberine (THB), and l-stepholidine (l-SPO) are three homologues of tetrahydroprotoberberine isolated from a Chinese herb, *Coptis chinesis* (12). They demonstrate a common antagonistic effect to the central dopaminic receptor. Any of these principles can potentiate the analgesic effect in rabbits that are given EAP at the HoKu locus; the duration of action was greatly prolonged. The THP- or EAP-induced analgesia is markedly attenuated by icv injection of either DA or apomorphine. The injection of SKF-38393, a selective D_1 agonist, can produce the same attenuation effect.

However, the injection of Quinpirole HCl, a selective D_2 agonist, can enhance the analgesic effect induced by either THP or acupuncture. Neither DA, apomorphine, SKF-38393, nor quinpirole will influence the baseline pain threshold (34). When the D_2 receptor antagonist, domperidone or sulpiride, is injected ICV into rats, an enhancement of the acupuncture-induced analgesia has been observed (30).

When J. L. Dai and S. L. Xu (4,5) injected chlorpromazine (CPZ), an antidopaminic agent, into a conscious rabbit, it significantly attenuated the EAP-induced analgesic efficacy, with a marked increase of DA metabolites in the CSF. This suggests that the activation of the DA system was unfavorable to the acupuncture analgesic action. It is unclear whether such effect is through the opioid peptides system or not.

NE exhibits the same action as DA. It has been found that EAP can lower the NE content of the central nervous system, especially in the PAG and NRM areas (40). But the 5HT and 5HIAA content of these areas and in the spinal cord was found to be markedly higher. Conversely, the administration of NE directly into the brain can reduce the acupuncture effect. Reports show that the icv injection of dihydroxyphenylserine (DOPS), a precursor directly synthesized to NE that bypasses the DA step, can increase NE concentration in the brain and has been noted to attenuate acupuncture-induced analgesic effects by approximately 65 percent. The icv injection of either 6-hydroxydopamine (6-OHDA), a NE biosynthesis blocker, or an α-adrenergic blocker into rats' ventricles can augment acupuncture-induced analgesia. Such an effect was not seen when a ß-adrenergic blocker was administered (27). Figure 7-3 presents the results of these studies with rats. A similar result has been obtained by injection of 6-OHDA into the preoptic area of a rabbit; a decrease of NE content coincided with an observed augmentation of acupuncture analgesic (41).

Analgesia was induced in rats after they were acupunctured at the acupoints Zusanli and Sanyinjiao bilaterally for thirty minutes. An intraperitoneal administration of clenbuterol, a ß2-adrenergic activator, causes a 85 percent reduction of the analgesic effect (25).

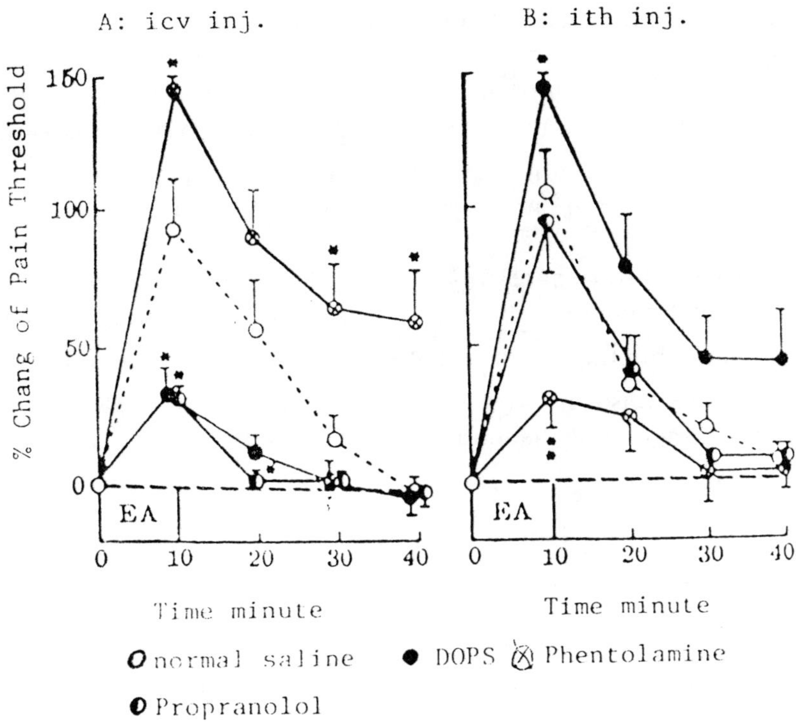

Figure 7-3. Analgesic Effect of Electro-acupuncture (EAP)

(3 V for 10 Minutes) during (A) Intracerebro-

ventricular or (B) Intrathecal Injection of:

(o) Normal Saline; (o) Dihydroxyphenylserine;

(o)Phentolamine; or (o) Propranolol

mean ± S.D. of 5-9 animals

* $p<0.05$ compared with the control value

(From Xia (27))

Experiments were done on the rats with chronic implantation of a cannula in the lateral ventricle or subarachnoid space, who were given EAP. It was found that the NE concentration of the collected CSF was reduced by 29±8 percent, and the concentration of its metabolic product, 3-methoxyl-4-OH-phenylglycol sulfate was increased by 48 to 56 percent. If the EAP to the animal was continued to six hours long, a tolerance to acupuncture analgesia was produced. The concentration of NE metabolic product was further increased to 197 percent of the control level (1, p. 419; and 27).

Other studies have shown that the destruction of the preoptic catecholaminergic terminal can enhance the acupuncture-induced analgesic effect in animals (17,41). Experimentation with monkey, cat, rat, and human subjects has shown that locus coeruleus (l.c.) plays an important role in pain modulation (37). Lesion of l.c. can cause a fall in NE level in the spinal cord and a reduction in morphine-induced analgesic effects. Stimulation of l.c. or EAP can produce a significant reduction in the nociceptive response of dorsal horn neurons of the spinal cord. This reduction in nociceptive response was not affected by the lesion of the NRM, nor by administration of naloxone. However, the reduction in response can be enhanced by administration of clonidine, a α_2-adrenergic agonist, or reduced by administration of phentolamine, an α_1-adrenergic antagonist. Data suggest that the effect of l.c. stimulation or EAP on the nociceptive response of spinal cord dorsal horn neurons is mediated by 2 receptors.

Experiments in rats have shown that HARN and l.c. play an important role in pain modulation and acupuncture analgesia. Stimulation of l.c. could shorten the duration of noxious response of HARN unit, resulting in an inhibiting effect on HARN. Clonidine (an α_2 agonist) and phenoxybenzene (an α_1 antagonist) can raise the average rate of discharge of HARN while ß-agonist and ß-antagonist have no effect, suggesting that both l.c. and HARN might be mediated by the adrenergic alpha receptors (38).

GABA and Cholecytokinin

Other investigators have administered acupuncture to rats bilaterally at the Shousanli (LI 10) and Huantiao (G 30) acupoints. They found a notable increase in 5HT content in the medulla and midbrain, an increase in LEK in the striatum, and higher levels of DA in the brain stem and diencephalon (31). Additionally, the pain threshold of the animals increased. When the animals were pretreated with Bicuculine, a GABA blocker, no increases in 5HT, LEK, or DA were observed. This suggests that the GABA receptors in the central nervous system play an antagonistic role in the antinociceptive mechanism. Still other studies have reported that the administration of a GABA transaminase inhibitor can increase GABA levels in the brain and suppress acupuncture-induced analgesia (22).

L. R. Watkins, et al., (33) reported that cholecystokinin octapeptide (CCK-8) can act as a physiological antagonist against the opiate analgesia. They suggested that CCK blocker may be clinically useful in enhancing acupuncture-induced analgesia, which may be mediated by the release of endogenous opioid peptides in the central nervous system.

J. S. Han and his coworkers studied the behavior of rats and showed that cholecystokinin octapeptide (CCK-8) can antagonize the opioid peptides in both the brain and spinal cord; angiotenin II (A II) can antagonize the opioid peptides in the brain, but not in the spinal cord (11). They also showed that CCK-8 blocks the analgesic effect elicited by morphine, endorgenous opioid peptides, µ-receptor agonist, PLO-17, and NDAP-500 (a kappa receptor agonist), but not analgesic effects induced by DPDEE, a δ-receptor agonist. The analgesic effect elicited by intraaccumbens injection of morphine can be significantly attenuated by the injection of a GABA-receptor agonist, muscinol, and enhanced by a GABA-receptor antagonist, Bicuculine, into the same brain area. The authors suggested that the analgesia elicited by intraaccumbens injection of morphine is mediated by the suppression of GABA-ergic inhibitory neurons, which are located in the Nucleus accumbens.

In their recent article (3) Han's team demonstrated that the cholecystokinin octapeptide (CCK-8) has a potent antiopiate activity by blocking the morphine analgesic effect in rat. They postulated that such effect is mediated by CCK-B receptor in CNS. When CCK-8 antagonist L-365260, was injected ICV to the rat, it markedly potentiated the EAP-induced analgesic effect. Such potentiation depended upon the frequency of EAP used: the greater the frequency, the better the potentiation. They also found that EAP at higher frequency more easily increased the release of CCK-8 in CNS as compared with the low-frequency EAP.

Further, it has been reported that analgesia induced by EAP can be augmented by the injection of 3-mercaptopropionic acid (3-MP), an inhibitor of both GABA synthesis and release; it can be reversed by aminooxyacetic acid (AOAA), an inhibitor of GABA transaminase (GABA-T), which results in a retardation of GABA degradation (22). Similar effects can be observed in cases of morphine-induced analgesia. When the GABA content of the brain tissue was measured thirty minutes after injection of 3-MP, levels were significantly lower in the brain stem, spinal cord, and cerebellum, but not in the forebrain or diencephalon.

Figure 7-4 illustrates the effect of 3-MP on the analgesia induced either by EAP or by morphine.

An increase in GABA content obtained by AOAA injection has been observed to suppress acupuncture or morphine analgesia. This suppression can be reversed by administration of bicuculline methochloride or isoniazid, a GABA biosynthesis inhibitor. This is additional evidence indicating that the GABA system in the brain exerts an antagonistic effect on acupuncture- or morphine-induced analgesia.

Muscinol, a GABA agonist, or nipecotic acid, a GABA uptake inhibitor, was injected directly into the dorsal Raphe nuclei of rat, resulting in an increase in the pain threshold and an enhancement of acupuncture analgesia; the analgesic effect lasted over two hours. When bicuculline, a GABA antagonist, or 3-mercaptopropionic acid, a GABA biosynthesis inhibitor, was injected into the same area, no significant change of the pain threshold was found. However, the acupuncture-induced analgesic effect declined significantly. This indicates that GABA in the dorsal Raphe nucleus plays an important role in the modulation of pain transmissions (35).

Studies in rats by Y. M. Zhao, et al., (39) have shown that the stress-induced hypertension and hyperviscosity can be inhibited either by EAP at the Zusanli point, or by icv injection of GABA. The antihypertensive effect of EAP is believed mediated through the GABA-A receptor, not the GABA-B receptor, because the icv injection of a GABA-B antagonist could not block the EAP effect.

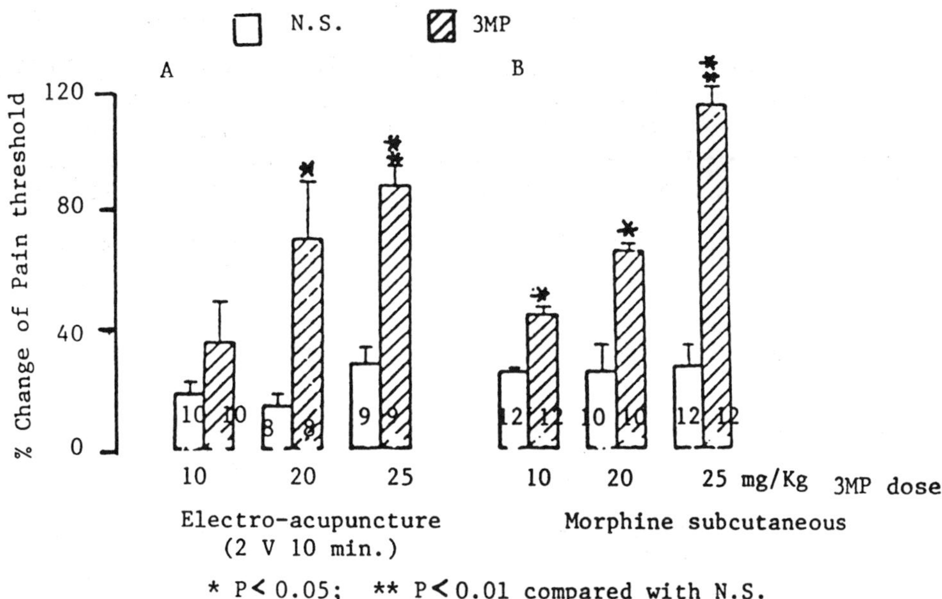

Figure 7-4. Potentiation of 3-Methylcaptopropionic Acid on the Analgesic Effect of Electroacupuncture (A) or Morphine (2 mg/Kg Subcutaneously) (B) in Rats

(From Qiu et al. (22))

Acetylcholine (Ach)

It has been shown in experiments with animals that the administration of Ach in small doses may have little effect on the pain threshold. When physostigmine, an acetylcholinesterase inhibitor, is injected, however, the pain threshold has been observed to increase, and a potentiation of analgesia induced by acupuncture has also been observed (13). As shown in table 7-1, such effects are dose-dependent. Metoclopramide, an antidopaminic and anticholinesterase agent, was given to patients who received thyroidectomies under EAP anesthesia, showing a synergistic effect with the acupuncture anesthesia (28).

Cyclic-AMP and Others

A correlation between analgesia induced by opioid peptides and the cAMP level in brain tissues has also been demonstrated (1, p. 429, and 10). The icv administration of cAMP into rats produces an antagonist effect to analgesia induced by morphine or acupuncture, while the injection of cGMP augments such analgesic effects. The antagonistic effect of cAMP to acupuncture analgesia is dose-dependent (20). Acupuncture analgesia in rats has been suppressed by icv injection of aminophylline, an inhibitor of phosphodiesterase, and augmented by the injection of imidazol, an activator of phosphodiesterase. These effects are illustrated in figure 7-5.

Table 7-1. Effect of Physostigmine on Acupuncture-Induced Analgesia in Rats

	Dose	Physostigmine Alone				Physostigmine + Acupuncture			
		No. of animals	Pain thres-hold	Ach. Content N. caud-atus	Hypo-thal.	No. of animals	Pain thres-hold	Ach. Content N. caud-atus	Hypo-thalamus
	mg/Kg		mA	µg/g.tissue			mA	ug/g.tissue	
Control (n.s.)		51	0.044± 0.038	2.022	1.57	29	0.200± 0.007	2.45	1.927
Physostimine	0.125	9	0.124± 0.038			15	0.192± 0.063		
	0.25	25	0.149± 0.024			39	0.513± 0.157		
	0.50	42	1.26± 0.284	3.437	2.019	42	2.071± 0.246	3.571	2.099

(Data modified from Kuan et al. (13))

X. C. Qui and J. S. Han reported that cAMP can attenuate acupuncture-induced analgesia, while the icv administration of aminophylline can further decrease such analgesic effects. However, imidazole can augment acupuncture analgesia (21). Rats were treated with low-frequency (4 Hz) or high-frequency (220 Hz) EAP for thirty minutes daily for a total of three weeks. Both the Na-K ATPase and Achase activity of the brain tissue increased. Such increase was only partially blocked by intraperitoneal administration of naloxone prior to acupuncture treatment. This suggests that other neurotransmitter pathways besides the opioid peptides are involved in the modulation of pain sensation (14).

Activity of Other Endocrines

Recently, C. Y. Song, et al., (23,24) reported that the icv injection of oxytocin (OXY) into rabbits or arginine-vasopressin (AVP) into rats can raise their pain threshold 28 to 33 percent higher than the control value. Oxytocin can enhance EAP analgesia in rats between 139 and 234 percent of the control value. Administration of anti-OXY or anti-AVP serum does not change the pain threshold but significantly decreases the analgesic effect induced by EAP. The icv injection of anti-ß-endorphin serum (AEPS) prior to oxytocin does not block the oxytocin-enhancing effect, while injection of antidynorphine $A_{1\text{-}13}$ serum (ADYNS) can reduce electro- acupuncture analgesia. If ADYNS is given prior to OXY, it results in a potentiation of OXY enhancement. Neither the anti-MEK nor the

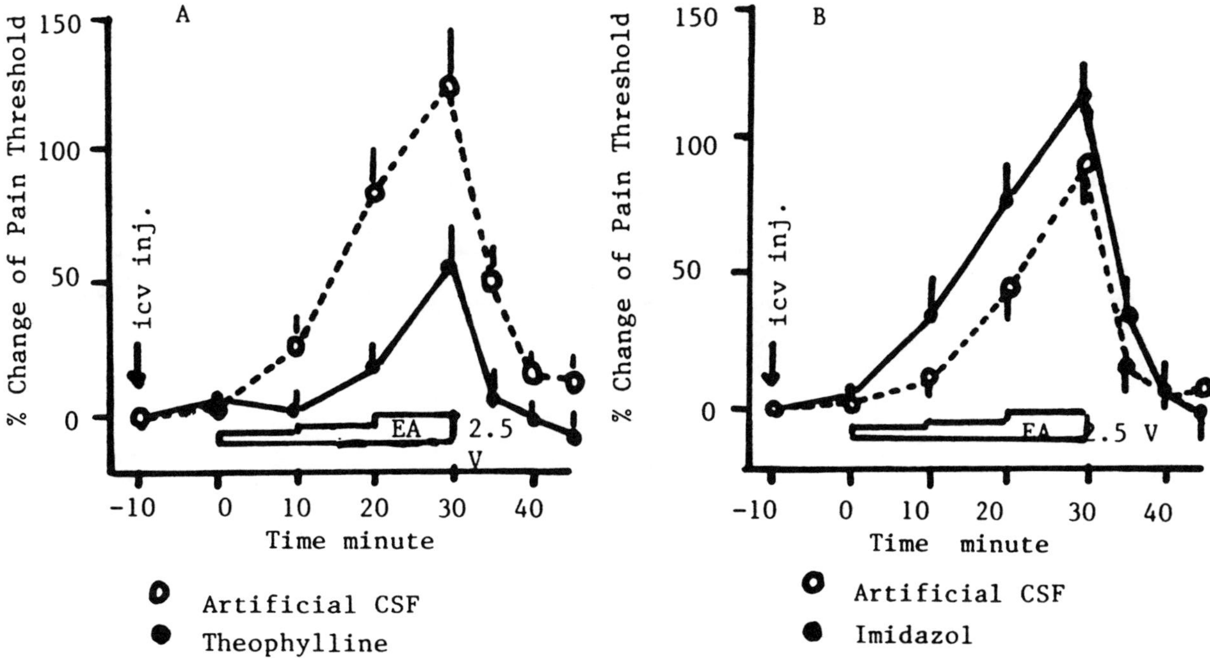

Figure 7-5. Analgesic Effect of Electroacupuncture (EAP) in the Presence of Theophylline (A) or Imidazol (B) in Rats

(From Qiu (21))

anti-LEK serum has an effect on OXY enhancement. Data suggest that OXY enhancement of EAP analgesia is not dependent on endogenous opioid peptides in the brain. It is unclear how this mechanism works. Experiments performed in rats showed that low-frequency (2 Hz) EAP or thermo stimulation can induce a significant increase of oxytocin in plasma and CSF, thirty to ninety minutes after the stimulation, which can be abolished by oxytocin antagonist. This suggests that the analgesic effect induced by nonnoxious sensory stimulation may in part be mediated through the activation of oxytocinergic mechanism (26).

Since the opioid peptides are the cleavage products of the prohormone, ß-lipotropin and the residues 47–53 of ß-lipotropin are identical to the residues 4–10 that are fractioned in adrenocorticotropine hormone (ACTH). Thus it is not surprising to find that acupuncture can increase the endorphin content of the pituitary, as well as the ACTH content. This has been confirmed in studies on human volunteers (16). A. Masula., et al., reported that EAP on human patients would raise the ß-endorphin and ACTH levels in the plasma. Such elevation was suppressed by pretreatment with cortisol. However, cortisol administration alone on nonacupuncture patients did not elicit such effects (19).

EAP can produce opiatelike antinociception and catalepsy in rats. Such analgesic effects cannot be produced in hypophysectomized rats, whereas adrenectomized rats show an increased sensitivity to the EAP. In intact rats, ACTH and dexamethasone effectively sensitize the animals to acupuncture analgesic effects; deoxycorticosterone, on the other hand, attenuates this effect. Spironolactone is also effective in potentiating the acupuncture analgesic effect (6). Table 7-2 summarizes the effect of drugs on acupuncture analgesia in rats.

Table 7-2. Effect of Hormones and Drugs on Acupuncture-Induced Analgesia in Rats

Pretreatment	Induction Period for Analgesia (minutes ± S.E.M.)	
	Intact Rats	Adrenalectomized Rats
Vehicle	12.5 ± 2.5*	2.5 ± 0.5
ACTH	3.5 ± 0.5 **	
Dexamethasone	2.5 ± 0.5**	2.5 ± 1.0
Deoxycorticosterone	29.0 ± 4.0**	24.5 ± 4.0
Spironolactone	1.5 ± 0.5 **	
Angiotensin II	25.5 ± 4.0**	2.0 ± 0.5
Captopril	6.0 ± 2.0**	

* $p < 0.001$ compared with the control adrenalectomized rats

** $p < 0.001$ compared with the control intact rats

(Extracted from Das et al.'s data (6))

H. S. Lee, et al., (15) have found that acupuncture did influence the plasma level of certain endocrines—for example, when needling at the acupoint Shenshu (B 23) could decrease the plasma level of atrial natriuretic peptide (ANP) and plasma renin activity (PRA), but needling at the Xinshu point (B 15) could cause an increase of plasma ANP and decrease of aldosterone, indicating that acupuncture in specific meridian points may have site-specific regulatory function for the hormone level. The acupoints B 23 and B 15 may have a control mechanism for the regulation in the body fluid and electrolyte balance.

References

1. All China Society of Acupuncture and Moxibustion. Second National Symposium on Acupuncture and Moxibustion and Acupuncture Anesthesia. Beijing: 1984.
2. Chen, B. Y., et al. Acta Physiol. Sinica 34:385, 1982.
3. Chen, X. H., and J. S. Han, et al. Chinese Medical Journal 107(2):113, 1994.
4. Dai, J. L., and S. L. Xu. Acta Physiol. Sinica 14:388, 1993.
5. Dai, J., and S. Xu. Acupuncture Electro-Therap. Res. 16:101, 1991.
6. Das, S., et al. Pain 18:135, 1984.
7. Dong, X. W., et al. Acta Physiol. Sinica 36:214, 1984.
8. Han, J. S., and G. X. Xie. Pain 18:367, 1984.
9. Han, J. S., et al. Neuropharmacol. 23:1–6, 1984.
10. Han, J. S., et al., in Chang, C. T., ed. Research on Acupuncture and Moxibustion Anesthesia. Beijing: Science Publisher, 1986, p. 179.
11. Han, J. S., et al. Acta Physiol. Sinica 42:219, 1990; 42:226, 1990; 42:277, 1990.
12. Huang, K. C. Pharmacology of Chinese Herbs. CRC Press, 1993.
13. Kuan, S. M., et al., in Chang, C. T., ed. Research on Acupuncture and Moxibustion Anesthesia. Beijing: Science Publisher, 1986, p. 251.
14. Lee, D. Z., and A. Y. Sem. Neurochem. Res. 9:669, 1984.
15. Lee, H. S., et al. Acupuncture Electro-Therap. Res. 16:111, 1991.
16. Lee, S. C., et al. American Journal of Chinese Medicine 10:62, 1982.
17. Li, K. Y., et al. Acupuncture. Electr-Ther. Res. 15:179, 1990.
18. Li, S. J, M. S. Wu, and J. S. Han. Acta Physiol. Sinica 35:454, 1983.
19. Masula, A., et al. Acta Endocrin. 103:469, 1983.
20. Omura, Y., et al. Acupuncture Electro-Ther. Res. 18:125, 1993.
21. Qiu, X. C., and J. S. Han. Acta Physiol. Sinica 35:340, 1983.
22. Qu, Z. C., et al. Acta Physiol. Sinica 35:401, 1983.
23. Song, C. Y., et al. Acta Physiol. Sinica 42:169, 1990; and 45:231, 1993.
24. Song, C. Y., et al. Chinese Journal of Applied Physiology 7:26, 1991.
25. Su, S. Y., et al. Acta Pharmacol. Sinica 5:82, 1984.
26. Uvnes-Moberg, K., et al. Acta Physiol. Scand. 149:199, 1993.
27. Xia, C. W., et al. Acta Physiol. Sinica 35:186, 1983.
28. Xu, Z. B., et al. Acup. Electro-Therap. Res. 8:283, 1983.
29. Xu, S. F., et al. Acta Physiol. Sinica 36:220, 1984.
30. Wang, H. H., and S. F. Xue. Acta Physiol. Sinica 45:61, 1993.
31. Wang, Y. J., et al. Journal of Traditional Chinese Medicine, in English 8:141, 1988.
32. Wang, Y. J., et al. Journal of Traditional Chinese Medicine, in English 5:297, 1985.
33. Watkins, L. R., et al. Brain Res. 327:181, 1981.
34. Wu, G., et al. Acta Pharmacol. Sinica 11:116, 1990.
35. Ye, M. L. and X. C. Feng. Acta Physiol. Sinica 38:123, 1986.
36. Yu, F. S., et al. Acta Pharmac. Sinica 4:232, 1983.
37. Yu, G. D., et al. Acta Physiol. Sinica 42:76, 1990.
38. Yu, G. D., et al. Acta Physiol. Sinica 37:120, 1985.
39. Zhao, Y. M., et al. Acta Acad. Med. Shanghai 21(2):158, 1994.
40. Zhu, C. F., et al. Acta Physiol. Sinica 36:220, 1984.
41. Zhu, J. M., et al. Acta Physiol. Sinica 42:135, 1990.
42. Zhu, S. P., and Z. H. Liu. Acta Physiol. Sinica 37:497, 1985.

8

Acupuncture Analgesia

Primitive man believed that illness was due to invasion of the body by evil spirits or demons. According to an old Chinese proverb, the best remedy against poison is poison, or a sword against evil. Therefore, stabbing a sharp instrument into the body was a way to chase away or kill the intruding demon. Trepanning of the skull was used by ancient Egyptians and is still used by some Pacific Island tribes. The Chinese developed needles made of stone, animal bone, or metal to serve a similar purpose. The method known as Zhen Djiu, which involved needling and burning, gradually developed into acupuncture in the "demonologic age," when people were plagued with pain, swollen tissues, and diseases. As recorded in the *Huang Ti Nei Chian,* the Yellow Emperor, Huang Ti, was the first to officialize the Zhen Djiu, or acupuncture, as a method for treating the suffering of his people.

Literally, *acupuncture* means "piercing with a sharp point or needle." Technically, it is a simple, inexpensive technique that has been in widespread use in China for more than four thousand years. In most rural areas of China, street peddlers still practice acupuncture in pulling teeth, relieving pain, and reducing swelling. In hospitals, the conventional manual acupuncture has been largely replaced by EAP. Historically, electric analgesia was first employed by Francis in 1858 as a method to electrically relieve pain in dental extraction and by Garratt in Boston as a method to produce electro-anesthesia (16). Studies have shown that electrical stimulation of different nerves can produce pain relief (105). Such electrically induced analgesia was later transformed into the technique of Transcutaneous Electric Nerve Stimulation (TENS). In a sense, the EAP is quite similar to TENS, except that TENS involves stimulation at the skin surface and requires a higher electric current, which might provoke an epileptic seizure. The electric current applied in acupuncture procedures is relatively low and can be delivered not only to cutaneous nerves, but also to deep structures such as muscles, neurovascular bundles, tendons, and bones. Selection of the right acupoint for puncturing is a key requirement for successful acupuncture, but not for TENS. Some scientists still view acupuncture a mysterious technique and consider its action uninterpretable. However, in the past fifty years, experiments with animals, human volunteers, and patients have shown definite positive effects of acupuncture, especailly the EAP, in relieving pain of various pathological causes. In a recent survey in Norway, medical students expressed their opinion that acupuncture already is, or at least should be, a part of ordinary health care and that it is especially useful in the treatment of migraine headache.

Clinically, acupuncture induces analgesia, which can be potentiated by the administration of D-phenylalanine (86,87,88). In the early 1920s Goulden reported that Dr. Davis had introduced the use of acupuncture in the treatment of sciatica and that over two decades more than one hundred cases of sciatica and other forms of neuritis had been treated with acupuncture. Only a small amount of current (3-6 mA) was used. The mechanism of action was said to involve induction of hyperemia of nerves. Acupuncture could not reverse the muscle wasting that frequently accompanied long-standing sciatica. The treatment was solely to relieve pain. For lameness and wasting of muscles, patients had to be taught to walk correctly and received massage with electrical stimulation. It was reported that a fifty-year-old man suffering with sciatica obtained complete pain relief with acupuncture (56).

The effectiveness of acupuncture in relieving pain has been reviewed recently by H. Nissell (115). This chapter deals mainly with data reported in medical journals (mostly Chinese) published in the last two decades.

It has been reported that acupuncture at the acupoints Zusanli (S 36) and Feng Chi (G 20) can increase intracephalic blood flow due to increase release of 5HT. This neurotransmitter is thought to mediate the acupuncture-induced analgesia and antidepressive effects of acupuncture. (For details, see chapter 7.) Using segmental electric acupuncture (SEA) in eighty-five clinical physical disorders, A. Chen (23) reported that the patients had a remarkable 78.8 percent improvement in mental disorders and 77.1 percent improvement in physical disorders.

J. G. Lin, J. S. Han, and their coworkers (100) found that stimulation of the hind legs of rats at the acupoint Zusanli by using a square wave electrical stimulator can significantly increase pain threshold and that the effect can be partially blocked partially by naloxone, an opiate antagonist.

Studies on thirty five healthy volunteers demonstrated that acupuncture at the acupoint HoKu (LI 4) can raise the pain threshold by 27.1 percent. Administration of naloxone, 0.8 mg intravenously, could decrease the elevated pain threshold back to the placebo level (110). Other investigators (160) reported studies on a thirty five-year-old patient and nine healthy volunteers. Acupuncture increased pain threshold and produced an analgesic effect when the needles were applied bilaterally at the acupoints HoKu, Zusanli and Sanyinjiao, but no change was seen when acupuncture was performed at nonacupoints. Administration of naloxone reversed the analgesic effect in six of the nine volunteers.

D. J. Mayer, et al., (110) also reported that acupuncture can increase pain threshold and that the effect was reversed by administration of naloxone. Similar results were obtained in studies on subjects treated by auricular electrical stimulation (127).

Figure 8-1 illustrates the effect of acupuncture therapy on pain threshold and reversed of the effect by naloxone.

In twelve patients with terminal malignancies, a group of investigators at Shanghai HuaShan Hospital implanted a pair of electrodes in the caudate nucleus of the midbrain. They reported that electric stimulation of the head of the caudate nucleus can produce relief of intractable pain and an increased pain threshold. The analgesic effect persisted for some time even after cessation of the stimulation. The investigators also performed acupuncture in these patients at a certain acupoint and recorded a potential that contains a positive and negative component, from the caudate nucleus (2, p. 33).

H. Ashton, et al., (6) induced pain in forty-six young, healthy volunteers by immersing their hands in cold water and tested the effect of acupuncture and high-frequency (100 Hz) TENS. Acupuncture significantly increased the pain threshold, but TENS had no effect. In other studies of eight volunteers, pain induced by a cold pressure technique was attenuated by either hypnosis or acupuncture (112). Neither method of treatment produced any significant change in the plasma endorphin level.

In studies performed from 1978 to 1980, Shimohara, et al., (126) found that low frequency EAP produce a persistent satisfactory analgesic effect. The analgesic effect appeared on the first day, immediately after the treatment. It has also been shown that acupuncture was much more effective than infrared massage in relieving chronic pain (107). Patients not only obtained pain relief, but were able to perform their usual daily activities and return to work. If the patients were taking medications previously, after acupuncture it was possible to completely eliminate the drug or reduce the dose.

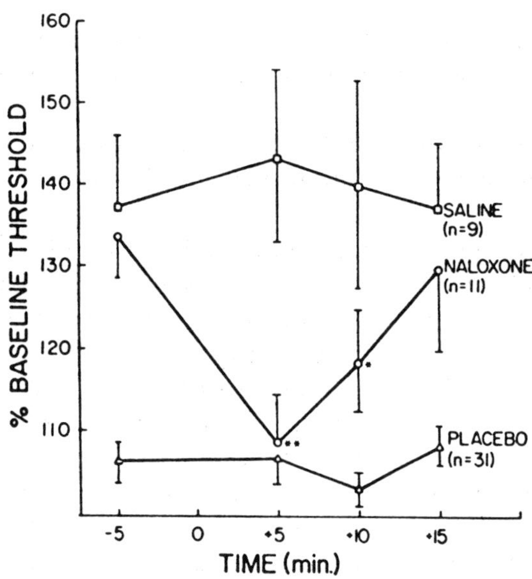

Figure 8-1. Effect of Acupuncture on Pain Threshold and the Reversal by Naloxone

(From Mayer et al. (110))

However, L. Grabow (57) evaluated the effectiveness of acupuncture-induced analgesia in postoperative patients and reported that acupuncture produced similar effectiveness to the placebo treatment. But he pointed out there is always a minority of the population who are completely satisfied with acupuncture as the sole treatment for pain.

Comparing the benefit of acupuncture and the drug pentazocine, E. Facco, et al., (47) reported that patients treated with EAP treatment had a net increase in vital capacity in addition to pain relief. The increase in vital capacity lasted three to four hours after stimulation. This effect was not seen in patients taking pentazocine.

Studies on eighty-one patients with chronic pain from a variety of causes have shown that acupuncture altered their thermographic picture, consistently producing an increase in infrared radiation (IRR) from the affected part of the body. There was no change or a slight decrease in pain-free volunteers (98).

Acupuncture is claimed to produce relaxation, vasodilatation, and stillness similar to the effects of quiet meditation (50).

The Needle and the Technique

In the application of acupuncture a needle made of very fine stainless steel in gauze from 26 (0.45 mm) to 32 (0.26 mm) and in length from 1 to 10 centimeters is inserted into the skin at a selected focus, the acupoint. (See chapter 4.) (The most commonly used needle has a gauze of 28 to 30 and a length of 1 to 2 centimeters.) The exact method of insertion of the needle depends on the skill and experience of the performer. Chinese acupuncturists suggest three ways to insert the needle—the perpendicular (ninety-degree angle to the skin), the oblique (forty five-degree diagonal to the skin), and the horizontal (approximately thirty-degree angle between the needle and skin).

The choice of technique depends on the desired depth of penetration and the thickness of the underlying tissue. For example, the horizontal method is commonly used in areas where the muscle layer is thin, such as in the head, face, and chest.

Locating the acupoint requires skill and practice and a knowledge of anatomy. A special instrument, a resistant meter, can be used in searching for the acupoint. This approach is based on reports that the resistance of the righteous acupoint is lower than the nonacupoint, which lies approximately two to four millimeters outside of the corresponding meridian channel. When the needle reaches the meridian via the right acupoint, within a few seconds a feeling of numbness, soreness, heaviness, and distension is sensed by the patient. This sensation is called Tai Qi by Chinese. The term implies the Qi is flowing along the corresponding meridian to reach the corresponding internal organ(s). The speed of such sensation feeling is especially important in acupuncture treatment, the quicker one feels the sensation the better acupuncture result.

After the Tai Qi is felt, the needle can be connected to an electrical stimulator, usually with a nine-volt D.C. battery unit, for stimulation at a varying frequency and intensity. The duration of acupuncture stimulation is five to thirty minutes. It has been reported that low-frequency stimulation, (1–5 Hz), was more effective than high-frequency stimulation (10–100 Hz) (4, 117). Also EAP with low frequency produced an analgesic effect that can be blocked by intravenous administration of naloxone. However, EAP at high frequencies (from 50 to 150 Hz) produced an analgesic effect that could not be reversed by naloxone. In acute pain, use of low-intensity, high-frequency, and short-duration electric stimulation is highly recommended, but in chronic pain, high-intensity, low-frequency, and long-duration stimulation is justified. The mechanism of differences in effects has not been explained.

J. C. Chan (22) used the bidigital O-ring test, derived by Y. Omura (116) (see chapter 4) as a guide to determine the best modality of treatment of pain conditions. He reported that the test can effectively determine whether a pathological state or problem suitable for acupuncture treatment exists.

It has been shown in man that auricular EAP can increase the pain threshold and reduce the amplitude of somatosensory potentials (5).

Headache

Headache has afflicted mankind universally and is one of the most common and distressing forms of suffering. The term *headache* describe a pain felt in or around the cranial circumference, including the neck and back of the head. There are sex and age differences. Females and young middle-aged people (thirty to fifty years old) complain of headache more often than males and older people. The source of the nociceptive stimulus may be localized close to the head, may come from the sense organs (eyes, nose, ears) or radiation from the teeth and jaws , or from sites distant to the head, and is affected by conditions such as hypertension, infection, trauma, cancer and cerebrovascular disorders. The traditional Chinese medicine describes the head as the junction of the Yangs, where the blood from all five *zhan* (the organs) and Qi from all six *fu* (the viscera) terminate. Therefore, any intruder from the outside ends up in the head, resulting in the symptom headache.

The pathogenesis of headache is manifold. Headache may be vascular or nonvascular. One of the biochemical mechanisms may be due to a large drop in opioid neuropeptides in the brain, as shown by J. E. Hardebo, et al., (62). In such cases, the relief of headache by acupuncture was associated with an increase in CSF methionine enkephalin (MEK) levels.

The treatment of headache varies from acupuncture and herbal medicines in China to mixtures of opium as prescribed in the ancient Egyptian pharmacopoeia. The mechanism of the acupuncture-induced analgesic effect has been thoroughly discussed in chapters 6 and 7. Similar to opiate analgesia, the acupuncture effect has been shown to be due to an increase in the opioid neuropeptides and/or a homeostatic balance of other neurotransmitters in the brain. The advantage of acupuncture is its lack of toxicity and dependence, which are often seen with opiates. Abundant clinical reports have indicated that acupuncture can produce a more favorable result than drugs in the treatment of headache. Furthermore, acupuncture can lower the dosage of analgesic drugs, indicating synergistic effect between acupuncture and the drug (51,93). The common acupoint for the treatment of headache is Feng Chi (G 20) of the Foot Xiao Yang–gallbladder meridian. (See Chapter 4.) This acupoint is particularly useful in the acupuncture treatment of occipital headache, vertigo, glaucoma, painful tinnitus, and rhinorrhea. Some acupuncturists also suggest the use of a second acupoint, Tai Yang (Extra), at the midpoint between the lateral end of eyebrow and the outer canthus of the ear. Recently a Korean acupuncturist reported a new, modified acupuncture technique for the treatment of headache. In this technique all acupoints are on the hand (45).

A typical case presented by a Chinese acupuncture clinic involved a female teacher who was treated with acupuncture (25). The patient suffered from chronic headache for ten years. Pain was localized to the right temporal lobe and become unbearable during the pre- and postmenstruation periods. She had a normal electroencephalogram (EEG) and no pathological findings involving the eyes and cardiovascular system. She was treated with acupuncture for one minute daily. After three treatments, the headache as well as all accompanying symptoms, which included nausea, vomiting, and disturbed vision, had resolved. She returned eight times for monthly treatments in the premenstruation period. The patient was apparently cured and did not have a recurrence over many years.

Surveying his eight years of studies on the acupuncture treatment of chronic headache, S. Y. T. Junnila (80) reported that long-term acupuncture therapy produces a high cure rate. Seventy-four percent of his patients had pain relief that lasted an average of twenty-two months without a recurrence. Some of the patients had used analgesic drugs prior to acupuncture treatment. In 75 percent of those cases it was possible to reduce the dose of medication by 50 percent or more. He also found that the drug metoclopramide had synergistic analgesic effect with acupuncture. Dowson, et al., (43) treated patients with chronic headache with acupuncture for six weeks and followed up these cases for six months. They reported a very satisfactory relief rate.

S. Sjoelhuand, et al., (128) also reported that eight of nine patients suffering from chronic pain had complete or partial pain relief after EAP treatment. Five of those patients' CSF endorphin levels were elevated, one patient failed benefit for acupuncture and had no changes in the CSF level of endorphins.

Tension-type headache (TTH) is a common illness among the general population (approximately 5 percent). None of the currently available treatment (e.g., drugs, biofeedback, or psychotherapy) demonstrates a clear superiority over the others. However, favorable results have been reported with acupuncture therapy. M. G. Biondi and G. Portuesi (13) reported that 30 percent of their patients obtained pain relief with acupuncture treatment. However, these researchers suggested that its actual value is difficult to assess and it should probably be reserved for particular cases. T. Tavola, et al., (138) reported on thirty patients with TTH treated by acupuncture or sham acupuncture. Effectiveness was assessed by reduction in the intensity, frequency, and duration of attack, "headache index," and analgesic consumption over a six-month period of observation. No difference between the acupuncture and placebo (sham acupuncture) groups was found, except that the acupuncture group had a lower analgesic drug consumption.

M. Sternfeld (133) injected a drug, voltaren, directly into the acupoint Feng Chi (G 20) in combination with acupuncture treatment. He found that this combination therapy relieved chronic tension headache. Other investigators (61) also reported a significant improvement of chronic tension headache with acupuncture therapy. The administration of an antidepressant, meprotiline, in a subtherapeutic dose can produce a synergistic effect with acupuncture in relieving pain, insomnia, and depression (93). In a report by H. J. Biedermann (14) acupuncture treatment alone provided relief from chronic myofascial pain in a sixty-three-year-old woman. However, when the patient was taking a tricyclic antidepressant, doxepin, for another medical reason, acupuncture no longer produced the analgesic effect. In patients with Horton's headache treated with EAP, 48 percent obtained complete pain relief and a prolongation of the interval between painful episodes. The interval was five to twenty times longer than before acupuncture treatment (53).

S. J. Yamaguchi (154) treated patients with chronic headache by acupuncture therapy and measured the pulse waves of the digital apical and shallow temporal arteries. Pulse waves were much lower during the headache attack than during the pain-free period. After acupuncture treatment the pulse waves returned to a higher level. He claimed that pulse wave measurements can serve as a criterion for diagnosis and an index for judging the efficacy of acupuncture therapy.

Other reports indicate that acupuncture therapy in chronic tension headache is less effective than physiotherapy (19).

Table 8-1 summarizes the clinical reports on the use of acupuncture in the treatment of headache.

Migraine Headache

Migraine, a vascular type of headache, is believed to be associated with increased vasodilator peptides, including calcitonin gene-related peptide (CGRP), Substance P (SP), and vasoactive intestine peptide (VIP), in external jugular blood. Acupuncture therapy has been used successfully in the treatment of this type of headache. In the early 1970s, after his visit to China, Chen (75, p. 3) reported on sixty-two patients suffering from a variety of pain problems, including migraine, cervical syndrome, osteoarthritis and peptic ulcer. They were treated with acupuncture at various acupoints depending upon the location of the pain. Fifteen patients (24.2 percent) obtained an excellent result, (100 percent relief of pain); another thirty-nine patients (62.9 percent) benefited from the treatment (50–75 percent pain relief).

W. Baisher (9) treated thirty patients suffering from chronic migraine headache with acupuncture. Sixty percent of the patients had substantial improvement. The subjective response rate was closely related to personality traits. Patients with high scores for extroversion and low scores for neuroticism had a better response. There was no relation between response and age, sex, or social status.

In a group of eighty-five patients with a history of migraine for more than two years J. Hesse, et al., (63) found that acupuncture therapy was equipotent to the drug metoprolol and was a valuable supplement to migraine prophylaxis, reducing the frequency and duration of attacks. Moreover, acupuncture was superior to medication in terms of undesirable side effects.

J. Boivie and G. Brattberg (15) observed a long-term benefit in migraine patients who received acupuncture treatments for six to eight weeks and were followed up for nine months. Migraine index has reduced to 39 percent and the number of days of headache reduced to 35 percent of pretreatment values. A. V. Markdova, et al., (108) claimed that acupuncture effectively relieved the pain of migraineous cephalalgia and raised the 5HT serum level. They suggested that the 5HT serum level can be used to access the effectiveness of acupuncture therapy. L. Loh (104) compared acupuncture and drug therapy in the treatment of chronic migraine in seventy-four patients. Patients treated with acupuncture had a 59 percent relief rate, but those treated with medications had only a 25 percent relief rate.

Table 8-2 summarizes the clinical reports on acupuncture treatment of migraine headache.

Chronic Pain and Other Varieties of Pain

Acupuncture was found to be quite effective in relieving some types of chronic pain, especially cases with cervical symptoms (92,107). Patients suffering from spinal pain syndrome for more than eight years have obtained relief with acupuncture treatments. Studies on chronic pain by R. M. Coan (40) have shown that acupuncture therapy produced an average of 40 percent reduction of pain and 68 percent reduction of pain hour per day in his patients. C. P. Carlsson and B. H. Sjoland (20) reported on 210 patients suffering from chronic pain with a duration longer than ten years. After an average of 7.8 acupuncture treatments, 85 of 202 patients (42.1 percent) experienced pain relief immediately after treatment. Followed up for six months, thirty five patients still experienced the symptom-free effect.

M. Bianchi, et al., (12) reported on the use of acupuncture in ten patients suffering from back pain. The concentration of endorphins in immune cells was increased and there was lymphocyte proliferation after treatment. The pain was improved.

Junnila reported a five-year trial of acupuncture therapy in the long-term treatment of chronic pain in Finnish NHS clinics. A total of 348 patients received EAP treatments; 41 percent had more than one course (average of ten daily treatments as a course). Significant relief of pain was achieved in myofascial syndromes affecting the head, neck, shoulder, and arm. Sixty-five percent of the patients who had taken medicine previously were able to completely discontinue drug therapy. Patients suffering from osteoarterosis and back pain responded less favorably (80).

R. X. Chen and Y. L. Zhao (24) reported a ten-year experience in treating 900 patients with painful heel with a combination of acupuncture and medication. Six hundred and fifty obtained complete relief—a "cure rate" of 72.2 percent. The other 27.8 percent of patients did not have any beneficial response.

In some cases, acupuncture has produced 95 to 100 percent relief of pain (36, 97, 99, 142), but in other cases the effective rate has been only 60–80 percent. Table 8-3 lists the literature on clinical application of acupuncture in treating chronic pain. Table 8-4 summarizes acupuncture therapy of lumbar pain and lumbar disc diseases. The effectiveness rate is quite remarkable. Japer reported one case of a fifty-four-year-old male suffering from lumbar and sciatic pain for seven years. After acupuncture treatment a complete vertebral realignment substantiated by X-ray examination was observed (74). R. Cheng and B. Pomerenz (32) obtained a 90 percent success rate in the treatment of musculoskeletal pain with acupuncture.

One hundred and ninety-two patients with spinal osteochondritis were treated with one of the following two procedures: high-frequency electrical stimulation of the nerve fibers (70 Hz; 0.1–0.2 minute duration) or receiving acupuncture such as epicutaneous electrical stimulation (7 impulses; 0.1–0.2 minute duration). Both procedures produced a prolonged analgesic effect (129).

Table 8-1. Clinical Data on Acupuncture Therapy on Headache

Source	Mode	Acupoint	Diagnosis	No. of Patients	Effectiveness %
Li (95)	AP*	Baihui (Du 20) Shou-sanli (LI 10)	Headache acute & chronic	1,100	99%
Huang (70)	AP	Fengchi (G 20) Zusanli (S 36)	Headache	132	45% cured and other 52% improved
Lee (75 p.11)	AP		Headache	57	40.7% completely relieved
Zhang (164)	EAP#	Zusanli	Neurotic headache	202	44% were cured
Zhang (165)	AP	Daihui (Du 14) HoKu (LI 4)	Headache	60	80% were cured
Zhang (167)	AP and Physiotherapy		Headache	120	85% markedly improved
Martina (109)	AP		Headache & shoulder pain	58	53% cured
	Hom. detox.@			58	34% improved
	AP + Hom.detox.			58	70% cured
Junnila (80)	AP		Chronic headache	88	74% cured and followed up for 22 months
Wang (144)	AP	Fengchi	Chronic headache	322	14% cured and other 34% markedly improved
Dowson (43)	AP		Chronic headache	48	all improved, followed up for 24 weeks
Hsu (66)	AP & Chinese Herb	Fengchi	Chronic headache	250	53.6% cured and other 30% markedly improved
Carlssen (19)	AP and Physiother.		Chronic tension headache	110	markedly improved
Hansan (61)	AP		Chronic tension headache	18	6 of them cured
Ahonen (1)	AP		Tension headache	22	Significantly reduce the muscle tension and pain.
Strauss (136)	AP		Tension headache	124	78% cured

Table 8-1. (continued)

Source	Mode	Acupoint	Diagnosis	No. of Patients	Effectiveness %
Seppo (123)	AP		Tension headache	128	67% cured after 3-4 treatments
Rozenberg (121)	AP		Headache after lumbar puncture		relieve all common side effects
Furiosi (51)	AP		Vascular headache	85	AP gave a higher prophylactic effect.
	Medication			39	Less effective than AP.
Chen (26)	AP	Zulinqi (G 41)	Temporal region headache	16	75% cured
Hardebo (62)	AP		Cluster headache	7	Significantly relieved. MEK level in CSF was elevated after AP
Gwan (84, p.546)	AP		Cluster headache	1	Symptom-free after 5 courses treatment
Ku (90)	Laser (HeNe)	Fengchi	Headache	45	82.2% were cured

* AP = Body Acupuncture
# EAP = Electro-acupuncture
@ Hom. detox. = homeopathic detoxication

Table 8-2. Clinical Data on Acupuncture Therapy on Migraine Headache

Source	Mode	Acupoint	Diagnosis	No. of Patients	Effectiveness %
Arseni (7)	AP*		Migraine	17	Markedly effective and reduce the dosage of drug medication
Batra (10)	AP		Migraine	20	30% excellent result, other 35% improved
Boivie (15)	AP		Migraine	25	40% effective and followed up for 9 months no recurrence
Cao (17)	AP	Taichong (Liv 3)	Migraine	78	53% cured after 1-2 treatments
Cha (20)	AP and bleeding	HoKu (LI 4)	Migraine	262	51% cured, no recurrence in 6 months
Chen (27)	EAP# (80-90 Hz)	Fengchi (G 20)	Migraine	40	43% control the attack 50% markedly improved.
Damyanova (40)	AP		Migraine	53	Improved
Gan (53)	AP	Xuanlu (G 5)	Migraine	31	95% effective
Hsu (67)	AP		Migraine	100	30% immediately effective
Ivanova (70)	AP		Migraine (one side)	19	Improve the vascular reactivity of the affected side
Kim (84' p. 527)	AP		Migraine	25	68% improved after 6 months treatment
Laitinen (84,p.542)	AP		Migraine prophylaxis	39	92% improved
Loh (104)	AP		Chronic migraine & muscle tension	48	59% effective after AP only 25% effective with medication treatment
Markdova (106)	AP		Migraineous caphalalgia	49	Effective
Mueller (111)	AP		Migraine		Highly effective and low risk

Table 8-2. (continued)

Source	**Mode**	**Acupoint**	**Diagnosis**	**No. of Patient**	**Effectiveness %**
Okazaki (84, p.532)	Ap-Ryodor-aku therapy	Fengchi & Houding (Du 19)	Migraine	20	15 of them (75%) showed excellent result
Wang (139)	AP	Sizhukong (SJ 23)	Vascular migraine	384	89% were cured
Wong (147)	AP and bleeding	HoKu	Migraine	38	71% cured with compl-eted remission

* AP = Body acupuncture
# EAP = Electro-acupuncture

Table 8-3. Acupuncture Therapy on Chronic Pain

Source	Mode	Acupoint	Diagnosis	No. of Patients	Effectiveness %
Dung (44)	AP*		General pain	221	Excellent improvement
Yang (156)	AP	Zusanli (S 36)	General pain	412	85.2% effective
Giannoni (55)	AP		Non-malignant acute & chron. pain	222	49.6% have a quick relief and a completed recovery of articular function.
Beebe (75 p.1)	AP		Chron. pain	18	62% obtain a relief
Chen (84, p.441)	AP		Chron. pain	556	62.4% excellent result
Kreitler (89)	AP		Chronic pain	30	33% excellent improved
Junnila (83)	AP		Chronic pain	128	67% cured after 4 treatments
Kepes (75 p.8)	AP		Chronic pain	82	68% relieved
Long (75, p. 39)	TENS#		Chronic pain	500	39% excellent; 28% benefited
Luis Gonzalaz (107)	AP Infrared massage		Chronic pain	80	Completely relieved
Kitade (86,88)	AP & Oral DPA@		Chronic low back pain	60	60% excellent
Wilber (84, p.465)	AP		Low back pain	23	19 of them completely relieved
			Arachnoiditis	4	no effect.
Matsumoto (75,p.19)	AP		Chron. musculoskeletal pain	50	80% relieved
Thomas (140)	EAP** (2 Hz or 80 Hz)		Chron. low back pain	40	2 Hz is the mode of choice, all patients were significantly improved
Ene (46)	AP		Low back pain & frozen shoulder		Excellent result, completely recovered
Batra (11)	AP & Medication		Chron. shoulder pain & back pain		Significantly improved

Table 8-3. (continued)

Source	Mode	Acupoint	Diagnosis	No. of Patients	Effectiveness %
Chen (24)	AP		Carpal tunnel syndrome	36	82.8% cured, averaged no recurrence in 5 yrs.
Petie (117)	AP		Neck pain	25	no improvement
Zwoelfer (169)	AP	Zusanli	Gonarthrolic pain	35	71% relief of pain
Chiu (36)	AP		Temporomandi-bular joint dysfunction	228	98.2% cured
Sternfeld (130)	Intra-acupoint inj. of NaOH		Musculoskel-etal pain	20	80% effective
Umeh (142)	Ear AP		Musculoskel-etal pain & stiffness;	55	20% effective
			Acute torti-collis	11	100 % effective
Cheung (34)	EAP	Fengchi	Painful contraction	204	74% significant reduction of pain
Moore (75, p.21)	AP		Benign intrac-table pain	69	78% relief of shoulder pain; 45% relief of cervical pain; 33% relief in low back pain.
Chen (23)	AP & medication		Painful heel	900	72.2% were cured, other 27.7 % not responded.
Li (95)	AP		Spasmodic torticollis	42	95% completely cured
Jewer (76)	Podiatric AP		Bunion pain & deformities		As a pre- and post-operative method to control pain
Lin (97)	Ear AP		Tooth pain	18	100% completely relieved
Au (8)	AP	Yanglingquan (G 34)	Postherpes neuralgia	43	90% cured after 3-5 courses of treatment
Shi (123)	AP & intra-acu-point inj. of Vit. B_{12}	Around affected area	Postherpes neuralgia	16	100% cured after 2-8 courses treatment
Wu (151)	AP with a plum-blossom needle		Postherpes neuralgia	23	100% cured after 1-4 courses treatment

Table 8-3. (continued)

Source	Mode	Acupoint	Diagnosis	No. of Patients	Effectiveness %
Lewith (94)	AP		Low back pain & sciatica	151	70% obtained relief
Miyamate (111)	AP		Low back pain shoulder pain knee joint pain	1,823	69.5% improved
Garvey (54)	AP	Trigger point	Low back pain	63	63% effective
	Lidocaine & steroid				42% effective
Han (60)	Heating needle AP	Vertebra	Back pain	61	93.4% cured
Coan (40)	AP		Spine pain (over 8 yr.)	30	80% improved after 12 wks treatment
Huang (70)	AP	Fengchi	Shoulder pain	75	55% cured
Fischer (49)	AP		Cephalalgia and other functional disorders	971	Significantly improved
Arseni (7)	AP		Craniofacial pain	50	Improved and reduced the drug supplement
Hillman (64)	AP		Craniofacial pain	34	80% obtain relieved, better than steroid therapy
Petelin (118)	AP		Acute closed craniocerebral trauma	117	Normalization of the vegetovascular dysfunction
Cao (18)	Heating needle AP	Shenmen (H 7) Yingxiang (LI 20)	Facial myospasm	23	14 of them cured
Delmzec (42)	EAP		Fibromyalgia	70	Significantly improved
Johnsson (78)	AP		Facial muscular pain	45	Significant reduction of symptoms and clinical signs of stomatogmetis system.

* AP =Acupuncture; # TENS Transcutaneous electrical stimulation
** EAP = Electro-acupuncture ; @ DPA = D-phenylalanine

Table 8-4. Acupuncture Therapy on Lumbar Pain

Source	Mode	Acupoint	Diagnosis	No. of Patients	Effectiveness %
Chen (30)	AP*	Huoxi (SI 3)	Acute lumbar sprain	300	81.6% completed disappearance of symptoms
Chen (29)	AP	Chengshan (B 57)	Lumbar sprain	124	100% recovered and painless
Chu (39)	AP	Yanglao (SI 6)	Lumbar sprain	45	60% cured after one treatment; 22% cured at the end of 2nd treatment.
Chu (37)	AP	Jizhong (Du 6)	Lumbar sprain	40	90% were cured
Liu (107)	AP	Yanglao	Lumbar sprain	155	89% were cured
Wang (3, p.76)	AP	Weizhong (B 40)	Acute lumbar sprain	343	50% were cured after one treatment, totally 94% cured after continued 3 treatments.
Wang (149)	AP	Fengchi (G 20) Dazhui (Du 14)	Acute lumbar sprain and other joint and kee pain	5,401	76.1% clinical cure
Zhang (163)	AP	Yanglao	Lumbar sprain	145	83% cured after 1-3 treatments, patients can go back to work
Wang (147)	AP	Renzhong (Du 26)	Back sprain	36	50% cured after one treatment, 25% after the 2nd and another 25% after the 3rd treatment.
Won (150)	AP	Vertebrae L2-L3 area	Acute lumbar injury	130	55% cured, and other 42% improved.
Fang (48)	AP and tapping		Lumbago	74	50% cured and other 31% markedly improved
Japer (74)	AP		Lumbar & sciatic pain	1	completed vertebral realignment and X-ray confirmed the result
Takase (137)	Modified AP method		Lumbar pain		100% improved

Table 8-4. (continued)

Source	Mode	Acupoint	Diagnosis	No. of Patient	Effectiveness %
Zhang (166)	AP	Dachangshu (B 25) Qihai (Du 6)	Lumbar disc	383	66% cured and other 29% markedly improved
Chin (35)	AP	Vertebrae	Lumbar disc	2,009	99% effective to relieve pain
Liu (101)	AP and massage	Huoxi	Lumbar disc	956	89% were cured
Wang (146)	AP		Lumbar disc	100	82% cured; less effective in patients suffer over 2-3 months long.
Wang (148)	AP		Acute prolapse of lumbar disc	118	94% cured, other 6% improved, no failure
Zhang (161)	Moxib.#	Vertebrae at C6-C7	Lumbar disorders	58	39.6% cured and 43% markedly improved.
Cheng (31)	AP	Neck vertebrae	Spinal pain; vertigo and headache	206	92.3% were cured
Song (129)	AP		Soft tissue injury in lumbar region	1,000	61.9% were cured and other 21.9% improved.
Laitinen (84 p.458)	AP		Sacrolumbalgia & ischialgia	50	58% obtained relief
	TENS@			50	46% obtained relief
Lobzin (103)	AP		Postoperative lumbar spinal osteochondriosis	130	much more effective than using physical therapy or medication

* AP = Acupuncture
# Moxib. = Moxibustion
@ TENS = Transcutaneous electrical stimulation

Based on his twenty-five years of experience with acupuncture therapy in many nervous system diseases, B. R. Khudaidatov reported that use of ear acupuncture as a type of reflexotherapy to relieve pain is highly effective, with efficiency rates of 90 percent or higher (85).

Reports also showed that eighty patients suffering for heel pain were treated with acupuncture. Twenty-nine were cured after one treatment, twenty-three were cured after two treatments, eighteen after three treatments, and ten after four or more treatments (159).

H. Sprott, et al., (130) reported the studies on thirty patients suffering from generalized tendomyopathy (floromyalgia) who received the treatment of acupuncture. There was an increase of pain threshold and a decrease of positive "tender points."

M. Sternfeld and J. Hod (135) reported a case involving a woman who had suffered back pain for ten years after an accident on the road. A foreign body was found over her left scapula. After unsuccessful conventional treatment, she received acupuncture therapy. The needle was inserted directly to the scar. After a few sessions the foreign body disappeared and the pain was relieved.

Using acupuncture therapy as noninvasive physical therapy has been found to be effective in treating cervical spondylosis. C. T. Jackson and M. Nordin (73) reported that 80 percent of patients had a remission after acupuncture therapy, as compared to only 30 percent in the control group treated with other methods. Also, acupuncture therapy provided significant long-term improvement in 64.9 percent of the patients suffering from chronic neck and shoulder pain.

Studies in patients suffering from neck and chronic pain have shown that the patients who responded well to acupuncture treatment with a significant relief of pain had an average change of finger temperature of 0.55 C. Those who did not obtain significant relief of pain had a finger temperature change of only 0.22 C, indicating that the beneficial effect of acupuncture involved a somatic sympathetic vasomotor activity (139).

Recently some Chinese acupuncturists advertised a modified acupuncture technique involving the injection of some herbal extracts or vitamin solutions into a specific acupoint and claimed excellent results. For example, T. Zhong (169) reported that 210 patients suffering from postabdominal operation pain were treated by injection of eight milligrams of vitamin K3 into the Zusanli acupoint. Fifty-nine percent had a remarkable improvement in symptom. If the vitamin was injected intramuscularly, no improvement was observed. In another studies, Chinese herbs were prepared as a paste that was applied on the Zusanli acupoint. The paste reportedly produced an excellent curative effect in children suffering from abdominal pain (145). In 250 patients with various types of pain, such as headache, neuralgia, and back pain, an extract of *Radix angelica sinensis* was injected into the acupoint Feng Chi (G 20) or Dachangshu (B 25). After one to ten treatments, 95.2 percent of the patients had a very satisfactory improvement, including a 53.6 percent curative rate (67). In 120 patients suffering from sciatic neuralgia, two mililiters of angelica extract was injected into the Kunlun (B 60) acupoint; after ten treatments fifty-three (44 percent) were completely cured and another sixty-one (51 percemt) were markedly improved (106).

Table 8-3 summarizes the data on acupuncture treatment of various chronic pains.

Table 8-4 summarizes the acupuncture treatment of lumbar pain and lumbar disc disorders.

Table 8-5 summarizes the acupuncture treatment of spondylitis.

Neuralgia

There are abundant literature reports on the success of acupuncture in the treatment of neuralgia, especially trigeminal neuralgia. S. H. Gu, et al., (59) reported on 1,500 cases of trigeminus neuralgia treated with acupuncture at the acupoints Yushin (9) and Xiaguan (S 7) daily or every

Table 8-5. Acupuncture Therapy on Spondylitis

Source	Mode	Acupoint	Diagnosis	No. of Patients	Effectiveness %
Ga (52)	Scalp AP*	Neck vertebrae	Cervical spondylosis	46	63% markedly effective and other 33% improved
Junhasa-vasdikul (79)	AP		Cervical spongylitis	33	85.6% improved
Li (96)	AP and Moxib.#	Vertebrae	Cervical spondylosis	58	48% markedly effective and other 45% improved
Lin (3, p.74)	AP		Cervical spondylitis	138	15% were cured and other 80% improved
Tsuai (141)	AP & massage or medication	Fengchi (G 20)	Spondylitis	138	26% were cured
Yang (157)	Operation under AP anesthesia		Cerebral spondylitic myelopathy	500	74% excellent result, follow-up for 1 yr.
Yen (158)	EAP@	Huatuojiaji (Extra 15)	Hyperplastic spondylitis	105	65% were cured and other 31% improved

* AP = Acupuncture
\# Moxib. = Moxibustion
@ EAP = Electro-acupuncture

Table 8-6. The Effectiveness of Acupuncture Therapy on Neuralgia

	Total Number of Patients	Pain Symptom: Severe	Pain Symptom: Moderate	Pain Symptom: Mild
Patients received AP treatment	1,500	652	553	295
Cured (pain completely disappeared)	815	399	261	155
Percentage of cured	(54)	(61.2)	(47.2)	(52.5)

(From Gu et al. (59))

Table 8-7. Acupuncture Therapy on Neuralgia

Source	Mode	Acupoint	Diagnosis	No. of Patients	Effectiveness %
Chu (38)	AP*		Trigeminus neuralgia	150	45% effective
Gu (59)	AP	Yushin (B 9) Xiaguan (S 7)	Trigeminus neuralgia	1,500	54% were cured
Grechko (58)	AP		Trigeminus neuralgia	82	Only the patients with peripheral genesis are responded to the treatment satisfactory
Hon (65)	AP	Xiaguan	Trigeminus neuralgia	25	40% were cured and other 32% markedly improved
Xu (2, p. 80)	AP	Xiaguan	Trigeminus neuralgia	225	33.4% were cured and other 65% improved
Xu (3, p. 41)	AP	Yuyao (Extra 5)	Idiopathic trigeminal neuralgia	1,000	54% were cured, follow-up for 5 yrs. 40% no recurrence
Xu (153)	AP		Primary trigeminal neuralgia	300	46% completely relieved and other 34% markedly improved
Yin (84, p.564)	AP	HoKu (LI 4) Yaoyan (Extra 21)	Trigeminus neuralgia	378	88.1% excellent result
			Intercostal neuralgia	88	90.9% excellent result
Nakagawa (114)	.AP		Occipital neuralgia	43	52% excellent improved
Xia (152)	AP		Supraorbital neuralgia	61	Very encouraging
Yamashiro (155)	EAP#		Ophthalmic neuralgia (left side)	1	Completedly relieved, but not by nerve blockage or ganglion blockage
Wen (84, p.559)	AP		Acute central cervical spinal cord syndrome	12	Pain gradually disappeared, shortened the hospital stay
Huang (71)	AP	Fengchi Danshu (B 19)	Cervical neuralgia	37	46% cured and other 32% improved

Table 8-7. (continued)

Source	Mode	Acupoint	Diagnosis	No. of Patients	Effectiveness %
Zheng (168)	AP	Yanglingquan (G 34)	Ischialgia neuralgia	191	58% cured and other 40% improved
Cheng (33)	AP	Intercostal area	Intercostal neuralgia	56	60% cured after one treatment, another 25% cured at the end of 3rd treatment
Zhou (172)	AP	Neiguan (P 6) Yanglingquan	Intercostal neuralgia	308	90.9% cured after one treatment
Hsu (68)	AP	Dachangshu (B 25) Huantiao (G 30)	Sciatic neuralgia	200	76% were cured
Jiang (77)	AP		Sciatic neuralgia	106	Results were very satisfactory especially in those patients who had the neuralgia less than 1 month old.
Qi (120)	AP	Shenshu (B 23)	Sciatic neuralgia	145	42.5% cured, totally 95.7% effective
Shen (124)	AP	Zusanli (S 36)	Sciatic neuralgia	398	91.6% showed effective
Zhang (162)	Ear AP & Body AP		Sciatic neuralgia	450	51% were cured
Zhou (170)	AP	Dachangshu	Sciatic neuralgia	246	55% were cured and other 42% improved
Zhou (171)	AP	Weizhong (B 40) Yanglingquan	Sciatic neuralgia	37	29.7% were cured and other 56% greatly improved

* AP = Acupuncture
# EAP = Electro-acupuncture

other day. After ten treatments, which constituted a course, came a three to five day rest period, followed by a second course if needed. Patients were grouped according to the severity of neuralgia. The results are summarized in table 8-6.

In follow-up studies they reported that the recurrence rate was 15 percent after the first year, 24 percent after the second year, 29 percent after the third year, and about 50 percent after the sixth year. EAP has been used to treat patients with painful radicular syndrome caused by unilateral lesions of the root S1 resulting from L5-S1 disc pathology. After acupuncture treatment, vessel spasm and venous congestion subsided, and the blood supply was increased. Forty-eight percent of the patients achieved a complete absence of pain, 40 percent had a decrease in pain, and 12 percent had no improvement (142).

In a review article, K. L. Rosenkopf (122) described the effects of acupuncture therapy on trigeminal neuralgia as very promising.

Table 8-7 lists the literature reports on acupuncture therapy of neuralgia.

References

1. Ahonen, E., et al. Acupuncture Electro-Ther. Res. 9:141, 1984.
2. All China Society of Acupuncture and Moxibustion. First National Symposium on Acupunture and Acupuncture Anesthesia. Beijing: 1979.
3. All China Society Acupuncture and Moxibustion. Second National Symposium on Acupuncture and Moxibustion and Acupuncture Anesthesia. Beijing: People Health Publisher, 1984.
4. Andersson, S. A., and E. Holmgren, American Journal Chinese Medicine 3:311, 1975.
5. Arefeva, V. V., et al. Anesteziol Reanimatol 0(3):21, 1986.
6. Ashton, H., et al. J. Psychosom. Res. 28:301, 1984.
7. Arseni, A., et al. Rev. Roun. Med. Neurol. Psychiatr. 26:85, 1988.
8. Au, Y. C., and K. H. Yu. New Journal of Traditional Chinese Medicine 26(2):29, 1993.
9. Baisher, W. Wiener Klinisch. Wochenschr. 185:200, 1993.
10. Batra, Y. K., American Journal of Acupuncture 14:135, 1986, 15:153, 1987.
11. Batra, Y. K., et al. American Journal of Acupuncture 13:69, 1985.
12. Bianchi, M., et al. American Journal of Chinese Medicine 19:101, 1991.
13. Biondi, M. G., and G. Portuesi. Psychother. Psychosom. 61:41, 1994.
14. Biedermann, H. J. Med. Hypothesis 19:397, 1986.
15. Boivie, J., and G. Brattberg. American Journal of Chinese Medicine 15:69, 1987.
16. Bonica, J. J., in Management of Pain. Philadelphia: Lea Febiger, 1990, p. 1850.
17. Cao, L. N. Shanghai Journal of Acupunture and Moxibustion 12(4):157, 1993.
18. Cao, W. H., et al. Journal Chinese Acupuncture and Moxibustion 13(3):17, 1993.
19. Carlsson, J., et al. Cephalalgia 10:131, 1990; 10:123, 1990.
20. Carlsson, C. P., and B. H. Sjoland. B. H. Clin. J. Pain 10:290, 1994.
21. Cha, T. Y. Journal of Chinese Acupuncture and Moxibustion 13(5):28, 1993.
22. Chan, J. C. Acup. Electro-Ther. Res. 13:41, 1988.
23. Chen, A. Acup. Electro-Ther. Res. 17:273, 1992.
24. Chen, B. X. and Y. L. Zhao, Chinese Medical Journal 98:471, 1985.
25. Chen, G. S. American Journal of Acupuncture 18:5, 1990.
26. Chen, J. R., et al. American Journal of Acupuncture 15:321, 1987.
27. Chen, J. R., et al. American Journal of Acupuncture 16:217, 1988.
28. Chen, T. and C. S. Zhou. Shanghai Journal of Acupuncture and Moxibustion 13(1):17, 1994.
29. Chen, W. C. New Journal of Traditional Chinese Medicine (in Chinese) 25 (5):36, 1993.
30. Chen, Z. L., and X. F. J. Zhou. Journal of Traditional Chinese Medicine 4:93, 1984.
31. Cheng, P. E. Journal of Traditional Chinese Medicine (in Chinese) 34(10):589, 1993.
32. Cheng, R. and B. Pomerenz, Chinese J. Pain 2:143, 1987.
33. Cheng, Y. M. Shanghai Journal of Acupuncture and Moxibustion 12(1):18, 1992.
34. Cheung, J. Y. T. American Journal of Chinese Medicine 13:33, 1985.
35. Chin, P. Y., et al. Shanghai Journal of Acupuncture and Moxibustion 13(1):22, 1994.
36. Chiu, L. C., et al. Crano 5:260, 1987.

37. Chu, G. T. New Journal of Traditional Chinese Medicine 25(5):35, 1993.
38. Chu, K., and S. M. Tang. Shanghai Journal of Acupuncture and Moxibustion 10(4):373, 1987.
39. Chu, Y. Z. Journal of Traditional Chinese Medicine, (in Chinese) 34(8):466, 1993.
40. Coan, R. M., et al. American Journal of Chinese Medicine 9:326, 1981.
41. Damyanova, G. M., et al. Probl. Nevrol Psikhiatr. Nevrkhir. 14:47,1986.
42. Delmze, C. and T. L. Vischer. Rheumatologie 45:119,1993.
43. Dowson, D. I. et al. Pain 21:35, 1985.
44. Dung, H. C. American Journal of Acupuncture 14:345, 1986.
45. Eckman, P. American Journal of Acupuncture 18:135, 1990.
46. Ene, E. E. American Journal of Chinese Medicine 11:106, 1983.
47. Facco, E., et al. American Journal of Chinese Medicine 9:243, 1981.
48. Fang, J. G., et al. Journal of Chinese Acupuncture and Moxibustion 14(1):8, 1994.
49. Fischer, M. V., et al. Acupuncture Electro-Therap. Res. 9:11, 1984.
50. Freed, S. Acupuncture Electro-Therap. Res. 12:113, 1987.
51. Fuliosi, D., et al. Riv. Pathol. Clin. 41:237, 1986.
52. Ga, Y. L. Shanghai Journal of Acupuncture and Moxibustion 12(3):113, 1993.
53. Gan, Z. Y., et al. Journal of Traditional Chinese Medicine 6:21, 1986.
54. Garvey, T. A., et al. Spine 14:961, 1989.
55. Giannori, A., and G. Angeloli Gazz. Med. Ital. Arch. Sci. Med. 150:139, 1991.
56. Goulden, E. A. British Medical Journal 1:523, 1921.
57. Grabow, L. Arneimittel Forschung 44:554, 1994.
58. Grechko, V. E., et al. ZH Neuropatol. Psikhiatr. I M S S Korsakova 86:515, 1986.
59. Gu, S. H., et al. Journal Traditional Chinese Medicine 28:213, 1987.
60. Han, X. J. Journal Chinese Acupuncture and Moxibustion 13(4):23, 1993.
61. Hansan, P. E., and J. H. Hansan, Cephalalgia 5:137, 1985.
62. Hardebo, J. E., et al. Headache 79:494, 1989.
63. Hesse, J., et al. Journal of Internal Medicine 235:451, 1994.
64. Hillman, L., et al. Anesth.-Pain-Control-Dent. 1(2):85, 1992.
65. Hon, S. J., and J. Kao. Shanghai Journal of Acupuncture and Moxibustion 13(1):18, 1993.
66. Hsu, J. Y., et al. Journal of Acupuncture and Moxibustion 13(4):28,1993.
67. Hsu, J. Y., et al. Journal of Chinese Acupuncture and Moxibustion 13(4):23, 1993.
68. Hsu, T. Y. Journal of Chinese Acupuncture and Moxibustion 13(5):15, 1993.
69. Hsu, Z., and J. M. Lu, Shanghai Journal of Acupuncture and Moxibustion 12(3):97, 1993.
70. Huang, C. H., Journal of Chinese Acupuncture and Moxibustion 13(2):17, 1993.
71. Huang, P. New Journal of Traditional Chinese Medicine 26(4):32, 1994.
72. Ivanova, L., et al. Probl. Nevrol. Psikhiatr. Nevrokhir. 12:94, 1984.
73. Jackson, C. T., and M. Nordin. Orthopedic Clinic of North America 23:435, 1992.
74. Japer, W. K. American Journal of Acupuncture 17:135, 1989.
75. Jenerick, H. P., ed. NIH Acupuncture Research Conference. DHEW 74-165, 1973.
76. Jewer, G. N. American Journal of Acupuncture 14:147, 1986.
77. Jiang, Y. G., et al. Journal of Traditional Chinese Medicine 4:183, 1984.
78. Johnsson, A., et al. Acta Odontol. Scand. 49:153, 1991.
79. Junhasavasdikal, B., and N. Junkasavasdikal, Siririg Hosp. Gaz. 36:689, 1984.
80. Junnila, S. Y. T. American Journal of Acupuncture 14:351, 1986.
81. Junnila, S. Y. T. Acupunture Electro-Ther. Res. 12:23, 1987.
82. Junnila, S. Y. T. Acupunture Electro-Ther. Res. 11:269, 1986.
83. Junnila, S. Y. T. American Journal of Acupuncture. 11:345, 1983.
84. Kao, F. F., and J. J. Kao, eds. Recent Advances in Acupuncture Research. Institute for Advanced Research in Asian Science and Medicine, Garden City, NY: 1979.
85. Khudaidatov, B. R. Soobschch Akad-Nank Greuz. SSR 122:173, 1986.
86. Kitade, T., et al. Acupunture Electro-Ther. Res. 15:121, 1990.
87. Kitade, T., et al. American Journal of Chinese Medicine 9:243, 1981.
88. Kitade, T., et al. Journal of Osaka Med. Coll. 45:28; 1987. 45: 219, 1986.
89. Kreitler, S., et al. Pain 28:323, 1987.
90. Ku, K. G., et al. Journal of Chinese Acupuncture and Moxibustion 11(5):5, 1991.
91. Kwasuchi, J. et al. Wiad. Lek. 42:1119, 1989.
92. Lehmann, T. R., et al. Spine 8:625, 1983.
93. Lewenberg, A. American Journal of Acupuncture 14:47, 1986.
94. Lewith, G. J., et al. American Journal of Acupuncture 12:21, 1984.
95. Li, C. S. Shanghai Journal of Acupuncture and Moxibustion 10(2):22, 1991.

96. Li, K. C. Shanghai Journal of Acupuncture and Moxibustion 12(3):112, 1993.
97. Li, J. Y. Chinese Medical Journal 96:591, 1983.
98. Liao, S. J., and M. K. Liao. Acupuncture Electro-Ther. Res. 10:41, 1985.
99. Lin, C. I. American Journal of Acupuncture 12:239, 1984.
100. Lin, J. G., and J. S. Han, et al. Int. J. Neurosci. 64:15, 1992.
101. Liu, M. D. Journal of Chinese Acupuncture and Moxibustion 10(2):3, 1990.
102. Liu, M. H., and S. Y. Lin. New Journal of Traditional Chinese Medicine 25(9):33, 1993.
103. Lobzin, V. S., et al. Zh. Neuropatologii Psikhiatrii IM S S Korsakova. 92(3):13, 1992.
104. Loh, L., et al. Journal of Neurol. Nerosurg. Psychiatry 47:333, 1984.
105. Long, D. M. Arch. Surg. 112:884, 1977.
106. Lu, C. M. Shanghai Journal of Acupuncture and Moxibustion 12(1):19, 1993.
107. Luis Gonzalez Roig. J. Rev. Cubana Med. 27:84, 1988.
108. Markdova, A. V., et al. ZH Nevropatol. Psikhiatr. I M S S Korsakova 84:1313, 1984.
109. Martina, R. M. American Journal of Acupuncture 17:131, 1989.
110. Mayer, D. J., et al. Brain Res. 121:368, 1977.
111. Miyamato, T., et al. J. Jpn. Assoc. Phys. Med. Balneol. Chimatol. 50:139,1987.
112. Moret, V. Pain 45:135, 1991.
113. Mueller, D. Z. Klin. Med. (Berl.) 45:653, 1990.
114. Nakagawa, S. and M. Takeda. Jpn. J. Clin. Ophthalmol. 42:1130, 1988.
115. Nissel, H. Acupuncture Electro-Ther. Res. 18(1):1, 1993.
116. Omura, Y. Acupuncture Electro-Ther. Res. 13:153, 1988.
117. Omura, Y. Acupuncture Electro-Ther. Res. 1:157, 1975.
118. Petelin, L. S., et al. ZH. Nevropatol. Psikhiatr. IM SS Korsakova 85:1166, 1986.
119. Petrie, J. P. and B. L. Hazleman, Brit. J. Rheumatol. 25:271, 1986.
120. Qi, L. Y., et al. Journal of Traditional Chinese Medicine 5:179, 1985.
121. Rosenberg, B., et al. American Journal of Acupuncture 15:255, 1987.
122. Rosenkopf, K. L. Cranio 7(4):302, 1989.
123. Seppo, T. and Y. Junnila. American Journal of Acupuncture 11:345, 1983.
124. Shen, P. C. Journal of Chinese Acupuncture and Moxibustion 11(1):11, 1991.
125. Shi, C. J., and S. L. Zhang. Journal of Chinese Acupuncture and Moxibustion 13(4):19, 1993.
126. Shinohara, S., et al. Acupuncture Electro-Ther. Res. 11: 101, 1986.
127. Simmons, M. S., and T. D. Oleson. Anesth.-Prog. 46:14, 1993.
128. Sjoehund, S., et al. Acta Physiol. Scand. 100:382, 1977.
129. Song, C. G. Journal of Chinese Acupuncture and Moxibustion 11(4):1, 1991.
130. Sprott, H., et al. Aktuelle Rheumologie 18:132, 1993.
131. Starobinets, M. K., and L. D. Volkova. ZH. Nevropatol. Psikhiatr. IM. S.S. Kovsakova 85:350, 1985.
132. Steidl, L., et al. Acta Univ. Paladi Olomuc. Fac. Med. 116:373, 1987.
133. Sternfeld, M., et al. American Journal of Chinese Medicine 14:14, 171, 1986.
134. Sternfeld, M., et al. American Journal of Acupuncture 19:117, 1991.
135. Sternfeld, M., and I. Hod. American Journal of Chinese Medicine 16:96, 1986.
136. Strauss, S. American Journal of Acupuncture 9:73, 1981.
137. Takase, K. American Journal of Acupuncture 14:243, 1986.
138. Tavola, T., et al. Pain 48:325, 1992.
139. Thomas, D., et al. Clinical Rheumatol. 11:55, 1992.
140. Thomas, M., and T. Lundeberg. Acta Anesthesiol. Scand. 38:63, 1994.
141. Tsuai, S. K. Journal of Chinese Acupuncture and Moxibustion 11(6):5, 1991.
142. Umeh, B. American Journal of Chinese Medicine 16:67, 1988.
143. Wang, C. Y. Journal of Chinese Acupuncture and Moxbustion 11(1):25, 1991.
144. Wang, H. K. Journal of Chinese Acupuncture and Moxibustion 11 (4):5, 1991.
145. Wang, H. and L. Tianjin. Journal of Traditional Chinese Medicine 11(2):10, 1994.
146. Wang, J. L. Journal of Chinese Acupuncture and Moxibustion 13(2):19, 1993.
147. Wang, L. S., and C. H. Xan. New Journal of Traditional Chinese Medicine 26(4):34, 1994.
148. Wang, M. L., et al. Journal of Chinese Acupuncture and Moxibustion 11(3):15, 1991.
149. Wang, W. Y., et al. Beijing Journal of Traditional Chinese Medicine. February (1):39, 1993.
150. Won, Y. S. Tianjin Journal of Traditional Chinese Medicine 15(4):174, 1994.
151. Wu, C. L. New Journal of Traditional Chinese Medicine 26(2):35, 1994.
152. Xia, S. Z. et al. Journal of Traditional Chinese Medicine 7:116, 1987.
153. Xu, B. R., and S. H. Ge. Journal of Traditional Chinese Medicine (in English) 1:51, 1981.
154. Yamaguchi, S. J. Jpn. Assoc. Phys. Med. Bal. Med. Climatol. 50:207, 1987.
155. Yamashiro, H., et al. Jpn. J. Anesthesiol. 39:1239, 1990.
156. Yang, M. L. Journal Chinese Acupuncture and Moxibustion 11(2):29, 1991.

157. Yang, R. Q. et al. Chinese Medical Journal 98:1, 1985.
158. Yen, S. F. Journal of Chinese Acupuncture and Moxibustion 13(3):23, 1993.
159. Yew, K. C. Beijing Journal of Traditional Chinese Medicine Oct(5):36, 1993.
160. Yoon, S. H., et al. American Journal of Chinese Medicine 14:179, 1986.
161. Zhang, H., et al. Journal of Chinese Acupuncture and Moxibustion 14(1):21, 1994.
162. Zhang, J. G. Journal of Chinese Acupuncture and Moxibustion 10(4):7, 1990.
163. Zhang, J. M., and J. F. Qao. New Journal of Traditional Chinese Medicine 25(7):30, 1993.
164. Zhang, L. F., and L. M. Li. Journal of Traditional Chinese Medicine (in Chinese) 34:602, 1993.
165. Zhang, T. J. Chinese Acupuncture and Moxibustion 14(2):22, 1994.
166. Zhang, W. S., et al. Journal of Chinese Acupuncture and Moxibustion 13(5):17, 1993.
167. Zhang, Y. I., et al. Journal of Chinese Acupuncture and Moxibustion 10(3):11, 1990.
168. Zheng, Y. G. Beijing Journal of Traditional Chinese Medicine Feb(1):48, 1993.
169. Zhong, T. New Journal of Traditional Chinese Medicine 25(6):31, 1993.
170. Zhou, H. H. Journal of Chinese Acupuncture and Moxibustion 11(1):19, 1991.
171. Zhou, J. N. Journal of Chinese Acupuncture and Moxbustion 13(6):36, 1993.
172. Zhou, S. C. Journal of Acupuncture and Moxibustion 13(3):37, 1993.
173. Zwoelfer, W., et al. American Journal of Chinese Medicine 20:325, 1992.

9
Acupuncture Anesthesia in Surgery

In the late 1950s China was isolated from the West and the Soviet Union. There was a great shortage not only of food, but also of medical supplies. The Chinese medical professionals were forced to use their ingenuity and talent to overcome the difficulties created by such shortages. In operation rooms, acupuncture anesthesia was introduced in 1958 to replace a large proportion of the commonly used general anesthetic agents. Up to the year 1986 more than 2 million patients were operated on in China using the method of acupuncture anesthesia. It received surprising recognition from Western scientists and the medical profession during President Nixon's visit to China in 1972.

It has been well defined in textbooks that the stages of anesthesia induced by many general anesthetic agents include the stages of analgesia, delirium, surgical anesthesia and paralysis of the medulla, and death due to apnea and asystole. Acupuncture anesthesia reaches only the stage of analgesia; it does not produce a narcotic effect on the cortex, spinal cord, or medulla and, therefore, does not cause delirium or apnea. The mortality rate is very low, and when deaths occur they are not due to anesthetic paralysis of the medulla, but to other unforeseen complications.

The mechanism of acupuncture anesthesia is similar to that of acupuncture-induced analgesia, which has been discussed in detail in the previous two chapters. A. Masala, et al., (35) reported on ten patients who were operated under auricular acupuncture anesthesia. The plasma concentration of ACTH and ß-endorphin was elevated significantly during acupuncture anesthesia. ACTH increased from 20.31 ±6.21 pg/ml to 70.31 ±13.51, and the ß-endorphin level rose from 5.70 ± 2.29 pmol/l to 23.53 ±9.38 after thirty minutes of anesthesia. In another five patients, pretreatment with an intravenous injection of hydrocortisone completely suppressed the increased ACTH and ß-endorphin in response to the EAP. However, in all fifteen patients, regardless of whether they received hydrocortisone pretreatment, the same stage and planes of anesthesia were achieved and maintained under acupuncture throughout the surgery. Therefore, the researchers postulated that in addition to the release of opioid neuropeptides, acupuncture anesthesia has an effect on other neurological systems, such as the serotoninergic (5HTergic) system.

Acupuncture anesthesia was widely applied in China for almost every type of surgical case. From 1965 to 1986, it was tried in more than two hundred different types of operation, but its use gradually subsided to no more than two dozen types of surgical cases in which it is considered effective and safe. In some of these cases, acupuncture anesthesia has become a standard procedure. At present, acupuncture anesthesia is commonly used in thyroidectomy, neurosurgery, open-heart surgery with extracorporal circulation, and abdominal surgery, including cesarean section and tubal ligation. Acupuncture was performed with electric stimulation, so called EAP, and occasionally it was assisted with a reduced dose of narcoleptic agent, especially in operations lasting an hour or longer. In general, a better success rate was obtained in operations on the head, neck, and chest. According to a report from a Chinese public health official (7, p. 1), in 4,466 cases of brain surgery the success rate reached 76.6 percent, in 9,375 cases of thyroidectomy over 80 percent were successful, in 350 cases of open heart surgery involving repair of septal defects and section of mitral stenosis over 70 percent were successful, and in more than 2,000 cases of laparotomy 80 percent were successfuly.

The most remarkable result was obtained in tubal ligation: in 23,554 cases the success rate was 85.5 percent. The acupuncture technique was simple and risk-free. In appendectomy operations the success rate of acupuncture anesthesia was low (60–70 percent).

Early investigators (31,39) tried the technique on animals first, especially cats and dogs. Laporatomy in cats under acupuncture anesthesia was very successful. The abdomen was opened with perfect analgesia, muscle relaxation, and little hemorrhage. Normal physiological function was restored promptly after operation, and there were no postoperative complications.

Wang (3, p. 204) reported details of 1,293 surgical operations including success rate, according to the type of operation, under acupuncture anesthesia. Surgical procedures included resection of cerebroma, thyroidectomy, tonsillectomy, cesarean section, and tumor resection. A 67 percent excellent result rate and an average 90 percent success rate were observed.

Characteristics

There are four characteristics of acupuncture anesthesia considered to be advantageous over general anesthesia with anesthetic agents. First, the patient remains conscious and awake throughout the operation. Except for reduced or dulled pain sensation, other sensations (vision and hearing) are normal. Few physiological functions are disturbed by acupuncture; for example, blood pressure and cardiac and respiratory functions remain relatively stable. In a survey of fifty cancer patients operated on under acupuncture anesthesia, only one patient (2 percent) had a decrease in blood pressure of greater than 20 mmHg, compared with another fifty cases operated under general anesthesia in which thirty-two patients (64 percent) had a greater than 20 mm Hg drop in blood pressure. Another advantage of acupuncture anesthesia is that the patient can cooperate with the surgeon and report sensation during the operation. This is especially beneficial in surgical removal of cancerous tissue in the nervous systems minimizing damage to surrounding nerve fibers. It is safe, can reduce the operation time, and decreases "guessing" whether a structure can be safely cut. For example, L. D. Gao, et al., (18) reported on surgical removal of pituitary adenomas under acupuncture anesthesia. The patients remained conscious and were able to communicate with the surgeon, thus avoiding any damage of vital structures such as hypothalamus. Also, some unpleasant side effects frequently occurring with general anesthetic agents can be avoided. No acute cerebral tissue expansion caused by anoxia occurs during acupuncture anesthesia. In series of abdominal operations under acupuncture anesthesia, the gastrointestinal tract maintained a normal peristasis tone and the surgeon was able to observe the cavity clearly and finish the operation promptly. The patient recovered quickly after operation; this is an especially beneficial effect in elderly patients. Further, there is no hangover effect with acupuncture anesthesia.

Second, the procedure doesn't produce any intoxication or side effects as often observed with general anesthetic agents. Patients may be hypersensitive to certain drugs, but not to the acupuncture needle. Acupuncture does not potentiate the effects of antihypertensive drugs. Conditions such as shock or major organ dysfunction (heart, liver, kidney) greatly increase the risks of general anesthetic agents, but are less of a problem with acupuncture anesthesia. Respiratory infection is a frequent complication after general anesthesia but is observed much less frequently after acupuncture anesthesia. A team in Shanghai Hospital (3, p. 127; 7, p. 663) reported that the postoperative pneumonia rate was 10.5 percent (35 out of 333 cases) after operations in cancer patients under general anesthesia, but only 2.8 percent (9 out of 311 cases) after operation under acupuncture anesthesia. In the case of open heart surgery with extracorporal circulation, it was reported that 18 percent (11 out of 60 cases) of patients developed pneumonia after general anesthesia, but only 3 percent (5 out of 155 cases) developed pneumonia under acupuncture anesthesia (13,40).

Third, postoperatively patients usually complain less of pain and suffer no nausea or vomiting, as is often seen with general anesthetic agents. Many patients can get up from the operating table without assistance and do not have to spend time in the intensive care unit for recovery. The patients start to eat sooner and quickly gain weight and resume their activities. Acupuncture can also enhance body immunity, which speeds recovery. Studies of patients' blood substantiate the claim that phagocytosis and leucocyte activity are accelerated after acupuncture anesthesia. Another benefit of acupuncture anesthesia relates to narcotics-addicted patients, who respond to acupuncture well, with no need to increase the dosage of narcotic agent during the procedure. Acupuncture anesthesia is thus an especially useful alternative for drug addicts or recovering drug addicts.

Fourth, from an economic standpoint, acupuncture anesthesia does not require special, elaborate equipment and the expenses are minimal. This is an especially important consideration in rural areas of China and other developing countries.

Another advantage of acupuncture anesthesia is its antiemetic effect. Acupuncture not only reduces the vomiting caused by some preanesthetic medications, but also reduces postanesthetic vomiting, which is frequently observed with general anesthetics (6). These effects reduce the risk of postoperative aspiration pneumonia. Dundee and associates (15) reported that acupuncture therapy at the acupoint Neiguan (P 6) is a potent postoperative antiemetic, especially in women undergoing minor gynecological surgery and receiving premedication with opiate analgesics. They also found that acupuncture effectively reduced emetic symptoms in patients undergoing chemotherapy for testicular or ovarian tumor (17).

Recently a Canadian team reported that acupuncture anesthesia for surgical operations can accelerate patient recovery in comparison to general anesthesia (20).

It is also claimed that EAP is effective in promoting healing and preventing bacterial infections after surgical operations (1).

During acupuncture anesthesia procedures on twenty-eight patients, Lou and coworkers (3, p. 245) measured pulse rate, stroke volume, the impedance plethysmogram and blood pressure. Total peripheral resistance decreased 24 percent during acupuncture anesthesia, while stroke volume and heart rate increased 1.2 percent and 4 percent respectively. Cardiac output increased 5.7 percent, but the blood pressure remained at the pre-anesthetic level.

Recently, G. S. Shen (36) reported on a patient with tuberculous pleuritis and chronic bronchial asthma who needed a thoracic operation. Tracheal intubation was difficult to perform, even after administration of an analgesic agent. Finally, acupuncture at Neiguan (P 6) was applied for six minutes—the patient became calm and relaxed; no further hoarseness was heard.

There are some disadvantages in using acupuncture anesthesia. It has been reported that 15 percent of the patient population does not respond to acupuncture. Also, this technique has not yet successfully produced complete muscular relaxation and painlessness, especially for splanchnic pain, nor has it been able to control the reflex response of internal visceral organs. For example, during abdominal operations, pulling the internal organs could cause the patient to feel pain and discomfort. During the opening of the chest, if without the help of a respirator, patient would feel the chest stuffing and an uncomfortable difficulty in breathing. Strict selection of the right acupoint(s) for the corresponding operation, attention to the length of electrical stimulation, and careful psychological preparation of the patient, as most Chinese acupuncturists emphasize, could partially overcome such handicaps. Thoma and his colleagues have devised a special telemetric method to record the cardiovascular activity during the acupuncture anesthesia–induced operation (28, p.485). They reported that the patients were still not completely free from restlessness and showed slight excitation to weariness and drowsiness. They also stated that it is not true the acupuncture has a stabilizing effect on the circulation.

Further, acupuncture anesthesia is not satisfactory for operations on adhesion tissue or operations requiring extensive exploration, particularly those involving the abdomen. Acupuncture anesthesia is contraindicated in pregnant women and in patients suffering with malignant or acute dermatitis, hemophilia, or diseases producing choleiform movement.

Selection of Acupoints

There are two types of acupuncture anesthesia, auricular and body acupuncture anesthesia. In the latter, Chinese surgeons select no more than ten acupoints, usually in the arm and leg, where the meridian converts closely to the terminal of four limbs. For example, HoKu (LI 4), Zusanli (S 36), and Taichong (Liv 3) are used frequently for body acupuncture anesthesia. They claim that these acupoints can reach the five *zhan* (organs) and six *fu* (viscera). They are strong believers in the Zhan-Fu theory and meridian principle, which work as an entity in the human body. The other acupoints often used are: Gongsun (Sp 4), Li Gou (Liv 5), Fenglong (S 40), Neiguan (P 6), and Waiguan (SJ 5).

The surgeons select the acupoint according to syndrome differentiations. For example, HoKu is used for facial operations, dental extractions and sinusotomy, and is chosen as the acupoint of the adjacent segmentation for thyroidectomy. Acupoints Zusanli and Fenglong are used for GI tract surgery; Taichong and Li Gou for cranial surgery; Neiguan for cardiovascular surgery and to "tranquilize the heart," "sedate the mind," and "regulate the Qi."

Preanesthetic Medication

In certain types of surgery—for example, Fallopian tubal ligation—acupuncture anesthesia alone can produce excellent results without the use of any medication. However in many cases, especially in operations lasting more than an hour or when extensive exploration of the internal organ is required, a combination of acupuncture and some medication has often produced satisfactory synergistic effects in inducing maximal pain-free anesthesia and reducing complications due to discomfort and visceral reflex. The combination is also mutually beneficial. Acupuncture can lower the dosage of the drug required in general anesthesia by 50 percent or more. Commonly used supporting medications including central sedative or analgesic agents, such as barbiturates, given orally thirty minutes before the acupuncture anesthesia procedure, haloperidol, meperidine, fentanyl, and atropine given by parenteral administration. Also, the local anesthetics lidocaine and procaine are used for infiltration.

Preoperative Preparation

It is important that the patient be fully informed and educated about the value and characteristics of acupuncture, the methods, and details of the procedure. Such preparation enhances the patient's trust in the surgeon. The patient's physiological functions may be affected by his or her anxiety and degree of cooperation. With good preoperative preparation the patient can be mentally relaxed and able to cooperate during the operation. The patient also should practice slow and deep abdominal breathing before the operation. It helps relieve the feeling of chest stuffiness and dyspnea after the chest is opened and to reduce muscular spasm and nausea and vomiting caused by retraction of the visceral organs, especially during abdominal surgery.

Thyroidectomy

Chinese surgeons highly recommend acupuncture anesthesia as a substitute for general anesthesia in operations on the thyroid gland. This is probably the most successful one among the surgical operations in which acupuncture anesthesia is used, with low risk and less complication. In a survey covering the year from 1975 to 1976, a total of 9,375 thyroidectomies were performed in China (7, p. 684). There were more females than males, and the ages ranged from eight to eighty-two years. The etiologies of the diseases included thyroid tumor, goiter, and hyperthyroidism. Acupuncture anesthesia gave 74.2 percent excellent results and 95.4 percent total success rate of operations. Some used auricular acupuncture (21.7 percent) while other used body acupuncture on the acupoints HoKu (LI 4) and Neiguan (P 6). During the operation, patients' blood pressure remained stable; only 19 percent of the cases had a fluctuation above or below 20 mmHg in their preanesthetic value. Pulse was maintained at 70 ±20 beats/min. Among the 9,375 operations, 402 patients did not require any preanesthetic sedation. The others were given a smaller than usual oral dose of pentobarbital to reduce anxiety and augment the analgesic effect. Fourteen percent of the operations lasted less than one hour and the success rate was 98 percent. Twenty-four percent of the operations lasted one to two hours and 16 percent lasted two to four hours. Only 25 percent required a longer period (over four hours); in these cases the success rate was reduced to 68.7 percent.

Postoperative complications were minimal after acupuncture anesthesia, especially in the case of surgery for hyperthyrodism. For example, in a total of 1,204 cases of Graves' disease that were operated under acupuncture anesthesia, an excellent result rate of 82.6 percent and a total success rate of 95.2 percent were observed. Physiological functions of the patients rapidly returned to the control value after the operation. (Both T3 and T4 were significantly decreased.) The only disadvantage or adverse effect after the operation was the patients' complaining of numbness and lack of strength in their hands, which would last for more than a couple of days, probably due to excessive electrical stimulation at the Hoku point during a long period of operation. When operations were performed under auricular acupuncture, an infection of the ear resulting in atrophy of the helix regions was the major adverse effect. It has been reported that acupuncture anesthesia was very beneficial in operations for Graves' disease. The risk of evoking a cardiovascular crisis was much smaller than in operations under general anesthetics. As shown by H. P. Chen, et al., (10), thyroidectomy under acupuncture anesthesia gave an excellent result in both Graves' disease and Hashimoto's thyroiditis. The results are summarized in Table 9-1. Similar results in eighty-four cases of hyperthyroidism treated with conservative acupuncture therapy (not surgery) were reported by J. S. He, et al. (23).

A team from Beijing Hospital reported a total of 1,038 cases of thyroidectomy under acupuncture anesthesia; a success rate of 93 percent was obtained (7, p. 689). Compared with 101 cases of thyroidectomy under general anesthesia, five patients had postoperative vocal cord paralysis, five had postoperative pneumonia, two had accidental tracheal incision, and one died. The mean postoperative complication rate was 13 percent. But in 220 cases operated on under acupuncture anesthesia only two had postoperative vocal cord paralysis and ten had temporary postoperative hypocalcemia. The results indicated that acupuncture anesthesia for thyroidectomy was superior to the use of general anesthetic agents.

Wan, et al. (4, p.183) reported their 1,240 cases of thyroidectomy. One thousand and twenty-four were operated on under acupuncture anesthesia, 149 under epidural local anesthesia, and 67 under general anesthesia. The incidence of hypotension was 12.8 percent in the acupuncture group, 47.6

Table 9-1. Thyroidectomy under Acupuncture Anesthesia

Type of Disease	No. of Patients		Plasma Concentration T_4 ng/ml	T_3 ng/ml	TSH U./ml
Graves Disease	46	Before	225.28± 10.44	4.38± 0.25	1.86±0.22
		After	126.9 ± 7.81	2.30± 0.18	4.71±0.60
Hashimota thyroiditis	33	Bef.	66.71± 6.62	0.94± 0.51	22.83±24.1
		Aft.	87.5± 32.8	1.48± 0.60	8.9±0.63
Healthy volunteers	38		98.4± 4.42	1.48± 0.07	9.0±0.56

(Data abstracted from Chen et al. (10))

percent in the epidural group, and 79.1 percent in the general anesthetics group. Postoperative complications such as respiratory infection, phrenospasm, and laryngismus were observed in only 4 of 1,042 cases under acupuncture, 6 of 149 under epidural anesthesia, and 4 of 67, including one death under general anesthesia.

The electrophysiological functions of the patients under EAP anesthesia remained very stable during the operative period (38).

A report from the surgical team of Shanghai Hospital showed that in 340 cases of thyroidectomy, using meperidine as preanesthetic medication gave a better result than using other preanesthetic agents. However, acupuncture anesthesia in combination with the narcoleptic agent droperitol could increase the success rate of operations (3, p. 216). H. G. Kho, et al., (29) reported on twenty patients receiving thyroidectomy under acupuncture anesthesia supplemented with a small dose of meperidine (forty-five milligrams subcutaneous). During the surgery there was an increase in the plasma level of catecholamines, growth hormone, cortisol, antidiuretic hormone, and ß-endorphin, but a decrease in immunoglobulin (IgA, IgG, and IgM). There was an increase in lymphocyte count and falls in eosinophils and neutrophils. In the postoperative period, the concentration of norepinephrine and ß-endorphin remained high. J. Wang, et al., (41) operated on fifty patients' thyroid glands under acupuncture anesthesia in combination with a nonnarcotic analgesic, AP-237, and found that AP-237 can potentiate the anesthetic effect of acupuncture anesthesia better than other narcotic analgesics.

The other clinical reports on thyroidectomy under acupuncture anesthesia are summarized in table 9-2.

Z. R. Xue, et al., (43) found that metoclopramide, a drug with antidopaminergic and anticholinesterase actions, can synergize the acupuncture analgesic effect in both animals and humans, especially in patients undergoing thyroidectomy operations

Table 9-2. Surgical Operation of Thyroid Diseases under Acupuncture Anesthesia

Source	Mode	Acupoint	Diagnosis	No. of Patients	Effectiveness %
Chen (4, p.180)	EAP*	HoKu (LI 4) Neiguan (P 6)	Thyroid cyst Thyroid adenoma Nodular thyroid Hyperthyoidism Adenocarcinoma Others	2,283 5,931 2,813 1,538 322 427	Total Effective rate 85.3%; there was no significan change in cellular RNA:DNA ratio during & after operation
			Total	13,314	
Dong (14)	EAP & Ear AP	HoKu Neiguan	Varieties of thyroid diseases	73	71% excellent result
Sichuan Hosp. Team (3,p.141)	AP# Ear AP	HoKu	Varieties of thyroid diseases	9,375	84.5% were cured total success rate 95.4%
Huashan Hosp.Team (3,p.145)	AP Ear AP	HoKu	Thyroidectomy	685	70% success
		Futu (S 32)			92.8% success
		HoKu + Futu			81.6% success
Jiangsi Hosp.Team (3,p,146)	EAP	Taichong (Liv 3)	Thyroidectomy	1,227	98.1% success
Qi (4, p. 180)	EAP	HoKu Neiguan	Thyroidectomy	1,000	57.2% excellent result, 7.7% failed
Sichuan Hosp.Team (3,p.146)	EAP	Hoku + Futu	Thyroidectomy	103	99.1% success
St Thuyen (40)	EAP		Thyroidectomy	90	Successful
Wang (3, p.214)	EAP		Thyroidectomy	278	80% excellent result, used preanesthetic agent would give a better effect.
Wuhan Hosp.Team (3,p.143)	EAP	HoKu Futu	Thyroidectomy	268	99% success
Yan (4, p.180)	EAP	HoKu Neiguan	Thyroidectomy	822	47% excellent result, total success rate 81.9%

Table 9-2. (continued)

Source	Mode	Acupoint	Diagnosis	No. of Patient	Effectiveness %
Zhang (3, p.142)	EAP	HoKu	Thyroidectomy	220	Very successful, no postop. pneumonia
	Gen. Anesthesia			110	5 patients had postop. pneumonia
Chen (10)	AP + Moxib.@		Hyperthyroidism	46	Excellent result
			Hashimoto thyroiditis	33	Excellent
Ge (19)	EAP	Futu Ermen (SJ 21)	Exophthalmic hyperthyroidism		90% obtained excellent result
He (4,p.27) &(23)	EAP	Neiguan Zusanli (S 36)	Hyperthyroidism	51	33% excellent and other 23% improved
Li (4, p.24)	EAP	Neiguan Zusanli	Hyperthyroidism	112	64.3% cured and other 27% improved
Yin (45)	AP	Ah-shi	Hyperthyroidism	50	80% excellent and other 6% improved
Akitomo (2)	EAP (1 Hz)		Nodular thyroid *	14	excellent result, there was no different betwee these two groups
	Narcoleptic			8	
Guo (21)	EAP		Benign nodular thyroid	65	95.4% success
Quo (4, p.26)	EAP	Neiguan	Benign nodular thyroid	48	38% cured and other 23% improved
Starr (38)	EAP		Thyroid cancer	5	Success
Zhang (4, p.181)	AP and Ear AP	HoKu	Thyroid carcinoma	129	47.6% successful and 78.1% success when combined with preanesth agent.
Song (37)	AP		Thyroid adenoma	46	97.8% cured

*EAP = Electro-acupuncture
#AP = Body acupuncture
@Moxib. = Moxibustion

Neurosurgical Operation

Successful operation on the brain under acupuncture anesthesia was first reported in 1965 by a team of Chinese surgeons. The Shanghai Hua-shan Hospital has compiled data on 7,469 neurosurgical cases from 1965 to 1978, in which 4,466 were operated on under acupuncture anesthesia. Eighteen hundred and sixty-five cases involved surgery on the anterior fossa, in which the success rate was 78 percent; in 1,594 cases of tempor-parieto-occipital surgery, the success rate was 73.5 percent; in 1,007 cases of posterior fossa surgery, the success rate was 78.9 percent. There was no mortality and very few postoperative complications (3, p. 127, and 7, p. 663). Among 311 cases of neurenoma operated on under acupuncture anesthesia, only 9 patients had postoperative pneumonia. However, in another 333 cases operated on under general anesthetic agents, 35 patients developed pneumonia. The blood pressure of the acupuncture group usually remained stable during the operation and there was no change in respiratory rate. In the group operated on under general anesthetic agents, a higher percentage developed hypotension or slow respiration.

The data were further compiled. During the years 1965 to 1978, in twenty-four neurosurgical departments in China, there were a total of 10,635 cases of neurosurgical operations performed under acupuncture anesthesia and the success rate reached 95 percent (9). Table 9-3 summarizes the effect of acupuncture anesthesia on the cortical-evoked potential amplitude, pain threshold, and endorphin concentrations.

Sum (4, p.165) of Beijing described a fourteen-year-old old girl with a pituitary adenoma who had symptoms of progressive acromegaly for five years. She was operated on under acupuncture anesthesia at the acupoints Jinmen (B 63) and Taichong (Liv 3). No preanesthetic medication and no blood transfusions were required. The patient remained conscious and had no complaints during the operation. The postoperative recovery was excellent. She resumed her activity quickly after the operation.

In twelve craniotomy procedures performed under acupuncture anesthesia, Chen, et al., (4, p.170) measured intracranial pressure of their patients before and after section of the dura mater. It was 34±13 torr predural–opening and 24±8 torr post–dural opening. The mean arterial pressure remained stable during the operation.

Table 9-4 summarizes the other clinical reports on neurosurgical operations under acupuncture anesthesia.

Table 9-3. Effect of Acupuncture or Amygdala Stimulation on Cortical Potential and Endorphin Concentration

Mode of Treatment		Corticoal Evoked Potential (mV)	Pain Threshold		Endorphins Conc.	
			mA	% Change	ng/ml	% Change
Control (Sham)	Before	29.3				
	After	28.1				
Acupuncture	Before	27.2	0.53		0.65	
	After	15.7	1.13	+113	5.96	+815
Amygdala	Before		1.63		0.43	
stimulation	After		1.90	+17	0.56	+30

Table 9-4. Neurosurgical Operation under Acupuncture Anesthesia

Source	Mode	Acupoint	Diagnosis	No. of Patients	Effectiveness %
Chen (8)	EAP*	HoKu (LI 4) Futu (LI 18)	Anterior cranial fossa	242	Excellent result, safe and causes very little disturbance of physiol. functions.
Guo (18)	EAP	Yuyao (Extra 5) Shangguan (G 3)	Pituitary adenoma	43	93% excellent result
Jueda Hosp.Team (3,p.130)	EAP	Futu	Posterior cranial fossa	417	77.2% excellent
Lin (4, p.168)	EAP		Craniotomy	80	45% good
Luo (4, p.166)	EAP	Shenman (H 7)	Acoustic neuroma	117	54% excellent, other 34% good, one died.
Ma (4, p.223)	EAP	Hoku, Futu, Waiguan (SJ 5)	Anterior root of cervical spine	600	91.5% success
Xiao (4, p. 167)	EAP		Craniotomy	285	77.3% excellent
Wang (3, p.214)	EAP		Resection of cerebroma	147	72% excellent
Yang (44)	EAP		Multilateral discectomy	214	74% good result, follow-up for 4 yrs. all maintained in good health

* EAP = Electro-acupuncture

Open Heart and Open Chest Surgery

According to a report from the Shanghai Hospital (3, p.17 and 7, p.705), covering the period 1972–78, a total of 230 cases of open heart surgery were performed under acupuncture anesthesia. The patients ranged in age from ten to forty-eight years. The surgery included repair of ventricle septal defects, pulmonary valvotomy, mitral commissurotomy, aortic sinusal aneurysm section, and artificial valve replacement. The anesthetic results were reported as 18.3 percent excellent, 50.9 percent good, 22.7 percent fair, and 8.2 percent poor. There were eleven mortalities, but none was related to acupuncture anesthesia. Patients remained conscious during the whole operation, which included the procedure of extracorporal circulation. EKG, EEG, arterial pressure, and arterial pO2 were closely monitored. The duration of extracorporal circulation averaged from five to forty minutes, but in seventy-two cases it lasted over 60 to 132 minutes. The majority of the cases involved no tracheal intubation. In some cases, when the pO_2 was low, oxygenation was supplied with a mouth mask. The postoperative complications were few. Five among 155 cases operated on under acupuncture had respiratory complications. Most of the patients did not have a cough or increased sputum production after operation. In comparison with fourteen cases of open heart operation under general anesthesia, nine patients suffered pulmonary infections, pleuritis, and pneumonia.

But in another hospital's report (7, p.711) the surgeons claimed that tracheal intubation was beneficial in maintaining a high arterial pO2. They reported that the lung collapse occurred often in nonintubation cases when the chest was opened (89.2 percent), but in patients operated on with tracheal intubation, lungs remained expanded in 77.5 percent. G. Litarczek, et al., (33) performed open heart surgery involving valve prosthesis and correction of congenital defects under EAP anesthesia. Totally 110 cases were done with successful results. In eleven patients cardiac output remained normal during the critical moments of operation. This was credited to the lack of toxic effects of general anesthetics on the myocardium and blood vessels.

A team from the Beijing Tuberculous Institute reported on 1,048 cases of lung resection (7, p. 695). Eight hundred and fifty-six patients had pulmonary tuberculosis, 107 had lung abscesses, and 85 had lung cancer. The operations performed under acupuncture anesthesia included lobectomy (78.2 percent), partial lung resection (17 percent) and total lung resection (4.8 percent). Totally, a success rate of 97.2 percent was observed and only 2.4 percent of the patients had a drop in their blood pressure during the operation, as compared with 14 percent in patients receiving general anesthetic agents.

A report on 473 patients undergoing lung resection with acupuncture anesthesia technique showed that there is a direct correlation between skin electrical voltage fluctuations and success of the operation (7, p. 786). The authors measured skin electrical voltage with a special instrument and compared the ratio of the electrical voltage between the needling period and the rest period. It was found that 74 percent of the patients who had an excellent operative result showed a magnitude of skin voltage fluctuation of less than 0.9 volt. Only 5 percent had a fluctuation of greater than two volts, and this occurred in patients having a less satisfactory operative result. The success of the operation under acupuncture can also be judged by fluctations in pulse and respiratory rate. Generally, the pulse was stable and rarely fluctuated by more than 20 percent after the needle was placed on the acupoint(s). Also, the better result was related to the stability of the respiratory rate. In some cases, in which the respiratory rate increased by over 25 per minute after starting acupuncture, an unsatifactory operative result can be predicted. Therefore, the surgeon claimed that the continuous measurement of skin electrical voltage and pulse and respiratory rate can be used as a prognostic judgement of the operative outcome.

Table 9-5 lists the clinical reports on open heart and open chest surgery under acupuncture anesthesia.

Table 9-5. Open Heart and Open Chest Surgery under Acupuncture Anesthesia

Source	Mode	Acupoint	Diagnosis	No. of Patients	Effectiveness %
Hunan Med. College (3,p.151)	EAP*	Hoku (LI 4)	Mitral commissurectomy	215	54% excellent result, other 33% good, another 9% moderately good.
Feng (3, p.154)	EAP	Hoku	Mitral commissurectomy	66	95.5% successful
Shanghai Med. Coll. (3,p.152)	EAP		Mitral commissurectomy (severe)	100	70% excellent, no mortality
Shanghai Thoracic Hos. (7,p.711)	EAP	Hoku Neiguan (P 6)	Mitral commissurectomy		
			non-severe	123	71.5% excellent
			severe:	100	70% excellent result
Shao (4, p.187)	EAP	Hoku Neiguan	Mitral commissurectomy	600	96.1% successful, 7 cases suffered cerebral embolism and one died.
Zhang (3, p.153)	EAP	Hoku Neiguan	Mitral commissurectomy	95	96% excellent
Hollinger (28,p.427)	AP# Ear AP	Hoku Shenmen (H 7)	Coronary By-pass	87	92.1% satisfied
Hsu (25)	EAP (2 Hz) and Lidocaine	Neiguan	Intracardiac & extracorporal circulation	44	91% success
Zhen (3 p.148)	AP and Lidocaine	Hoku	Repair ventri. septal defect	27	26 of them successful (96%)
Zeng (3, p.149)	AP and preanesth. medication	HoKu Neiguan	Congenital heart defect	48	47 of them successful (98%)
Hunan 2nd. Hosp. (3,p.155)	EAP	Hoku	Pericardectomy	128	84% excellent result
Feng (3, p.164)	EAP	Futu (S 32) Jiexi (S 41)	Intrathoracic operation	268	84.7% excellent, the longest operating time was 6 hrs. & 25 min.

Table 9-5. (continued)

Source	Mode	Acupoint	Diagnosis	No. of Patient	Effectiveness %
Beijing Hosp. (3,p.158)	EAP	Sanyangluo (SJ 8)	Pulmonectomy	478	80% excellent
Shanghai Hosp. (3,p.156)	EAP	Hoku	Lobectomy	1,067	13.1% excellent,other 69.3% good, 3.9% failed
Beijing Med. Coll. (3,p.9) &(2,p.695)	EAP	Sanyangluo	Lobectomy	1,048	78.1% excellent result; total effective rate 97.2%
Li (3, p. 165)	EAP		Lobectomy	195	excellent
Xian Hosp. (3,p.188)	EAP		Lobectomy	800	80% success, no side effect and no accident
Wang (3, p.214)	EAP		Lung & eso-phagus surgery	45	58% excellent and other 40% good

*EAP = Electro-acupuncture
#AP =Body acupuncture

Gastrointestinal Surgery

Subtotal and total gastrectomies have been performed under acupuncture anesthesia since 1965. But the incomplete muscle relaxation and reflex responses of the internal organs during retraction of the GI tract have created many unpleasant difficulties for the patients and surgeons. The most common symptoms observed include pain, nausea and vomiting, palpitations, coolness of the extremities, and sweating. According to a report on 100 cases of gastrectomy under acupuncture anesthesia (7, p. 718), the blood pressure fluctuated by more than 20 mmHg and a slow heart rate was observed. This was mirrored by a low success rate of the operation. The surgeons considered it is important to maintain a good sympathetic control and to select the correct acupoint in order to get a successful operation.

The success of gastrectomy under acupuncture anesthesia was first demonstrated in animal experimentation. S. Zhou, et al., (46) tried this technique on ninety-three dogs and reported a 54 percent excellent result rate, 29 percent good rate, and 17 percent poor rate. In the fifty animals that responded excellently to acupuncture anesthesia, arterial and venous blood pressure remained stable throughout the operation. The plasma DA-ß-hydroxylase concentration fell significantly, but the content of NE and 5HT in the resected stomach was very high.

A team from Shanghai Traditional Chinese Hospital reported their results on gastrectomy in 1,100 patients who suffered from gastric or duodenal ulcer or carcinoma (7, p .729). They claimed a success rate of 95.9 percent for acupuncture anesthesia. Zusanli was the acupoint chosen for acupuncture and gave a good analgesic effect. Patients with intestinal peristalsis recovered quickly after the operation.

As showed by Chen, et al., (7, p. 736), pulling the greater curvature of the stomach during gastrectomy produces a greater increase in pulse rate; in many cases the pulse rate was double the preoperative value. Nausea and vomiting were observed in around 20 percent and 11 percent, respectively, of the acupuncture group, but still lower than rates observed in operations in the epidural anesthesia group (94 percent and 70 percent, respectively). It is surprising the authors found that gastrectomy under auricular acupuncture procedure did not produce such unpleasant responses due to retraction of the stomach and only one in thirty eight cases experienced vomiting (2.6 percent).

V. F. Markelova, et al., (34) found that during the surgical operation on biliary tract under EAP anesthesia the sympathetic activity of the patients remained quite stable. There was no change in urinary catecholamines or the blood nonesterified fatty acid concentration.

Peng and Zhu (4, p. 199) practiced subtotal gastrectomy on fifty-four dogs under acupuncture anesthesia and obtained a 44.4 percent excellent result rate. The animals had a high 5HT plasma level. Sun, et al., (4., p. 208) performed splenectomy in twenty-five dogs under acupuncture anesthesia at the acupoints Neiguan and Erman. They were totally successful, without a single failure.

The clinical reports on gastrectomy under acupuncture anesthesia are summarized in table 9-6.

Other Surgical Operations

Acupuncture anesthesia has been used very successfully in gastroscopic and colonoscopic procedure and appenectomy. Results are presented in table 9-7.

Recently H. G. Kho, et al., divided their patients for abdominal operation into three groups, one under acupuncture and TENS anesthesia, another under fentanyl anesthesia, and the last under a combination. They found that acupuncture anesthesia leads to an increase of ß-endorphin without change of the hemodynamics of the patients. The acupuncture group was doing as well as the other two groups, and acupuncture produced no adverse effect on the cardiovascular system during laryngoscopy and intubation (30).

In breast cancer operations Li of Beijing reported fifty-seven cases under acupuncture anesthesia (3, p. 163). HoKu was chosen as the acupoint, and pentobarbital and meperidine were used as preanesthetic medication. Extended radical mastectomy was done on two cases, with a poor result. In forty-five cases of conventional radical mastectomy eight of them (18 percent) showed an excellent result, twenty-two (49 percent) were good, thirteen (29 percent) were poor, and two failed. Ten cases were operated on by modified radical or simple mastectomy. Two of them had good results, six poor, and two failed.

Table 9-8 summarizes the miscellaneous surgical cases operated on under acupuncture anesthesia.

Table 9-9 summarizes the oral-facial surgery under acupuncture anesthesia.

Table 9-6. Abdominal Surgery under Acupuncture Anesthesia

Source	Mode	Acupoint	Diagnosis	No. of Patients	Effectiveness %
Beijing Hosp. Team (7,p.743)	EAP*	Zusanli (S 36)	Gastrectomy	51	65.2% excellent
Nanjing Hosp. Team (3,p.170)	EAP		Subtotal gastrectomy	1,434	95.1% success
Cheng (3, p.171)	EAP		Subtotal gastrectomy	142	31% excellent, and other 57% good, 12% failed
Liaoning Hosp.Team (3,p.171)	EAP	Zusanli	Subtotal gastrectomy	148	87.2% success
Sichuan Hosp. Team (3,p.116)	EAP	Zusanli	Subtotal gastrectomy	100	21% excellent, other 77% good, 2% failed
Wang (3, p.214)	EAP		Subtotal gastrectomy	96	63% excellent, total 84% success
Wang (4, p.195)	EAP	Zusanli	Subtotal gastrectomy	67	very successful
Zhang (3, p.167)	EAP		Subtotal gastrectomy	1,100	16.7% excellent
Zhang (7, p.729)	EAP	Zusanli	Peptic Ulcer	1,017	61.5% excellent total 95.9% success
			Stomach cancer	83	
			Total	1,100	
Donchenko (13)	EAP		Abdominal lapartomy	200	Result very good, with little postoperative complication.

* EAP = Electro-acupuncture

Table 9-7. Other Abdominal Surgery and Diagnosis under Acupunture Anesthesia.

Source	Mode	Acupoint	Diagnosis	No. of Patients	Effectiveness %
Fan (16)	EAP*	Zusanli (S 36)	Appendectomy	179	62.4% excellent
Cheng (11)	AP#	Zusanli Hoku (LI 4)	Gastroscopy	200	98.5% success
	Lidocaine			65	Satisfied but with some side effect
Wang (41)	Ear AP		Gastroscopy	150	94% success, 1.3% failed
	Local anesthesia			150	23.3% success
Li (32)	AP	Zusanli Hoku	Colonoscopy	36	Pain was significantly reduced
Jwakoshi (27)	AP		Colonoscopy	43	very successful, less discomfort than the group with medication

* EAP= Electro-acupuncture
\# AP = Body acupuncture

Table 9-8. Miscellaneous Surgeries under Acupuncture Anesthesia

Source	Mode	Acupoint	Diagnosis	No. of Patients	Effectiveness %
Li (3, p. 163)	EAP*	HoKu (LI 4)	Conventional radical mastectomy	45	8 excellent; 22 good result; 13 poor; 2 fail
			Simple mastectomy	10	2 good result; 6 poor; 2 failed
			Fxtensive radical mastectomy	2	poor
			Total	57	
Wang (3, p.214)	EAP	Zusanli (S 36) Gongsun (Sp 4)	Resection of tumor tissue	55	42% excellent; totally 80% effective
			Tonsillectomy	22	91% excellent
			Meniscectomy	43	47% excellent; total 81% effective
Heilungiang Hosp. Team (3,p.202)	EAP		Surgery of extremities	486	82.9% effective
Lei (3, p.201)	EAP		Surgery of upper extremities	72	63.9% excellent; total 93.6% success
Xu (4, p. 224)	EAP	Tianding (LI 17) Jiquan (H 1) of affected side	Orthopedic surgery of extremities	90	78.9% effective
Wang (3, p. 424)	EAP		Handamputation	2	Successful, no complication
Wuhan Hosp. Team (3,p 200)	EAP		Surgery of extremities	455	74.3% excellent, total 96.9% effective
Zhang (3, p.198) and (5,p.763)	EAP	Ciliao (B 32)	Prostatomy	150	70% effective with 10% suffered of postop. complication
	Epidural anest.			150	very high postop. complication
Zhang (4, p.227)	EAP	Zusanli Futu (LI 18)	Battle wounds	50	Result was better than used local anesthesia

Table 9-8. (continued)

Source	Mode	Acupoint	Diagnosis	No. of Patients	Effectiveness %
Beijing Hosp. Team (7,p.767)	EAP & Ear AP	Hoku (LI 4) Neiguan (P 6)	Surgery of cervical vertebrae	255	92.7% effective
Cao (5)	AP# combined with other analgesia		Carotid artery resection for head and neck tumor	21	very successful, with low complication, safe
Kao (28 p. 425)	AP	Zusanli Tienshu(S 25)	Herniorrhaphy	2	Completely successful
Koo (7, p.775)	EAP	Yinmen (B 37)	Meniscus resection	385	62.2% excellent; other 30.7% good result
Wang (42)	AP and Cryosurgery		Tongue carcinoma	80	77 patients were cured (96.2%), follow-up for 7 yrs. no recurrence

* EAP = Electro-acupuncture
# AP = Body Acupuncture

Table 9-9. Oral-Facial Surgery under Acupuncture Anesthesia

Source	Mode	Acupoint	Diagnosis	No. of Patient	Effectiveness %
Qiu (3, p. 135) and (7,p.678)	EAP*	Hoku (LI 4) Neiguan (P 6) Taichong (Liv 3)	Remove cysts and tumors; repair lip; resection of enlarged checkbone	1,802	90% success; the operating time lasted from 1-4 hrs., no different to the result.
Xu (7, p. 674)	EAP	Hoku Sibai (S 2)	Sinus maxillaris surgery	1,965	57% excellent, total 97.3% effective

* EAP = Electro-acupuncture

References

1. Abulapie, A. J. A. Veterinar. 16:27, 1985.
2. Akitomo, M., et al. Jpn. J. Anesthesiol 34:156, 1985.
3. All China Society of Acupuncture and Moxibustion. First National Symposium on Acupuncture and Acupuncture Anesthesia. Beijing: 1979.
4. All China Society of Acupuncture and Moxibustion. Second National Symposium on Acupuncture and Moxibustion and Acupuncture Anesthesia. Beijing: 1984.
5. Cao, Z. Z., et al. Chin. Journal of Clinical Oncology 20:262,1993.
6. Catteo, A. D., et al. Acta Anesthesiol. Ital. 38:683, 1988.
7. Chang, H. T., et al., eds. Research of Acupuncture and Moxibustion and Acupuncture Anesthesia. Beijing: Science Publisher, 1986.
8. Chen, G. B., et al. Journal of Traditional Chinese Medicine 4:189, 1984.
9. Chen, G. B., et al. American Journal of Chinese Medicine 14:86-95, 1986.
10. Chen, H. P., et al. Journal of Chinese Acupuncture and Moxibustion 11(6):33, 1991.
11. Cheng, T., et al. Journal of Chinese Acupuncture and Moxibustion 11 (5):27, 1991.
12. Department of Acupuncture Anesthesiology, Beijin Med. Univ. Chin. Medical Journal. 93: 287, 1980.
13. Donchenko, V. S., et al. Anesteziol. Reanimatol. 0(1):25, 1989.
14. Dong, P. J. Chinese Acupuncture and Moxibustion 10(6):22, 1990.
15. Dundee, J. W., et al. British Medical Journal 293(6547): 583, 1988.
16. Fan, Y. K., and L. C. Zhang. Chinese Medical Journal 96:491, 1983.
17. Fitzpatrick, K. T. J., et al. Irish J. Med. Sci. 157:29, 1988.
18. Gao, L. D., et al. Chinese Medical Journal 96:469, 1983.
19. Ge, T. Y., et al. Journal of Traditional Chinese Medicine 8:85, 1988.
20. Gemina, H., et al. Canad. J. Anesthesiol. 40:1224, 1993.
21. Guo, X. Z., et al. Journal of Traditional Chinese Medicine 4:261, 1984.
22. Hagege, J. C. Ann. Chir. Plast. Esthelique 33:277, 1988.
23. He, J. S., et al. Journal of Traditional Chinese Medicine 8:79, 1988.
24. He, J.S., et al. Journal of Chinese Acupuncture and Moxibustion 10(6):19, 1990.
25. Hsu, S. Y., et al. Journal of Chinese Acupuncture and Moxibustion 11 (4):24, 1991.
26. Huang, H. N., Chinese Medical Journal 98:417, 1985.
27. Jwakoski, K., et al. Gastroenterol. Endosci. 26:224, 1984.
28. Kao, F. F., and J. J. Kao, eds. Recent Advances in Acupuncture Research. Garden City, NY: Institute for Advanced Research in Asian Science and Medicine, 1979.
29. Kho, H. G., et al. Acta Anesthesiol. Scand. 34:563, 1990.
30. Kho, H. G., et al. Europ. J. Anesthes. 10(3):193, 1993.
31. Kumac, R., et al. Indian J. Vet. Surg. 6:124, 1985.
32. Li, C. K., et al. Deutsch Med. Wochenschr. 116:367, 1991.
33. Litarczek G., et al. Rev. Chir. Oncol. Radiol. ORL Oftalmol. Stomatol. Ser. Chir. 37:63, 1988.
34. Markelova, V. F., et al. Anesteziol. Reanimatol. 0:36, 1985.
35. Masala, A., et al. Acta Endocrin. 103:469, 1983.
36. Shen, G. S. Journal of Clinical Anesthes. (in Chinese) 9(2):80, 1993.
37. Song, L. C., et al. Europ. J. Surg. Suppl. 574:79–81, 1994.
38. Starr, A., et al. Arch. Neurol. 46:1010, 1989.
39. Stiel, J. American Journal of Acupuncture 15:155, 1987.
40. St. Thuyen, D., et al. Acupuncture Electro-Ther. Res. 13:25, 1988.
41. Wang, J., et al. Journal of Chinese Acupuncture and Moxibustion 11(2):35, 1991.
42. Wang, J. Y., et al. Shanghai Journal of Acupuncture and Moxibustion 12(1):8, 1993.
43. Xu, Z. B., et al. Acupuncture Electro-Ther. Res. 8:283, 1983.
44. Yang, K. Q., et al. Zhong Hua Guke Zazhi (in Chinese) 5:130, 1985.
45. Yin, H. H., and K. C. Tam, in Kao, FF, Kao ed. Recent Advances in Acupuncture Research, Garden City, NY: Institute for Advanced Research in Asian Science and Medicine, 1979, p. 564.
46. Zhou, S., et al. Journal of Traditional Chinese Medicine 3:251, 1983.

10

Acupuncture and Acupuncture Anesthesia in Gynecology and Obstetrics

Since the technique of acupuncture anesthesia has become popular in many surgical operations in Chinese hospitals and clinics after 1958, it has also been recognized as being beneficial in the treatment of women's diseases. Actually, Chinese acupuncturists have used this technique for thousands of years to induce labor and to relieve pain in childbirth, especially in the rural areas where Western physicians were not available. At the present, acupuncture is also in widespread use in correction of fetal abnormal position, in cesarean section, in Fallopian tubal ligation, and in hysterectomy. For example, data obtained from Chinese hospitals and clinics during the years 1978–83 showed that 2,069 cases of fetal abnormal position in the twenty-ninth to fortieth gestation week were treated with moxibustion at the acupoint Zhiyin (B 67). Eighty-six percent of the patients were corrected after one to four treatments. The rest received continued treatment an additional five to ten times, and the effectiveness rate reached 90 percent (6, p. 2).

In another report from Jiangxi Hospital, among 2,041 cases of abnormal fetal position there were 1,869 cases (90.3 percent) categorized as breech presentation and 28 cases of acromion presentation; all were corrected after acupuncture therapy. The rest of the patients failed to be corrected because either the fetus head was fixed under the costal margin or the abdomen muscle of the mother was in a tense condition (2, p.6).

Cesarean Section

Acupuncture anesthesia was found to be very successful in cesarean section. According to a recent report from the Beijing Woman's Hospital (4 and 6, p. 746) 1,000 cases of cesarean section were performed during the years 1966–78. Either these patients either had a narrow pelvis, the fetus was in an abnormal position with failed attempts at correction by other methods, or their previous pregnancy had ended in a cesarean section. The success rate was remarkable, reaching 98.4 percent. The reasons for such a high efficiency rate are the stability of blood pressure and heart rate during the operation and the delivery of the baby and the minimal loss of blood. The time from the induction of anesthesia to the end of the operation is also important. Generally a shorter time, about thirty minutes, was required to finish the operation and gave an excellent result. When the operation time was over ninety minutes, a success rate of 53 percent was obtained. The acupoints Neiguan (P 6), Zusanli (S 36), Taichong (Liv 3), and Sanyinjiao (Sp 6) were chosen in their report. They also described that sixty-four patients with toxic eclampsia were controlled under medication and then operated on with acupuncture anesthesia. Ninety-eight percent were successful, 68.8 percent of results were considered to be excellent. Blood pressure was closely monitored. There was greater fluctuation, especially in systolic pressure, than observed in noneclampsia cases. The average blood loss of all patients under acupuncture anesthesia was 268±22 ml. Only one of sixty-four patients went into shock, and five babies were born in an asphyxic stage.

In the same report the results of cesarean section operation under acupuncture anesthesia were compared with those under epidural anesthesia, which included 237 cases during 1966. There was more blood loss in the epidural anesthesia group, averaging 390 ±37.2 ml, as well as more postlabor pain and a higher incidence of postoperative complications.

Table 10-1 lists the clinical trials of acupuncture anesthesia in cesarean section and correction of fetal abnormal position.

Fallopian Tubal Ligation

Another excellent record of acupuncture anesthesia is in the operation of Fallopian tubal ligation. A survey of clinical data from all Chinese hospitals and clinics showed that from 1975 to 1977 there were 23,554 cases of such operations under acupuncture anesthesia. The success rate was 97.9 percent, and 85.8 percent were considered to be excellent. Auricular, body acupuncture or even acupuncture on the lip was used. For body acupuncture commonly the acupoints Sanyinjiao (Sp 6) and Renzhong (Du 26) were selected. The report indicated that body acupuncture gave a better result than the other two methods (6, p.759). In 6,268 cases operated on under body acupuncture anesthesia technique, 65–80 percent of the patients exhibited calmness during the operation, no pain and no complaints, and fewer than 1 percent of the patients had a feeling of terrific pain during exploration of the internal organs. The report also showed that acupuncture in combination with the preanesthetic medication meperidine (50 mgs) gave a higher effectiveness rate (93.3 percent) as compared to the rate (84.6 percent) in a group without medication.

Hysterectomy

The success of acupuncture anesthesia in the hysterectomy operation is still debated among some gynecologists. For example, P. A. Christensen, et al., (8) compared the results of hysterectomy under EAP anesthesia and general anesthesia. They found there was no difference in terms of postoperative pain among these patients.

But in their studies of hysterectomy under acupuncture anesthesia, Hsu, et al., from the Shanghai International Peace Maturity Clinic (6, p. 754), reported 674 cases and an 83.1 percent success rate. Three acupoints on the *du* meridian channel were chosen, including Yaoshu (Du 2), Jizhong (Du 6) and Ming Men (Du 4). The technique was quite comparable with spinal local anesthesia. The acupuncture needle was held directly on the intervertebral space and penetrated into the outside of the dura. The position of the needle could be verified by X-ray examination. The needle was then connected with an electrical stimulator and stimulation was applied. The intensity of the current was 10–15 mAmp, which is safe and would not cause any influence or damage to the spinal nerve fibers.

Li and Li (32) applied electrical acupuncture anesthesia to ninety-seven patients who had a rupture resulting from an ectopic pregnancy. The acupoints Renzhong (Du 26) and Chengjiang (Ren 24) were chosen. An 87 percent excellent result rate was obtained. Ten cases failed.

Table 10-2 summarizes the clinical reports on the use of acupuncture anesthesia in Fallopian tubal ligation and other gynecological operations.

Table 10-1. Gynecological Surgery under Acupuncture Anesthesia

Source	Mode	Acupoint	Diagnosis	No. of Patients	Effectiveness %
Beijing Hosp. Team (4) (6, p. 746)	EAP *	Sanyinjiao (Sp 6) Zusanli (S 36)	Cesarean section	1,000	98.2% effective
Beijing Gyn. & Obs. Clinic (3,p.212)	AP**	Sanyinjiao	Cesarean section	174	Very successful
Beijing Clinic (2,p.189)	EAP	Sanyinjiao	Cesarean section	458	79.1% effective
Jiang (2, p. 186)	EAP		Cesarean section	193	82.9% excellent result; total effective rate 95.8%
Lin (3, p. 214)	AP	Sanyinjiao	Cesarean section	128	Successful, 7 newborns had a low neurobehavior sign;
	Gen. Anesth.#			125	25 newborns had a low neurobehavior sign;
	Epidur. anesth.@			129	6 newborns had a low neurobehavior sign.
Wang (2, p. 214)	EAP		Cesarean section	612	64% excellent result; totally 92% success
Zhang (2, p. 188)	EAP	Sanyinjiao	Cesarean section	421	83% excellent result; 10 stillborn
Zongqing Hosp. Team (2,p.188)	EAP	Sanyinjiao	Cesarean section	85	87.1% excellent result; total effective rate 95.3%
Jiangxi Hosp. Team (2,p.192)	EAP	Sanyinjiao	Tubal ligation	698	77.8% excellent result; total effective rate 98.6%
Shanghai Internat. Clinic (2,p.193)	EAP and Ear AP	HoKu (LI 4)	Tubal ligation	8,000	97.2% successful
Shi (2, p. 196)	EAP	Ciliao (B 32)	Tubal ligation	120	Very successful

Table 10-1. (continued)

Source	Mode	Acupoint	Diagnosis	No. of Patient	Effectiveness %
Wang (2, p. 190) (6,p.759)	EAP	Sanyinjiao	Tubal ligation	23,554	85.8% excellent result; total effective rate 97.9%
Xiu (2, p.190)	EAP	Renzhong (S 17)	Tubal ligation	3,346	85.2% excellent result; total effective rate 90%
Zhou (2, p.194)	EAP		Tubal ligation	245	Highly successful
Zongqing Hosp. Team (2,p.191)	EAP	HoKu	Tubal ligation	2,047	90% success
Xian Hosp. Team (2, p. 182)	EAP	Yaoshu (Du 21) Sanyinjiao	Hysterectomy	100	50% excellent result
Beijing Hosp. Team (2,p.184)	EAP	Zhongjio (Ren 3)	Hysterectomy	95	22.1% excellent; total effective rate 95.7%
Shanxi Hosp. Team (3,p.218)	EAP	Ciliao Zhongjio	Hysterectomy	62	82.3% excellent
Xu (2, p. 181) (6,p.754)	EAP	Sizhong (Du 6)	Hysterectomy	674	36.8% excellent; total effective rate 83.1%
Yu (2, p. 183)	EAP	Mingmen (Du 4)	Hysterectomy	140	34.6% excellent; total effective rate 71.2%
Wang (55)	EAP	Qugu (Ren 2) Sanyinjiao	Hysteromyotomy	1,006	70.7% excellent; other 18% good

* EAP = Electro-acupuncture
** AP = Manual acupuncture
# Gen. Anesth. = General anesthesia
@ Epidur. anesth. = Epidural anesthesia

Artificial Abortion

Acupuncture anesthesia has also been used in artificial abortion, especially in rural areas in China. According to a report by Y. Wang (57), abortion was performed by auricular acupuncture technique in 618 cases. The acupoint Shenmen area was punctured. The patients were in the first trimester of pregnancy and were discharged home after the operation. In 43.3 percent of patients the results were recorded as excellent and in 20.2 percent the acupuncture failed.

Labor Induction

The effectiveness of acupuncture in inducing labor has been debated by two different groups. Chinese practitioners have claimed that the time to apply the acupuncture and the intensity of stimulation probably account for the different results. S. Lyrenas, et al., (39) reported on thirty-two primiparous women who received repeated acupuncture treatments during the month prior to term. There was no benefit as compared with the nonacupuncture group of women. Both groups of patients experienced successively rising pain during labor. In their early studies on fifty-six primiparous women, the researchers treated patients repeatedly with manual acupuncture during the month prior to parturition. Acupuncture caused a lengthening of the pregnancy and prolonged the labor (38).

S. M. Shnider treated six women in labor with acupuncture and reported that two of them had moderate relief of pain in early labor, one had mild relief, and three had no relief (47).

Lyrenas, et al., (37) studied sixty-two primiparous women in term pregnancy. Fifty patients received acupuncture therapy in an antenatal preparation procedure. CSF fluid was collected in fifteen patients six months after delivery. It was found that the dynorphin A level in the CSF was higher in the acupuncture group than in the nontreatment group. The ß-endorphin level was 7.1 pmol/l in acupuncture group and 5.7 pmol/l in the nontreatment group. However, there was no difference in the CSF dynorphin A or ß-endorphin level between acupuncture and nonacupuncture groups in the late pregnancy period. The researchers speculated that there is a possible connection between the number of acupuncture treatments and the prolongation of labor contraction (37).

Chinese acupuncturists argued that the repeated acupuncture treatments may be the reason for such difference. P. A. Dunn, et al., (15) treated twenty postdated pregnancy women with EAP therapy (30 Hz) at the acupoints Sanyinjiao (Sp 6) and Taichong (Liv 3) and produced a significant increase of uterine contractions both in terms of frequency and strength, followed by delivery of the neonates. A. Dorr (11) tried acupuncture on sixteen pregnant women and induced labor in 13 of them with a remarkable analgesic effect and dilation of the uterine cervix.

Other clinicians have applied acupuncture therapy in women during the first pregnancy with very satisfactory results. They considered that acupuncture is a simple and harmless method inducing labor and it would not cause allergic reaction in the mother or newborn baby (19).

In a study of 771 women in the tenth month of pregnancy, acupuncture was performed to induce labor (6, p. 641). Six hundred and four cases involved the first pregnancy, and 167 involved multipregnancies. Acupuncture was applied on the acupoints HoKu and Sanyinjiao and employed electrical stimulation at a frequency of 300/min. and intensity of five to fifteen volts. There was a 72.1 percent success rate. Labor in another 118 cases was induced by oxytocin with a success rate of 70.3 percent. Among the acupuncture-induced labor group, 556 babies (2 were twins) were born in a healthy condition, and two died due to rupture of placenta vessels or umbilical strangulation. B. U. O. Umeh (53) tried acupuncture-induced labor in thirty Nigerian women and observed a clinically adequate analgesia in 12 (63.3 percent). Six women experienced no pain throughout the labor, which lasted an average of eight hours, but another eleven women (36.7 percent) did not

Table 10-2. Obstetric Operation under Acupuncture Anesthesia

Source	Mode	Acupoint	Diagnosis	No. of Patients	Effectiveness %
Hayashida (21)	EAP*	Zhiyin (B 67)	Abnormal fetal postion (breech presentation)	584	89.9% success, corrected to a cephalic presentation.
Cui (9)	P1** with Vaccaria seeds	Ear	Abnormal fetal presentation	124	95.2% corrected the position (7-8th month, 98.9%; 8-9th month, 86.7%; over 9th month, only 40%)
Jiangxi Hosp. Team (2,p.6)	EAP	Zhiyin	Abnormal fetal presentation (Breech)	2,041	90.3% corrected the position
			(Acronion presentation)	27	
			Total	2,068	
Jiangxi Trad. Med. Coll. (6, p. 560)	EAP		Abnormal fetal position (Breech)	111	71% corrected the position
Wong (58)	AP# with warmed needle	Sanyinjiao (Sp 6)	Abnormal fetal position	82	83% corrected the position
Li (32)	EAP	Renzhong (Du 26)	Ectopic pregnancy	97	89.7% excellent result
Li (30)	AP	Zusanli (S 36)	Artificial abortion	32	59% no pain and 38% had slight pain
Shen (44)	AP	Ear	Artificial aborption	200	91% markedly effective
Tran (25, p. 625)	AP		Artificial abortion	14	50% satisfactory; 28.6% partial satisfied
Wang (57)	AP	Ear	Artificial abortion	618	43.3% effective
Ying (60)	AP	Sanyinjiao Zhongfeng (Liv 4)	Artificial abortion	20	90% effective; Plasma HCG level was elevated in 12 patients

Table 10-2. (continued)

Source	Mode	Acupoint	Diagnosis	No. of Patients	Effectiveness %
Yuan (62)	AP	Lumbar L5	Early abortion	21	95.2% success
Zhang (2, p. 86)	AP	Ear	Artificial abortion	56	98.2% effective, uterus cervix was dilated

* EAP = Electro-acupuncture
** PL = Plaster
\# AP = Acupuncture

benefit from this treatment and had to rely on the analgesic agent meperidine for pain relief. In general, the cardiorespiratory function and uterine contractions of the mothers were not adversely affected by the acupuncture therapy and no adverse effect on mothers or neonates was observed.

Yip, et al., (25, p. 643) studied thirty-one pregnant women treated by EAP therapy at the acupoint Sanyinjiao (Sp 6) and reported that twenty-one (67.7 percent) had a successful labor contraction. The uterus started to dilate as soon as the patient felt the needle sensation of Tai Qi and it required a latent period as long as three hours for the onset of contraction.

Table 10-3 summarizes the clinical application of acupuncture in labor induction and abortion.

Other Gynecological and Obstetric Diseases

Besides its use as an anesthesia tool in gynecology and obstetrics, acupuncture is also widely used as a therapy to treat many women's diseases. In a recent review, M. C. and C. J. Hong (23) summarized their clinical experience with the use of acupuncture therapy from 1988 to 1991. They included the treatment of menstruation difficulties, such as dysmenorrhea, premenstrual tension, and stress, uterine hemorrhage, and pain; pregnancy difficulties, such as nausea and vomiting, miscarrage, abnormal fetal position; postlabor symptoms, such as oligogalactia, urine retention, and acute mastitis; infertility, uterine tumors, and breast hypertrophy. They considered acupuncture therapy beneficial in most of the diseases.

X. M. Wang (56) treated 100 cases of dysmenorrhea with acupuncture and moxibustion and reported that 54 of patients were cured, 27 were markedly improved, 15 were moderatedly improved, and 6 failed. The total effectiveness rate was 94 percent.

J. M. Helms (22) divided patients with dysmenorrhea into three groups. In one group, treated with acupuncture over a two-year period, ten of eleven patients (91 percent) showed a significant improvement in their symptoms and reduced the dosage of drugs they took to relieve the symptoms. The other two groups served as controls (no medication and no acupuncture) or placebo (random acupuncture at nonacupoint): only 10 percent and 36.4 percent improvement rates, respectively, were obtained. Table 10-4 lists the clinical application of acupuncture in various gynecological and obstetric diseases.

Table 10-3. Acupuncture in Labor Induction

Source	Mode	Acupoint	Diagnosis	No. of Patients	Effectiveness %
Chu (6, p. 641)	AP*	Sanyinjiao (Sp 6)	Normal labor delivery	771	72.1% excellent
	Oxytocin			118	70.3% excellent
Dorr (11)	AP	Sanyinjiao	Normal labor delivery	16	81.2% excellent
Dunn (15)	EAP** (30 Hz)	Sanyinjiao	Labor	20	Very effective
Huang (2, p. 86)	EAP	Ciliao (B 32)	Labor	100	70.0% spontaneous delivery , babies were born normal and healthy
Hyodo (25,p. 663)	AP		Normal delivery	32	60% in primapara and 90% in multipara, very satisfactory
Ito (24)	AP		Normal delivery	80	85% successful
Kubista (25 p. 630)	AP		Normal delivery	35	31 of them showed an increase of contractio intensity
Lin (35)	AP	HoKu (LI 4) Sanyinjiao	Normal labor	110	92.7% success
Umeh (53)	AP		Normal labor	30	63.3 % had a spontaneous delivery
Yip (25, p. 643)	AP	Sanyinjiao	Normal labor	31	67.7% excellent

* AP = Acupuncture
** EAP = Electro-acupuncture

Table 10-4. Acupuncture Therapy in Other Gynecological and Obstetric Diseases

Source	Mode	Acupoint	Diagnosis	No. of Patients	Effectiveness %
Feng (16)	AP*	Ear	Dysmenorrhea	120	37% were cured
Helms (22)	AP	Sanyinjiao (Sp 6)	Dysmenorrhea	11	10 of them improved and reduced the dose of other analgesic.
	Control (no AP)			11	2 of them improved
	Placebo	randomized non-acupoints		11	4 of them improved
Liu (36)	P1# with Vaccaria seeds	Ear	Dysmenorrhea	1,000	81.7% cured
Tin (52)	AP	Sanyinjiao	Dysmenorrhea	535	70% were cured
	IAc inj @ of Angelia extract			80	60% were cured
Wang (56)	AP and Moxi.**	Sanyinjiao	Dysmenorrhea	100	54% were cured; total effective rate 94%
Zhang (63)	AP		Dysmenorrhea	49	85.7% were cured
Chien (7)	AP	Sanyinjiao Tanzhong (Ren 17)	Infertility	30	57% were cured and became pregnant
Gerhard (14)	AP	Ear	Infertility	27	Very successful
Li (18)	EAP***	Ganshu (B 18)	Infertility	105	100% effective and became pregnant
Qian (41)	AP	Taichong (Liv 3) Sanyinjiao	Infertiligy	20	15 patients became pregnant
Si (48)	AP	Zusanli (S 36) Guanyuan (Ren 4)	Infertility	30	17 of them became pregnant
Tereshin (51)	AP		Chronic salpingo-oophoritis with infertility	64	39 of them were cured and became pregnant

Table 10-4. (continued)

Source	Mode	Acupoint	Diagnosis	No. of Patient	Effectiveness %
Li (29)	AP	At affected region	Chronic pelvitis and salpingitis	80	78% were cured
Liang (2, p. 96)	AP	Sanyinjiao	Cervical erosion	1,010	62.4% were cured and total effective rate 90.1%
Alieva (1)	AP		Polypous ovary	80	33.7% effective and became pregnant
Fong (17)	AP	Sanyinjiao	Uteroptosis (1st. degree)	21	95% were cured
Li (27)	EAP	Sanyinjiao	Post-labor hemorrhage	18	78% effective
Shi (46)	Pl with Vaccaria seeds	Ear	Functional uterine bleeding	54	59% were cured
Shi (45)	EAP	HoKu (LI 4) Tanzhong	Oligogalactia	40	94.7% effective
Guo (20)	AP	Multiple	Hyperplasia of Mammary glands	500	Improved
Dong (10)	AP and Cryot##		Mastitis	104	88% effective
Li (33)	AP	Huatuojaji (Extra 15)	Mastitis	553	96% effective
Tang (50)	AP	Jianjing (G 2) Ashi (Extra)	Mastitis	58	98.3% were cured
Xibin (54)	AP		Mammary fibrocystoma	57	45.6% were cured, total effective rate 91.2%
Yuan (61)	AP	Yingchuan (S 16) Tanzhong	Mastosis	110	30.9% excellent result
Li (31)	AP	Guangming (G 37)	Lactation mastitis	25	92% were cured
Zhang (63)	AP	Dazhui (Du 14)	Acute Mastitis	258	93% were cured

* AP = Acupuncture; ** Moxi. = Moxibustion
*** EAP = Electro-acupuncture; #Pl = Plaster; ## Cryot.= Cryotherapy
@ IAc inj. = Intra-acupoint injection

Kubista, et al., (25, p. 638) reported twenty cases of female urethral incontinence treated with EAP therapy. Seventeen patients (85 percent) showed a positive closing pressure of the urethra. It is possible that acupuncture could increase the tonus of the entire sphincter area of urethra and strengthen the muscles by increasing blood flow in the submucosal region of the urethra.

Acupuncture therapy has also been used in China effectively to treat reproductive disturbances. In their recent experimentation on anoestrous sows, J. H. Lin and his coworkers (34) demonstrated an effect of EAP causing reflex response of ovary and uterus via the CNS system. They found that three of four anoestrous sows, after acupuncture treatment in fourteen repeated daily doses, started to return their oestrus cycle with an accompanying increase in serum progesterone and cortisol levels and a fall of serum LH level. Three sows served as controls without acupuncture treatment and four sows received an intravenous dose of gonadotrophin-releasing hormone; only one of each group returned to the oestrus cycle. The data indicate that acupuncture is more effective in stimulating reproduction than the gonadotrophin-releasing hormone.

J. Gerhard and F. Fostneek (18) praised the beneficial effect of acupuncture in helping patients to combat oligo-menorrhea and luteal body insufficiency. They treated patients with auricular acupuncture and obtained very successful results, especially in cases of amenorrhea with a positive gestagen test and normal basal hormone levels. They stated that this technique has low toxicity, or low abortion rate, and a positive influence on the patients' general condition.

Infertility

S. H. Li, et al., (30) reported on 105 cases of infertility during the period 1982–89. The age of the patients ranged from twenty-five to thirty-five years. Diagnosis included chronic pelvitis, obstruction of oviducts, and underdevelopment of uterus. The acupoint Ganshu (B 18) was chosen for acupuncture, averaging in ten consecutive daily treatments. All patients were cured at the end of the treatment and subsequently conceived.

Yi, et al. (3, p.554) showed that EAP can stimulate ovulation in young women and elevate endogenous estrogen levels and skin temperature.

E. A. Alieva, et al., (1) treated eighty patients with polycystic ovary syndromes and excessive obesity with acupuncture and diet. Twenty-seven patients were cured and subsequently became pregnant.

In another European study acupuncture therapy was found to be very effective in the treatment of infertility in women (58).

Morning Sickness and Antiemetic Effect

Acupuncture prior to cancer chemotherapy has been reported to significantly reduce the emetic effect. The acupoint Neiguan (P 6) was chosen in such an antiemetic effect. Studies also showed that the antiemetic effect of acupuncture could be blocked by administration of local anesthetic agents (38,45).

A. O. Cattaneo, et al., (5) reported that in 200 cases that acupuncture not only prevented the nausea and vomiting which often occurred before gynecological surgery but also significantly reduced postanesthetic emetic symptoms. Twenty-four pregnant patients suffering from severe emetic toxicosis were treated with acupuncture (42). They had previously tried medications without success. After acupuncture, nineteen patients (79.2 percent) had stopped vomiting and others had symptomatic improvement. In all cases, the pregnancy developed normally and labor proceeded without difficulty.

Rempp and Bigler (43) reported their experience in the use of acupuncture therapy in 1,000 pregnant women, including 800 during the delivery period. The researchers found that acupuncture had a very satisfactory effect on a wide range of complaints, including morning sickness, pain during delivery, lactation problems, and postpartum depression. They advised the regular use of acupuncture in office visits for pregnant patients and in the delivery room.

C. L. Stone has described that using acupoint pressure waistbands in pregnant women can prevent nausea and morning sickness (49).

Oligogalactia

Generally, lactation starts twenty-four to forty-eight hours after the partuition as the pituitary gland starts to increase prolactin secretion. Mothers with reproductive difficulties, hormonal insufficiency, or emotional disturbance may suffer from oligogalactia symptoms. Several reports have demonstrated that acupuncture therapy produced a remarkable increase in lactation, especially in mothers who had such symptoms within twenty days after labor. It was ineffective in those mothers who had suffered oligogalactia for months. For example, in a Chinese clinic, forty cases of postlabor oligogalactia were treated with acupuncture at the acupounts HoKu and Tanzhong (Ren 17). Thirty-eight were cured (94.7 percent) and two failed (5.3 percent) (45). However, acupuncture did not affect prolactin secretion and had no effect on patients with galactorrhea (26).

Mammary Hyperplasia and Mastitis

Acupuncture therapy has also been used to treat nonmalignant mammary hyperplasia and mastitis. C. J. Guo and W. H. Zhang (20) treated 500 cases of mammary hyperplasia with acupuncture and reported good immediate and long-term curative effects. It was thought that acupuncture could probably improve cellular immunological function and correct the endocrinological disturbance.

In another report, acupuncture was used to treat 110 cases of mastosis at the acupoints Ying Chuan (S 16) or Rugen (St 18), Tanzhong (Ren 17), and Qimen (Liv 14). Thirty-four patients (30.9 percent) had complete disappearance of their lumps and pain, another sixty-five (59 percent) had a reduction in the size of the lumps and pain, and eleven showed no effect (61).

Acupuncture was used in combination with cryotherapy to treat the acute mastitis (10). The center of the lump was selected as the primary acupoint (stimulated thirty minutes daily), and Rugen (S 18) was the secondary acupoint (stimulated ten minutes daily). The temperature of the cryotherapy was from -10 to -15º C once a day for mild cases and -15 to -25° C twice a day for severe cases. Totally, 104 cases were treated, and 91 were cured (88 percent) after three to five days of treatment.

Another 553 cases of mastitis, including 53 cases in the suppurative stage, were treated with acupuncture at the acupoint Huatuojiaji (Extra 15) for twenty to thirty minutes. A 96 percent effectiveness rate was reported (33).

References

1. Alieva, E. A., et al. Acta Anesthesiol. Ital. 38:683, 1987.
2. All China Society of Acupuncture and Moxibustion. National Symposium on Acupuncture and Acupuncture Anesthesia. Beijing: 1979.
3. All China Society of Acupuncture and Moxibustion. Second National Symposium on Acupuncture and Moxibustion and Acupuncture Anesthesia. Beijing: People Health Publisher, 1984.
4. Beijing Acupuncture Anesthesia Unit. Chinese Medical Journal 93:231, 1980.
5. Cattaneo, A. D., et al. Acta Univ. Palacki Olomac Fac. Med. 126:233, 1990.
6. Chang, H. T., et al., ed. Research in Acupuncture and Moxibustion and Acupuncture Anesthesia. Beijing: Science Publishing Company, 1986.
7. Chien, S. E. Journal of Chinese Acupuncture and Moxibustion 14(2):15, 1994.
8. Christensen, P. A., et al. Brit. J. Anesth. 71:835, 1993.
9. Cui, S. H., and J. G. Zhang. Journal of Chinese Acupuncture and Moxibustion 13(6):11, 1993.
10. Dong, J. L., and C. H. Journal of Chinese Acupuncture and Moxibustion 11(4):13, 1991.
11. Dorr, A. American Journal of Acupuncture 18:213, 1990.
12. Dundee, J. W., et al. British Medical Journal 293 (6547):583, 1986.
13. Dundee, J. W., and C. M. McMillen. Acupuncture Electro-Ther. Res. 15:211, 1990.
14. Dundee, J. W., and G. Ghaly. Chinese Pharmacol. Ther. 50:78, 1991.
15. Dunn, P. A., et al. Obstet. Gyn. 73:286, 1989.
16. Feng, S. H. Shanghai Journal of Acupuncture and Moxibustion 12(3):117, 1993.
17. Fong, S. C. New Journal of Traditional Chinese Medicine 25(7):29, 1993.
18. Gerhard, I., and F. Fostneek. Geburtsch Frauenheilkd. 48:165, 1988.
19. Gevoikyan, S. M., et al. Zh. Eksp. Klin. Med. 29:433, 1989.
20. Guo, C. J., and W. H. Zhang. Journal of Traditional Chinese Medicine 8:157, 1988.
21. Hayachida, Y. J. Med. Soc.: Toho Univ. 34:196, 1987
22. Helms, J. M. Obstet. Gyn. 69:51, 1987.
23. Hong, M. C., and C. Hong. Journal of Chinese Acupuncture and Moxibustion 11 (3):34, 1991.
24. Ito, T. Jpn. J. Anesth. 23:10, 1974.
25. Kao, F. F., and J. J. Kao. Recent Advances in Acupuncture Research. Garden City, NY: Institute for Advanced Research in Asian Science and Medicine, 1979.
26. Komorowski, J. M., et al. Encokrynol Pol. 35:231, 1984.
27. Li, K. A. Shanghai Journal of Acupuncture and Moxibustion 12(3):108, 1993.
28. Li, M. H., et al. New Journal of Traditional Chinese Medicine 26(1):35, 1994.
29. Li, S. C., and S. S. Li. New Journal of Traditional Chinese Medicine 26(3):31, 1994.
30. Li, S. H., et al. Journal of Chinese Acupuncture and Moxibustion 11 (6):13, 1991.
31. Li, S. H. Shanghai Journal of Acupuncture and Moxibustion 12(4):168, 1993.
32. Li, Y. K., and S. L. Li. Journal of Chinese Acupuncture and Moxibustion 11 (6):29, 1991.
33. Li, Z. C. et al. Journal of Chinese Acupuncture and Moxibustion 11 (4): 13, 1991.
34. Lin, J. H., et al. American Journal of Chinese Medicine 16:117, 1988.
35. Lin, P. C., et al. Journal of Chinese Acupuncture and Moxibustion 14(1):29, 1994.
36. Liu, S. C. Journal of Chinese Acupuncture and Moxibustion 13(6):27, 1993.
37. Lyrenas, S., et al. Acta Endocrinol. 115:253, 1987.
38. Lyrenas, S., et al. Gyn. Obstet. Invest. 24:217, 1987.
39. Lyrenas, S., et al. Gyn. Obstet. Invest. 29: 118, 1990.
40. Pei, D., and Y. L. Huang. Journal of Traditional Chinese Medicine 5:253, 1985.
41. Qian, C. Y. Journal of Chinese Acupuncture and Moxibustion 14(2):15, 1994.
42. Raca, N., et al. Rev. Pediatr. Obstet. Ginecol. Ser. Obsetet. Ginecol. 36:83, 1988.
43. Rempp, C., and A. Bigler. American Journal of Acupuncture 19:305, 1991.
44. Shen, C. S., and Q. L. Hong. Journal of Chinese Acupuncture and Moxibustion 13(1):4, 1993.
45. Shi, S. M., ed. The Art of Chinese Acupuncture (in Chinese). Tianjin: Tianjin Science and Technology Publisher, 1992, p. 551.
46. Shi, T. C., et al. Journal of Chinese Acupuncture and Moxibustion 14(2):20, 1994.
47. Shnider, S. M., from Jenerick, H. P., ed., NIH Acupuncture Research Conference. DHEW 74-165, 1973, p. 87.
48. Si, C. D., and Y. P. Si. Shanghai Journal of Acupuncture and Moxibustion 13(1):15, 1994.
49. Stone, C. L. Nurse Pract. 18(11):15, 1993.
50. Tang, H. S. Journal of Chinese Acupuncture and Moxibustion 13(5):19, 1993.

51. Tereshin, A. T., and B. I. Levshin. Vestnik Dermatogii I Venerologii. 0(7):71, 1992.
52. Tin, C. G. Journal of Chinese Acupuncture and Moxibustion 14(2): 30, 1994.
53. Umeh, B. U. O. Acupuncture Electro-Ther. Res. 11:147, 1986.
54. Xibin, L., and X. F. A. Yutan. American Journal of Acupuncture 20:31, 1992.
55. Wang, L., et al. Journal of Chinese Acupuncture and Moxibustion 11(3): 11, 1991.
56. Wang, X. M. Journal of Traditional Chinese Medicine 7:29, 1987.
57. Wang, Y., and Y. H. Zhang. Chinese Acupuncture and Moxibustion 11 (3): 34, 1991.
58. Wong, J. Shanghai Journal of Acupuncture and Moxibustion 12(4):166, 1993.
59. Veroptovelyan, M. S., and P. N. Veroptovelyan, Zh. Eksp. Klin. Med. 23: 573, 1983.
60. Ying, Y. K., et al. Journal of Reproductive Medicine 30:530, 1985.
61. Yuan, S. et al. Journal of Traditional Chinese Med. 4:50, 1984.
62. Yuan, Y. P. Journal of Chinese Acupuncture and Moxibustion 13(6):11, 1993.
63. Zhang, S. Y. Shanghai Journal of Acupuncture and Moxibustion 12(2):65, 1993.

11
Acupuncture in Internal Medicine

Traditionally, there have been two types of practitioners of medicine in China. One was the scholar physician, whom the chinese called *Long Chong* or *Tai Fu*, who learned his trade from books or his parents or grandparents and considered medical practice as one of his habits or the honorable job of helping the masses and saving lives. The other group was the traveling practitioner, with a motto such as "have needle or herbs, will travel." They wandered the streets and bazaars, selling their products, which ranged from "tiger bone (some may even be *dinosaur* bone!)" to varieties of aphrodisiac. They also healed illness by using the needle for such procedures as dental extraction and stopping diarrhea. It is impossible to assess the success of acupuncture technique used for thousands of years in China. But the traveling practitioners still exist in the rural areas of China, even though many have been replaced by the barefoot doctors.

Alimentary Tract Diseases

Diarrhea and Dysentery

Besides pain, the most common illness the travelling practitioners treated was gastroenteritis, including diarrhea and dysentery, caused mainly by ingestion of unhygienic food or infections. Opium or opium tincture was not available centuries ago and was not described in the old Chinese pharmacopoeia. Acupuncture is the remedy which has been kept in used in China since 1960 when the shortage of medical supplies from the outside world became very acute. Liang's review (150) has placed the effectiveness rate of acupuncture in diarrhea at 94 percent, a remarkable result. In rural areas, infants often suffered from diarrhea. In Lin's report (155) 170 infants aged from one to nineteen months suffering diarrhea were treated with acupuncture at the acupoint Zusanli (S 36), once a day. After three treatments 151 were cured (89.8 percent). Their watery stool became formed and the frequency decreased to no more than two times a day. Only six of the infants failed to respond to the treatment (3.6 percent).

Some Chinese physicians claimed that they did not have to use a needle, but rather would only apply a herbal paste to the acupoint Shenque (Ren 8), the point right at the navel. They reportedly obtained a remarkable effect in acute diarrhea. In 328 cases, 316 were cured (96.3 percent) (293).

Zhang (313) studied the effect of acupuncture in fifty cases of infant diarrhea. It was applied on the acupoint Zusanli, once a day. One course of treatment averaged 5.08 days. At the end of one course, all patients were cured. Table 11-1 compares the effectiness of acupuncture therapy and Chinese herbal therapy. Results indicated that the acupuncture therapy is superior.

Table 11-1. A Comparison of Effectiveness on the Treatment of Diarrhea by Acupuncture and Herbal Therapy

	Acupuncture Group	Herbal Group
	Averaged Treated Days Required	
When patient's stool was 2 or less /day	2.08 ± 0.13	4.27 ± 0.28
When the terperature returned to normal	1.23 ±0.07	1.74 ± 0.08
When dehydration symptom disappeared	2.40 ± 0.05	3.36 ± 0.22
Total sick days	5.08 ± 0.72	7.60 ± 1.30

(From Zhang (313))

Bacterial dysentery was a widespread disease in most Chinese rural areas, especially in the summer months. The Huang Ti Nei Chian described such illness as "CH'ANG BI" (meaning "intestinal pecularity"). Other ancient medical texts called it "SHA LI"(meaning "down-pouring bowel movement"). Althougth they did not know it was caused by bacterial infection, acupuncture treatment of this illness was well described in the book ACUPUNCTURE ABC (published in A.D.265 by Huang Fu-mi). Qiu et al., (2, p.2 and 25, p. 561)] reported the clinical result of the acupuncture therapy in 926 patients who had been found by culture to have *Shigella* bacteria in their stool, and had symptoms of high temperature and frequent bowel movements. The patients were divided into two groups: 281 of them were treated with medication, and the other 645 were treated with acupuncture therapy. Results are summarized in Table 11-2.

Table 11-2. Acupuncture Therapy or Herbal Therapy on Shigella Dysentery

Treatment	No. of Patients with positive stool culture	Negative Stool Culture after treatment		
		No. of Patients		Average Days
Herbal Medicine	281	276	(98.2%)	4.3
Acupuncture	645	596	(92.4%)	5.12

(From Qlu et al. (24, p.561))

Half of the patients cured by acupuncture therapy were followed up for six months; only thirty-three patients had a relapse. The plasma level of IgG and IgA was also studied in those patients after acupuncture therapy; 43 percent had an increase in IgG and IgA levels (2, p. 2 and 5).

Data collected from all major clinics throughout China showed that acupuncture therapy in the treatment of 1383 cases of bacterial dysentery reached a 91.5 percent cure rate. The acupoints Tianshu (S 25), Qihai (Ren 6) and Zusanli were chosen and the average treatment was for 5.4 days. In 1090 cases treated with antibiotics instead of acupuncture, the curative rate was 82.8 percent. (142).

In a later report 114 cases of bacterial dysentery treated with daily acupuncture, repeated for seven days as a course, ninety-seven patients were cured (87.5 percent) and another nineteen were improved, while only two failed (287).

Hwang and Jenkins (102) induced enteropathogenic *E. coli* diarrhea in young pigs and treated them with acupuncture at the acupoints Zusanli and Baihui (Du 20), bilaterally. They obtained an 80 percent cure rate in term of disappearance of diarrhea symptoms. Acupuncture therapy is often used successfully in veternary medicine to treat piglet's diarrhea. (See Chapter 20.)

Table 11-3 lists the clinical reports of acupuncture therapy in diarrhea and bacterial dysentery.

Peptic Ulcer

Studies of acupuncture on gastric secretion had conflicting results. For example, Huang, et al., (2, p. 62) experimentally created an artifical gastric perforation in rabbits and treated the ulcer with EAP at the acupoint Zusanli. It was found that acupuncture therapy can enhance the absorption of blood from the peritoneal cavity and potentiate body resistance by stimulating the neutrophilocytosis. The perforated ulcer was closed by adhesion with the omentum and finally healed. Such healing occurred in 83.3 percent of animals treated with acupuncture and in only 33.3 percent in the placebo group. Studies on anesthetized cats also showed that EAP could inhibit gastroelectrical activity (196). In another study, acupuncture was found to have an inhibitory effect of gastric mobility in spinalized cats, which was not antagonized by the administration of naloxone (222).

However, H. Kurosake, et al., (130) studied both animals and human subjects and reported that acupuncture could increase gastric acid and lower pH. Their result was very controversial, because they also found that the secretion of gastrin was decreased. Gastrin is a hormone that is known to stimulate gastric acid secretion. In experiments on dogs, L. Zhou and Wm. Y. Chey (335) showed that acupuncture could stimulate gastric secretion by nonparietal cells, especially the secretion of bicarbonate, but that acid secretion was decreased.

Y. Li, et al., stated in their review article that no firm conclusions can be drawn on the effects of acupuncture therapy in gastrointestinal disorders, because of a lack of controlled trials (148).

In clinical practice, Lovacky, et al., (175) treated five male patients with duodenal ulcer with acupuncture for fourteen days and found a remarkable improvement in their symptoms. The plasma ß-endorphin immunoreactivity declined after the treatment. Other investigators also reported that acupuncture therapy produced a significant improvement in ulcer patients in terms of both their gastroduodenal symptoms and psychosomatic symptoms (70). Studies on thirty-eight healthy male subjects have shown that EAP can decrease the basal gastric acid output by decreasing the gastrin secretion, which is probably mediated through the naloxone-sensitive opioid neural pathways and vagal efferent pathways (253).

Table 11-3. Clinical Data on Acupuncture Therapy in Diarrhea and Dysentery

Source	Mode	Acupoint	Diagnosis	No. of Patients	Effectiveness %
Lin (153)	AP*	Zusanli (S 36)	Infantile diarrhea	170	88.8% were cured
Song (239)	AP	Ear	Diarrhea	28	All cured
Wong (276)	EAP#	Ear	Pediatric diarrhea	69	97.1% effective
	Medication			55	87.3% effective
Yang (293)	AP and Herbs	Shenque (Ren 8)	Acute diarrhea	328	96% were cured
Zhang (313)	AP	Zusanli	Infantile diarrhea	50	all cured
Zhang (319)	AP	Zusanli	Infantile diarrhea	40	16 of them (40%) cured after one treatment; another 19 (48%) were cured after 2 treatments; another 4 (10%) cured after 3 treatments.
Chang (2, p.39)	AP	Zusanli	Bacterial dysentery	134	89.4% were cured
Li (142)	AP	Tianshu (S 25) Qihai (Ren 6) Zusanli	Acute bact. dysentery	1,383	91.5% were cured
Qiu (2, p. 2)	AP	Qihai	Bact. dysentery	645	94.2% were cured, follow-up for 6 months 12% recurrence
Qlu (2 , p.567)	AP	Tianshu,Qihai	Acute bact. dysentery	645	92.4% were cured;
	Medication			181	98% were cured.

* AP = Body Acupuncture
\# EAP EAP = Electro-acupuncture

Other Alimentary Diseases

Four hundred and twenty patients suffering from chronic atrophic gastritis were treated with acupuncture therapy. Three different kinds of needle were applied and achieved a 45 percent effectiveness rate (280). Acupuncture was also used to treat indigestion in children. Xu and Zhao (3, p. 91) reported their trials on 250 cases and obtained a 72 percent curative rate.

Seventy cases of volvulus of the stomach, diagnosed by BaSO4 meal and X-rays, were treated with acupuncture at the Zusanli point, daily for thirty to sixty minutes. All patients were cured except two (159).

S. D. Tian, et al., (252) treated 140 cases of pediatric anorexia with daily acupuncture; one course consisted of twelve sessions. After two to four courses of treatment, the appetite of the children increased substantially and a gain in body weight was observed. The other malnourishment symptoms were greatly improved. In another report, acupuncture was found to increase the exocrine functions and secretions of the pancreas (200).

Acupuncture can relax the smooth muscles. In twenty-two patients suffering from esophageal achalasia, acupuncture therapy was applied; 12 had a significant decrease in lower esophageal sphincture tone and were successively able to swallow and eat. (201).

Three hundred and sixty-three cases of diaphragm contraction, hiccup, and gallbladder disease mainly due to gastrointestinal problems were treated with acupuncture at the Yongquan (K 1) point bilaterally. After one treatment 90 percent of the patients were relieved from hiccup, and the others were cured after two treatments (170).

Acupuncture has been used to treat gastroptosis (2, p. 60, 64, 65, and 66), childhood prolopse of the rectum (6), and ascariasis (2, (p. 45).

Table 11-4 summarizes the clinical reports on acupuncture therapy in other alimentary diseases.

Antiemetic and Anti–Sea Sickness:

C. McMillan, et al., (188) reported that the application of acupuncture at the Neiguan (P 6) point can enhance the antiemetic effect of antiemetic agents, such as metoclopramide, phenothiazines, and cyclizine. He and his colleague have discussed the promising antiemetic effect of both acupuncture and EAP in gynecological and cancer therapeutic applications (61). When acupuncture is given prior to preanesthetic administration, it can significantly reduce the vomiting effect caused by opiates and also minimize the postoperative sickness for six to eight hours. The most rewarding results they have found are in the prevention of morning sickness in early pregnancy by pressing the acupoint Neiguan (P 6) for five to six minutes and preventing emesis in cancer patients before taking cancer chemotherapy. The researchers also found that the antiemetic effect of EAP or acupuncture is superior to that achieved by TENS stimulation.

In a five-year period Liu, et al., (164) treated 300 cases of seasickness, including people who were sensitive to the smell of gasoline vapor, with the auricular paste technique in which the paste contained the Vaccaria seeds. Sixty-two percent of the patients obtained marked relief and another 34 percent were improved.

Table 11-4. Acupuncture Therapy in Other Alimentary Diseases

Source	Mode	Acupoint	Diagnosis	No. of Patients	Effectiveness %
Zhu (3, p. 54)	AP*	Zhongwen (Ren 12)	Peptic Ulcer	41	73% were cured (based on gastroscopic exam.)
Kravtsova (126)	Ap with a magnetic needle	Pishu (B 20) Zusanli (S 36)	Duodenal ulcer	66	Symptoms disappeared & ulcer was healed rapidly
(127)				86	Promote a regression of vegetable dystonia; symptoms disappeared and ulcer healing speed up.
Lovacky (175)	AP	Zusanli	Duodenal ulcer	5	Remarkable improved
Luo (182)	Catgut EM**	Pishu (B 20) Zusanli	Peptic Ulcer	245	100% effective; all clinical & physical symptoms disappeared
Wu (289)	EAP***	Zusanli	Perforated peptic & duod. ulcer	24	17.3% patients started to eat in the 2nd day; average 5.36 days can start to eat, about 3 days earlier than the surgical group.
Zhou (334)	AP	Weishu (B 21) Zusanli	Gastro-intes-tinal diseases including: 293 peptic ulcer, 270 duod. ulcer, 6 stomach cancer, 68 gastroptosis	863	70% clinical cure ; $BaSO_4$ meal showed that ulcer was gone; other 22% improved.
Chen (33)	AP	Zusanli Neiguan (P 6)	Chron. gastritis	53	89% were cured
Hong (90)	EAP	Zusanli	Chron. super-ficial gastritis	32	93.6% effective
Li (140)	IAc@ of Angelica extract	Zusanli	Chron. gastri-tis	70	69% were cured
Wu 285)	AP with warmed needle		Chronic atrophic gastritis	102	69.6% effective
Zhang (328)	AP	Taibai (Sp 3)	Atrophic gastritis	110	91.8% were cured

Table 11-4. (continued)

Source	Mode	Acupoint	Diagnosis	No. of Patients	Effectiveness %
Wu (3, p. 63)	AP	Danshu (B 19) Zusanli	Chronic cholecystitis	375	11% were cured.
Liang (3, p. 58)	AP	Dazhui (Du 14)	Acute & chron. ulcerative colitis	50	74% were cured and other 20% improved
Deng (55)	AP	Zhongwan (Ren 12) Qihai (Ren 6)	Gastroptosis	100	64% recovered to the normal condition
Zhang (326)	AP	Youman (K 21)	Gastroptosis	37	68% were cured
Liu (159)	AP	Zusanli	Volvulus of stomach	70	97% improved
Beijing Tradit. Med. Coll. (2,p.65)	AP	Juque (Ren 14)	Gastroptosis	108	39.1% excellent result another 50.8% improved
Chinese Tradit. Med. Academy (2,p.64)	AP		Gastroptosis	66	21.2% recovered to normal condition
Shanghai Hosp. Team (2, p.60)	AP	Zhongwan (Ren 12) Zusanli	Gastroptosis	176	32.4% recovered to normal conditon; other 30% improved.
Shenyand Hosp. Team (2, p.66)	AP	Zusanli	Gastroptosis	197	46.2% excellent result; other 39.6% improved
Wu (280)	AP	Geshu (B 17) Zusanli	Chronic atrophic gastritis	420	45% improved
Nosalini (201)	AP		Esophagal achalasia	22	55% improved
Xu (3, p. 91)	AP	Zusanli	Indigestion	250	72% were cured
Lin (2, p. 45)	AP	Daheng (Sp 15)	Pediatric ascariasis	472	36.9% had worms expulsion

Table 11-4. (continued)

Source	Mode	Acupoint	Diagnosis	No. of Patients	Effectiveness %
Lo (173)	AP	Danshu (B 19) Zhiyang (Du 9)	Ascariasis	63	Completely cured after 7-15 treatments.
Wu (284)	AP & Moxi#	Zusanli Mingmon (Du 4)	Ulcerative colitis	79	89.6% were cured;
	IAc @ of B_{12}	Zusanli		43	63% were cured;
	Catgut EM			120	74% were cured
	Aur. Pr##	Ear		120	94.4% effective
	Laser			44	66% were cured
	Medication			33	33% were cured
Liu (171)	IAc of B_{12}	Changqiang (Du 1)	Anal prolapse	40	95% were cured
Feng (74)	Aur. Pr.	Ear	Constipation	50	84% were cured.

* AP = Acupuncture
# Moxi. = Moxibustion
@ IAc = Intra-acupoint injection
** Catgut Em. = Catgut embedding
Aur. Pr. = Auricular pressing with plaster
*** EAP = Electro-acupuncture

Acute Appendicitis

In an article describing their medical experience of the last thirty years, Fan and Zhang recited many ways to treat acute appendicitis and concluded that acupuncture is a safe and effective, conservative remedy (71). According to their report, during the years 1958–67 they used acupuncture therapy to treat acute appendicitis and obtained a 67.4 percent curative rate; another 31.3 percent improved and only 6.3 percent failed. The follow-up of 461 patients from 1967 to 1980 showed that 179 patients (38.8 percent) retained their appendix without recurrence of symptoms and 272 patients did undergo appendectomy. The causes of operation were partially due to failure of acupuncture therapy or to recurrence; a couple of cases were a by-product due to operations for other abdominal diseases. Ten patients died in this period, but not from appendicitis or the operation. Other investigators have also used acupuncture to treat acute appendicitis by using blood-letting punctures and a cupping technique at acupoint Fusche (Sp 13); a 61 percent cure rate was achieved (163).

Cardiovascular Diseases

Acupuncture therapy has been used successfully to treat many cardiovascular diseases, such as angina pectoris, coronary heart disease, arrhythmia and hypertension. T. G. Thieman (249) claimed that acupuncture therapy effective in cardiovascular diseases was much superior to the standard medicated therapy, based on improvements in pulse rate and symptoms during an eight-week period of acupuncture treatment. Dr. Omura, an electrophysiologist in New York, has postulated that acupuncture can increase vasodilatation in the microcirculation, and because most acupoints are points with lower electrical resistance than surrounding areas (see Chapter 4), when they were needled and stimulated electrically, this generated a pattern of bioelectrical field and modified certain physiological function, resulting in improvements in the cardiovascular system.

P. J. Li (144) speculated that acupuncture can reduce sympathetic nerve discharge and lower blood pressure by activating endorphinergic and 5HT-ergic neurons in the brain. K. Yazawa (304) reported that acupuncture can cause bradycardia through the vagal and ß-adrenergic activity.

K. Itaya et al., (104) performed the experiments on rabbits, measuring the cutaneous microcirculation of the earlobe. Acupuncture was applied at the acupoint Geshu (B 17) for thirty minutes. It was clear that the microvascular blood flow increased markedly, parallel with augmenting spontaneous rhythm fluctuations in vessel diameter, and continued for two hours following the release of the needle. The diameter of the arterioles and venules can reach a level of 200–250 percent of initial values. This may explain the clinical efficacy of acupuncture in increasing blood flow or lowering blood pressure.

Angina Pectoris

Acupuncture therapy can relieve anginal pain remarkably and reduce the dose of medication required. During the years 1965–79, a medical team in Beijing treated 621 cases of angina pectoris with acupuncture and reported an improvement rate of 89.2 percent. About 93.6 percent of the treated patients had a 50 percent or greater decrease in nitroglycerin use (2, p. 1 and 45; 16). Be, et al., (2, p. 5) reported 140 cases of angina pectoris treated with acupuncture and obtained an 84.3 percent excellent result rate. W. P. and P. C. Fan (69) treated 100 cases of angina pectoris with acupuncture once a day for thirty to forty minutes and repeated for ten sessions; after a two day break the treatment could be repeated if required. Fifty-two patients were asymptomatic after treatment, forty-two were improved, and the other six failed to obtain a benefit.

A. Richter, et al., (217) treated twent-one cases of stable angina with acupuncture at the acupoints Neiguan, Tongli (H 5), Xinshu (B 15), and Zusanli. After treatment, anginal attacks were greatly reduced and the intensity of pain and ST segment depression on EKG at maximal workload were also lowered significantly. The patients had a sense of improvement and well-being and greatly benefited from the treatment.

Acupuncture therapy was used to treat twenty-six patients with severe stable angina pectoris who were resistant to medication treatment. Compared with the control group of patients, where a sham acupuncture was performed on nonacupoints at random, the acupuncture group improved in terms of cardiac work capacity (11).

Cardiac Arrhythmia and Other Heart Diseases

Myocardial ischemia was produced experimentally in rabbits by ligation of the left ventricular branch of a coronary artery for thirty minutes (189). Animals treated with EAP at the Neiguan point were compared with a group without acupuncture. The glycogen content in the myocardium was significantly depleted in the control group (down 66.7 percent) and in the EAP group (down 29 percent). The depletion of phosphorylase in heart muscle correlated with the depletion of glycogen. EAP resulted in a much better chance of recovery. In another investigation with similar experimental technique EAP was found to effectively promote recovery of reversible lesions and to improve blood circulation (22, 314).

A team from Zhuzhow People's Hospital in China (2, p. 54) reported on acupuncture treatment in 100 cases of cardiac arrhythmia and angina pectoris and obtained an 81 percent excellent result rate. The EKG record of these patients showed a 46.8 percent improvement. Another two groups of investigators found that acupuncture resulted in a 20 percent complete relief rate in arrhythmias and an overall effectiveness rate of 72.6 percent (2, p. 53 and 55). In another report, 120 cases of cardiac arrhythmia were treated with acupuncture: 85 had significant relief of their symptoms and 38 were improved (2, p. 3).

In the second symposium on acupuncture and moxibustion, held in Beijing in 1984, several articles were presented on the effectiveness of acupuncture therapy in coronary heart disease. The effectiveness rate ranged from 61 percent to 87.5 percent. The diagnosis was based on EKG records (3, p. 6 and p.7). Acupuncture therapy in rheumatic heart disease gave an effectiveness rate of 66.6 percent (3, p. 3). In experiments on rabbits, H. L. Zhang (314) ligated the ventricular branch of the left coronary artery for about ten minutes to produce acute myocardial ischemia. Animals were treated with acupuncture at the acupoints Weishu (B 21) and Ximen (P 4). There was a marked reduction in the development in myocardial injury and rapid recovery of the animal. Animals treated with acupunture at random at any nonacupoints did not have any improvement.

Using the REPP measurement technique on the skin area, which has a low electrical resistance, K. Saku, et al., (221) reported that there was a positive correlation between the positive REPP test and the presence of acute myocardial infarction or angina pectoris as compared with healthy volunteers.

Acupuncture therapy was applied to thirty patients with acute myocardial infarction. There was definite improvement, with a significant change in electric resistance in the ear at the Shenmen point and heart region, indicating that acupuncture could be used as a supplement in the diagnosis of heart diseases (205).

By measuring left ventricle ejection time (LVET) in twenty-one patients suffering from chronic coronary arteriosclerosis, S. C. Chen and C. X. Liu (31) reported there was a positive linear correlation between the acupuncture effect and the physiological states of the patients. The average LVET was 19.9 ±2.20 msec. before treatment and was reduced to 4.91 ±0.85 msec. after acupuncture.

Lin, et al., (3, p. 514) applied EAP to twenty-four patients suffering from chronic myocardial infarction and found that acupuncture can increase the coronary blood flow and oxygen supply and can also promote collateral circulation. Bao, et al., (13) reported on acupuncture therapy of thirteen patients suffering acute myocardial infarction. The acupoint Neiguan was needled bilaterally. Seven patients had their symptoms completely alleviated, and the other six were greatly improved immediately after the treatment. The blood cAMP level of twelve patients was studied: eight had showed a fall in cAMP to an average of 10.1 pmol/ml level, and two were unchanged. One patient died suddenly of ventricular fibrillation, and another developed a cardiogenic shock. Chen, et al., (34) treated twenty-four cases of hypertrophic obstructive cardiomyopathy (HOCM) and sixteen cases of congestive cardiomyopathy (CCM), while twelve normal subjects served as controls. The acupoints Neiguan and Shaofu (H 8) were chosen. DC current at a frequency of 120 per minute was applied for two minutes. EAP at the Neiguan point increased the cardiac contraction and benefited the heart failure in CCM cases, but not in HOCM cases. However, electrical acupuncture at the Shaofu point decreased cardiac contraction and benefited HOCM but not CCM patients.

Seventy cases of coronary heart disease were treated with acupuncture (49). As compared with a group of patients treated with nitrate and Ca^{2+} blockers, the acupuncture group showed a significant improvement in their symptoms. The EKG pattern was changed significantly toward normal and the microcirculation of the fingernail was noticeably improved to various extents, especially acceleration of blood flow velocity in the capillary loop. The improvement was much more significant in those patients receiving a second course of acupuncture therapy.

Table 11-5 summarizes the clinical data on the acupuncture treatment of angina pectoris and other heart diseases.

Hypertension

Acupuncture therapy is also widely used to lower blood pressure in hypertensive patients. Chen, et al., (3, p. 14) treated thirty-five patients with essential hypertension with acupuncture daily for thirty minutes. The acupoints Qu Chi (LI 11) and Fenglong (S 40) were chosen. Twenty-eight patients benefited from this treatment (79 percent). Their systolic pressure decreased an average of 34.2 mm Hg and the diastolic pressure decreased 19.2 mm Hg within thirty minutes after the therapy.

In another report thirty cases of hypertension were treated with acupuncture. Feng Shi (G 20) and Zusanli were the acupoints for needling. The average decrease in of systolic pressure was 20 mm Hg and the diastolic pressure decreased 13 mm Hg (92).

S. A. Radzievskii et al. (214, 215) reported on the hypotensive effect of acupuncture therapy in forty-nine patients with essential hypertension. Acupuncture improved and normalized myocardial contractity and produced a reversal of the myocardial hypertrophy and decreased the sympathetic influence. Y. V. Anshelevich, et al., (8) reported that acupuncture therapy had an excellent effect to bring a hypotensive reflex in their patients, without producing a significant change in the prostaglandins level.

Table 11-5. Acupuncture Therapy in Cardiovascular Diseases

Source	Mode	Acupoint	Diagnosis	No. of Patients	Effectiveness %
Ballegaard (10)	AP*	Zusanli (S 36)	Angina pectoris	33	67% improved, 84% of the patients had reducing the dose of nitroglycerin taking
Beijing Coop (2, p.1 & 45)	AP	Zusanli	Angina pectoris	621	89.2% improved and 92.6% reduced their dose of nitroglycerin
Fan (69)	AP	Zusanli	Angina pectoris	100	52 completely recovered; other 42 improved.
Liang (150)	AP	Zusanli	Angina pectoris	621	89% effective
Meng (2, p. 46)	AP	Neiguan (P 6)	Angina pectoris	123	69% improved
Richter (217)	AP	Neiguan	Stable angina	21	Significantly improved
Sternfeld (242)	AP		Angina pectoris	15	87% improved, patients had reduction of drug taking & their anxiety
Zhou (333)	AP		Angina pectoris	30	Marked improvement and marked reduction of plasma level of 5HT and 5-HIAA
Academy of Trad. Med. (2,p.52)	AP	Neiguan	Coronary heart disease	64	91.4% improved
Fang (3, p.6)	AP		Coronary heart disease	40	87.5% improved based on EKG diagnosis
Nanjing Hosp. Team (3, p.7)	AP	Zusanli	Coronary heart disease	61	61% improved
Liu (3, p. 514)	AP		Chronic myocardiac infarction	24	Improvement by increasing the coronary blood flow and promoting collateral circulation

Table 11-5. (continued)

Source	Mode	Acupoint	Diagnosis	No. of Patients	Effectiveness %
Geo (3, p.53)	AP	Neiguan	Cardiac arrhythmia	46	25% completely relieved another 38% improved.
Zhuzhou Hosp. Team (2,p.54)	AP	Xinshu (B 15)	Cardiac arrhythmia	100	90% improved (46.8% of them proved by EKG)
Lin (2, p. 55)	AP		Cardiac arrhthmia	112	72.6% improved
Gao (83)	AP + Moxi.#	Neiguan	Sinus bradycardia	54	65% markedly effective other 22% improved
Sternfeld (241)	AP		Ventricular tachycardia with Wolf-Parkinson-White syndrome	9	All had their sinus rhythm restored
Sternfeld (243)	AP	Neiguan	Recurrent paroxymal supraventric. tachycardia	22	54.5% completely recovered; 27.2% partial recovered; and 13.6% moderately improved.
Meng (191)	AP with Magnetic plum-blossom needle	Zusanli Sanyinjiao (Sp 6)	Varicosis in the leg	411	62.4% were cured;other 27.8% improved
Yang (300)	AP	Zusanli Sanyinjiao	Hyperlipemia	82	84.5% completedly effective to lower the cholesterol, TG and LDL-C, and HDL-C up.

* AP = Acupuncture
\# Moxi. = Moxibustion

Auricular acupuncture was used to treat twenty-nine patients with essential hypertension (197). The patients had deteriorated cardiac function and their total peripheral resistance was very high before the treatment. After three months of daily acupuncture a significant lowering of blood pressure, with a fall of the total peripheral resistance and a significant regression of the left ventricular hypertrophy, was observed.

S. Ballegaard, et al., studied the effect of acupuncture on twenty-three healthy male volunteers and claimed that acupuncture had the ability to enhance the regulatory mechanisms of the cardiovascular system and to maintain cardiovascular homeostasis in healthy condition (12).

Studies on spontaneously hypertensive rats (SHRS) reported acupuncture applied on the acupoints Zusanli, HoKu, or Taichong for fifteen minutes for fifteen continuous days. Blood pressure was significantly lowered and the microcirculation of the bulbar conjunctiva was improved (337).

Hypotension of conscious or anesthetized dogs was induced by intravenous infusion of nitroprusside at a constant rate (291). EAP was applied on the Zusanli or Neiguan point. A pressure effect was observed. The effect is mainly due to an increase in cardiac output and decrease in renal blood flow, suggesting that EAP could cause a "reset" phenomenon in the baroreflex system.

Table 11-6 lists the clinical application of acupuncture therapy in hypertensive patients.

Hypercholesterolemia

Acupuncture therapy has been claimed to lower the plasma ß-lipoprotein level and the atherosclerosis index (AI) and increase HDL concentration. Forty-six patients suffering from cerebral infarction had a very low serum HDL (average 41.7 mg/dl). After forty-five days of acupuncture therapy the HDL was markedly elevated and the LDL level was decreased (210). C. W. Kum (128) treated 110 hospitalized patients with hypercholesterolemia with acupuncture at the acupoint Zusanli. The results are summarized in table 11-7. Other investigators have also reported such lowering cholesterol effects by acupuncture (254, 272).

Thrombophlebitis and Varicosis

Acupuncture therapy was used to treat forty-two cases of thrombophlebitis and produced a significant reduction in the swelling, redness, local heat and pain at the end of three days in twelve cases. Eighty percent of treated patients had a total remission after three months of treatment (216). In another study, seventy-seven cases were treated with acupuncture at the Zusanli point twice daily for forty minutes continued for months. Fifty-two patients were cured (67.5 percent) and four failed (303).

In 417 cases of varicosis of the lower extremities a round magnetic plum-blossom needle was applied at the acupoint Zusanli. The age of the patients ranged from seventeen to seventy-six years and the duration of disease was one to thirty-five years. The total treatment lasted for two years (258). The results are summarized in table 11-8.

Sickle-Cell Anemia

In Nigera, J. Sodipo treated five cases of sickle-cell anemia with acupuncture (237) and obtained a remarkable effect. The patients were dramatically relieved of pain and fever. HoKu and Neiting (S 44) were chosen as the acupoints and stimulated electrically at 3–10 Hz frequency. The acupoint

Xuanzhong (G 39) was chosen for bone marrow stimulation, combined with Geshu (B 17) as an acupoint for blood. After several treatments, an increase in hematopoiesis was observed. The hemoglobin was increased by an average of 21.1 percent and the hematocrit was elevated an average of 18.9 percent (from 12.2 percent initially to 26.7 percent after treatment). Body weight was increased by an average three to seven kilograms.

Stroke and Paralysis

The general treatments or management of stroke and postapoplectic paralysis are prevention, restoration of cerebral circulation, and physical therapy and rehabitation. The Chinese physicians and physiologists have claimed that acupuncture can exert beneficial effects by promoting the circulation in the affected region, activating the neurons, and stimulating the release of certain neurotransmitters in the brain.

In a recent article, S. Y. Bei, et al., (17) compared acupuncture therapy and medication therapy in eighty-three stroke patients. The age of the patients ranged from forty-one to eighty-two years. The results are summarized in table 11-9.

Qiu, et al., (3, p. 13) reported their studies on thirty-four cases of apoplexia (including twenty-seven cases due to cerebral embolism) treated with acupuncture at the acupoints HoKu, Shidou (Sp 17), and Qu Chi (LI 11) for thirty minutes daily and continued for five days; after a two-day break the treatment could be continued if necessary. After an average of 6.83 days of treatment, the clinical symptoms were eliminated in 93.3 percent of their patients.

In a ten-year period, Shi, et al., (3, p. 18) treated 422 apoplexia patients with acupuncture. The acupoints Neiguan and Sanyinjiao were chosen. After treatment 58.23 percent of the patients were clinically cured, woke up from unconsciousness, and spoke clearly to their families.

Zeig, et al., (3, p.20) reported the effect of acupuncture therapy on forty comatose patients after stroke from three weeks to one half year. Nine patients showed excellent result after the treatment and eighteen improved. Those patients stayed in the hospital for an average of 52.5 days and went home recovered from the coma.

Bi, et al., (3, p. 21) reported 133 cases of apoplexia treated with acupuncture. Sixty of them showed a remarkable improvement and were able to go back to work. Sixty-two were not completely recovered but could handle themselves well in their daily activities. Nine failed to achieve any benefit.

In 500 cases of cerebral vascular hemiplegia, Sun, et al., (3, p. 20) reported that acupuncture therapy produced a 47 percent curative rate. Four hundred and seventy-eight patients out of 500 recovered their muscular energy and 87 of them were able to go back to work.

Y. H. Chen, et al., (37) treated 162 cases of stroke with acupuncture on the paralyzed side. Several acupoints along the large intestine meridian were chosen for needling. The age of the patients ranged from thirty-seven to eighty-three years. Their results are summarized in table 11-10.

The authors pointed out that the success of the acupuncture therapy depended upon the time lapse after the stroke; the longer the time, the less the effectiveness. In general, a better result was obtained if the treatment was started soon after the stroke.

Table 11-6. Acupuncture Therapy in Hypertension

Source	Mode	Acupoint	Diagnosis	No. of Patient	Effectiveness %
Akhmedov (4)	AP* and Psy.#		Essential Hypertension (early stage)	100	A significant improvement of both systolic and diastolic pressure
Berns (19)	Ear AP		Essential hypertension (Type I & II)	45	Both blood pressure and cardiac function were improved, peripheral resistance was down.
Chen (3, p. 14)	AP	Quchi (LI 11) Fenglong (S 40)	Essential hypertension	35	78.9% effectively improved.
Mitrovskaya (195)	AP		Essential hypertension	110	Very effective
Monaenkov (197)	AP	Ear	Essential hypertension	29	Significantly improved; TPR was down; regression of hypertrophic left ventricle.
Razievskii (214, 215)	AP		Essential hypertension	49	Effective
Weng (274)	EAP**	Fengchi (G 20) Taichong (Liv 3)	Essential hypertension	43	Both systolic & diastoli pressure were lowered.
Zhang (327)	AP	Zusanli (S 36)	Essential hypertension	34	83.3% improved
Dovgyallo (59)	AP and exercise		Borderline hypertension	63	42.4% had their blood pressure back to normal
Chen (27)	Moxi. @	Zusanli	Hypertension	318	72.6% effective in one week of treatment.
Hsu (92)	AP	Fengchi	Hypertension	30	Both systolic & diastolic pressure were lowered in all patients
Wang (270)	AP	HoKu (LI 4) Neiguan (P 6)	Hypertension	68	Blood pressure was falling and rheoencephalogram showed improvement
Zhou (336)	AP with plaster	Ear	Hypertension	135	83.3% effective
Anshelevich (7)	AP		Aldosteronism hypertension	65	Lower the blood pressure

* AP = Acupuncture; # Psy. =Psychotherapy; ** EAP= Electro-acupuncture
@ Moxi. = Moxibustion

Table 11-7. Anti-hyperlipemic Effect of Acupuncture Therapy

Serum Concentration	Before Acupuncture	After Acupuncture
Triglyceride mmol/L	2.06	1.66
β-Lipoprotein mg/dl	621.19	606.13
Cholesterol mmol/L	7.04	6.43

(From Kun (128))

Table 11-8. Effect of Acupuncture Therapy on Varicosis

Degree of Symptoms	Cases	Cured	Improved	Failed
Mild	107	90 (84%)	17 (26%)	0
Moderate	255	154 (60.4%)	81 (31.7%)	20
Severe	55	16 (29%)	18 (32.7%)	21
Total	417	62%	27.8%	9.8%

(From Wang (258))

Table 11-9. Effectivenss of Acupuncture Therapy or Herbal Therapy on Postapoplectic Symptoms

Postapoplectic Symptoms	Treatment	No. of Patients	Duration of Disease	Result of Treatment: Clinically cured	Improved	Failed
Paralysis	Acupuncture	44	9 months to 2 yrs,	28 (63.3%)	18 (41 %)	1
	Chinese Herbs	39	3 months to 6 months	12 (31 %)	17 (44 %)	12
Skill motor activity	Acupuncture	32		13 (40.6 %)	16 (50 %)	3
	Chinese Herbs	38		5 (13 %)	7 (18.4 %)	24
Speech difficulty	Acupuncture	24		13 (54.2 %)	11 (46 %)	
	Chinese Herbs	35		6 (17 %)	29 (83 %)	
Tongue movement	Acupuncture	12		7	5	
	Chinese Herbs	21		1	19	1
Facial paralysis	Acupuncture	21		13	7	
	Chinese Herbs	-				
Swallow difficulty	Acupuncture	10		7	3	
	Chinese Herbs	22		4	11	7

(From Bei et al. (17))

Table 11-10. Effectiveness of Acupuncture Therapy on Apoplexy

Apoplexy due to:	No. of Patients	Acupuncture Therapy: Cured	Improved	Failed
Cerebral embolism	87	28 (32.8%)	52 (59.8%)	7 (8%)
Cerebral hemorrhage	49	1	37 (75.5%)	11 (24.4%)
Cerebral thrombosis	18	3	13 (72.2%)	2
Subarach hemorrhage	8	-	2	6
Total	162	32 (19.7%)	114 (70%)	26 (16%)

(From Chen (37))

In another report, 207 cases of stroke were treated with acupuncture along the anterior and posterior parieto-temperal oblique lines (330). Thirty-three percent of the patients were cured and another 57 percent were improved; the total effectiveness rate was 73.4 percent. In comparison, in 84 cases treated with medication, there was a cure rate of only 16.7 percent, and a total effectiveness rate of 64.5 percent. T. Takahashi (246) applied acupuncture by holding a needle percutaneously to the facial nerve of patients and could relieve them from the hemifacial spasm for about six months without producing a facial palsy. A similarly successful treatment of facial paralysis by acupuncture was reported by L. P. Wang (264).

In fifty-two cases of paralysis of the common peroneal nerve, acupuncture therapy was performed once a day with a plum-blossum needle (302). Forty-six cases with foot-drop symptoms were cured (88.5 percent). The patients started walking in a normal step. Four cases were improved and two failed. The time of treatment to reach the curative effect averaged twenty-eight days.

H. H. Hu, et al., (94) treated thirty cases of acute apoplexia within thirty-six hours with acupuncture or medication and found that the acupuncture treatment group had a much better result. In another report of seventy-eight patients with severe poststroke hemiparesis, thirty-eight received acupuncture and the other forty served as controls. The acupuncture group showed a much quicker recovery than the control group, with a significant difference in body balance, mobility, quality of life, and days spent at the hospital/nursing home (117).

M. Zhang and S. C. Chen treated 400 cases of hemiplegia with acupuncture. The age of the patients was forty to seventy-eight years. They had the hemiplegia present for over one week to three months, which was caused by cerebral embolism or hemorrhage. EAP was applied for twenty minutes daily. A course of treatment consisted of ten days. After two to four courses of treatment, 130 were cured (32.5 percent), 211 were improved (53 percent), and 59 had failed (14.7 percent) (320).

In 188 cases of apoplectic hemiplegia treated with acupuncture, the patients appeared to achieve the positive immediate effect of ability to raise their paralyzed limb. Eighty percent of the patients were improved by restoration of the motor function of their paralytic limbs (47).

In 1,620 cases of apoplectic hemiplegia, C. C. Wong (275) divided patients into two therapeutic groups. Group 1 consisted of 972 patients treated with acupuncture on both the affected and nonaffected sides; group 2 consisted of 648 patients treated with acupuncture on the affected side only. Table 11-11 summarizes the results.

Table 11-11. Effectiveness of Acupuncture Therapy on Postapoplectic Hemiplegia

Duration of Hemiplegia	Acupuncture Therapy Performed on: Both Sides				Affected Side Only			
	No. of cases	Cured (Percent)	Improved (Percent)	Failed (Percent)	No. of cases	Cured (Percent)	Improved (Percent)	Failed (Percent)
Within ½ yr.	428	47.2	1.2	1.6	287	20.7	57.8	11.5
From ½ yr to 1½ yrs.	363	37.7	52.9	9.4	213	24.9	46.9	28.2
From 1½ yrs. to 3 yrs.	181	0	72.4	27.6	148	0	48.4	51.6

(From Wong (275))

Fifty-nine cases of paralysis due to traumatic injury of the spinal cord at T12,L1 and L2 were treated with acupuncture (292). The patients had paralysis, urinary retention, involuntary defecation, and lost sensation in the lower body. Acupuncture was applied at the acupoint Zusanli. The patients indicated there was a numb and distention feeling at the beginning of needling, which spread downward. Laminectomy was performed and confirmed that the spinal cord was compressed. One year after the operation, patients were able to sit upright and had restoration of voluntary urination and defecation.

Y. C. Jian (111) treated 160 cases of severe facial paralysis with acupuncture and external electrical stimulation on the facial area. Seventy cases were cured (43.7 percent), eighty-nine were improved (55.6 percent), and one failed. He also reported that the pulse wave of the patient's ear was lower on the affected side than on the healthy side. After acupuncture therapy the ear pulse wave of all patients except one had increased to the normal value, indicating that the local blood circulation was distinctly improved by acupuncture.

Y. H. Fon, et al., (76) studied sixty children suffering from infantile cerebral palsy. They all had a lower equilibrium rate along the twelve meridian channels than healthy children. A small dose of acetylglutamate was injected into the acupoints Zusanli and Shousanli (LI 10). An elevation of the equilibrium rate along the meridian channels was observed.

Table 11-12 summarizes other clinical data on acupuncture therapy in stroke and paralysis.

Table 11-13 summarizes the clinical data on acupuncture therapy in facial paralysis.

Other Neurological Diseases

Multiple Sclerosis

Twenty-eight patients with multiple sclerosis were treated with acupuncture. The results were very satisfactory, with a remarkable spontaneous remission. However, because of the various characteristics of the disease, the validity of the success of the treatment is difficult to evaluate. Sometimes patients were sensitive to the needling on the locus that would provoke spasm, clonus, and even tonic-clonic contraction of the extremity muscles (240). In another report (236), two cases of multiple sclerosis were received by acupuncture therapy and showed a substantial improvement.

Studies on thirty-three patients with cervical osteochondrosis showed that acupuncture therapy can improve the cervical circulation and decrease the angiospastic state of the vessels and vascular tone, resulting in an increase in cervical blood flow and intensification of the vessels' activities (255).

Intelligent Quotient Mentality

Prenatal care and routine obstetric delivery by physicians or midwives were almost nonexistent in many rural regions in China. Mental retardation and low IQs were not necessarily due to genetic defects, but quite often a result of mishandling during the delivery or a result of malnourishment (e.g., low iodine rock salt in endemic regions). T. L. Lin and L. Y. Zhou (154) reviewed the data on acupuncture therapy in the treatment of mental retardation of Chinese children and stated that approximately 1–3 percent of children in China suffered of a low IQ or mental retardation. This is unbelievably high. In the early 1960s acupuncture was used to treat such children and the results were found to be very promising. One child suffering from mental retardation due to asphyxia during delivery was improved greatly after forty-two acupuncture treatments. In another twenty-five

Table 11-12. Acupuncture Therapy in Stroke and Paralysis

Source	Mode	Acupoint	Diagnosis	No. of Patient	Effectiveness %
Chen (37)	AP*	Multiple	Stroke	162	19.7% were cured and other 70 % improved.
Ga (80)	AP	Multiple	Stroke	208	22.2% were cured and other 69.4% improved.
Huang (99)	AP		Stroke	34	32.4% were cured; total effective rate 97%
Qin (3, p. 17)	AP	Hoku (LI 4)	Stroke	34	Total effective rate 93.3%
Shi (3, p. 18)	AP	Neiguan (P 6)	Stroke	422	58.3% clinical cured.
Shu (231)	AP	Fengchi (G 20)	Stroke	61	42.6% cured
	Medication			41	14.6% cured
Zhou (330)	AP	Multiple	Stroke	207	33.9% were cured, effective rate 73.4%
	Medication			84	16.7% were cured, effective rate 64.5%
Wong (277)	AP	Scalp	Acute cerebral thrombosis	63	Significantly improved
Li (141)	AP	Sanyinjiao (Sp 6)	Cerebral hemorrhage	30	21 of them (70%) showed a completed absorption of the hemorrhage after one treatment
Jiang (112)	AP		Cerebral thrombosis & hemorrhage	102	80.4% effective, the motor function of the affected leg was improved
Jin (113)	AP	Fengchi Zusanli (S 36)	Cerebral infarction	105	63.8% cured; another 30.4% improved.
Academy of Trad. Med. (2, p.69)	AP	Zusanli	Cerebral thrombosis	209	16.3 % were cured and 13% failed, other improved.
Wang (260)	AP	Zusanli	Cerebral infarction	86	80% were cured
Wang (2, p. 70)	AP		Cerebral hemorrhage	283	18.9% recovered; other 28.3% improved

Table 11-12. (continued)

Source	Mode	Acupoint	Diagnosis	No. of Patients	Effectiveness %
Yang (294)	AP & Moxi. #	Zusanli	Cerebral infarction	100	50% were cured, other 38% markedly improved
Yu (306)	AP	Scalp	Cerebral infarction	60	17% cured, other 25% markedly improved
	IAc@ of B_{12}			60	23% cured, other 50% markedly effective
Zhou (332)	AP	Baiku (Du 20) Zusanli Sanyinjiao	Cerebral thombosis	79	Improved, and the superoxide dismutase activity increased to normal range
Bi (3, p. 21)	AP		Postapoplectic hemiplegia	133	45% markedly improved
Bao (14)	AP	Scalp	Hemiplegia	79	7.5% cured and 25% improved.
Chen (38)	AP	Shenmen (H 7)	Hemiplegia (included spastic paralysis)	162	19.7% were cured
Cheng (40)	AP		Hemiplegia	108	90.9% improved
Chu (47)	AP		Hemiplegia	188	80% effective
Cui (50)	AP	Fengchi Neiguan	Postapoplectic aphasia	63	31.8% basically cured; other 35% markedly improved.
Ding (56)	AP		Hemiplegia	14	71% greatly improved after 5 wks treatment.
Fan (70)	AP	Zusanli	Hemiplegia	108	27.3% were cured
Hu (93)	EAP **	Scalp	Hemiplegia	150	45% cured and other 16% markedly improved
Huang (98)	AP		Hemiplegia	34	32% cured and other 47% markedly improved
Huang (95)	AP	Multiple	Postapoplectic paralysis	358	23% were cured; total effective rate 97.1%
Ja (105)	AP	Scalp	Hemiplegia	238	23% completely cured and 55% markedly improved

Table 11-12: (continued)

Source	Mode	Acupoint	Diagnosis	No. of Patients	Effectiveness %
Liang (149)	AP	Shenque (Ren 8)	Hemiplegia	101	96% effective
Jin (114)	AP	Temporal region	Postapoplectic paralysis	108	27% basically cured and other 44 % markedly improved
Milanov (192)	AP	Yaoshu (Du 2) Yamen (Du 15)	Hemiplegia	30	Patients showed a reduction of spasticity, an increase of muscle tone and a decrease of motor activity.
Semenova (224)	AP		Spastic dysplegia	90	Very effective
Shi (228)	AP	Scalp and Baihui (Du 20)	Hemiplegia	100	45% basically cured and 38% markedly improved
Shi (227)	AP & IAc inj.	Zusanli Sanyinjiao	Hemiplegia	108	38% bascially cured and other 40% markedly improved.
Sun (3, p.20)	AP		Hemiplegia	500	47% were cured, 95.7% had recovered their muscle energy and strength
Wang (257)	AP	Zusanli Sanyinjiao	Poststroke muscle dysfunction	49	40% cured and 52% improved
Wong (275)	AP	Scalp	Hemiplegia	233	25% were cured
Yuan (307)	AP	Scalp	Hemiplegia	41	53.7% basically cured; other 29% markedly improved
Zeig (3, p. 20)	AP	Zusanli	Postapoplectic coma	40	22.5% showed an excellent improvement; total effective rate: 67.5%
Zhang (320)	AP		Hemiplegia	400	32.5% were cured; other 21% improved
Li (3, p. 72)	AP	Fengchi, Hoku	Traumatic paraplegia	107	83% improved

Table 11-12, (continued)

Source	Mode	Acupoint	Diagnosis	No. of Patients	Effectiveness %
Lu (177)	Acupoint pressure		Infantile cerebral palsy	318	73.2% received an excellent to good result
Qiu (3, p. 90)	AP	Dazhui (Du 14) Zusanli	Infantile paralysis	4,967	25.9% completedly recovered
Yuan (307)	AP with 7-star needle	Futu (LI 18)	Infantile paralysis	260	11% cured and 30% markedly effective
Xiang (290)	AP	Scalp	Cerebral palsy	18	28% completely cured; 17% markedly improved
Yuan (309)	AP		Hysterical paralysis	26	Completely cured

* AP = Acupuncture; *** EAP = Electro-acupuncture
# Moxi. = Moxibustion; @ IAc = Intra-acupoint inj.

Table 11-13. Acupuncture Therapy on Facial Paralysis

Source	Mode	Acupoint	Diagnosis	No. of Patients	Effectiveness %
Jian (111)	AP*	Fengchi (G 20)	Severe facial paralysis	160	43.7% were cured and other 55.6% improved.
Chan (24)	AP	Zusanli (S 36)	Facial paralysis	107	99% completely recovered
Li (136)	AP	HoKu (LI 4) Fengchi	Facial paralysis	274	83% cured and other 9.9% improved
Liu (3, p. 43)	AP		Facial paralysis	1,021	69.2% cured, other 30.2% markedly improv
Liu (165)	AP with Plum-blossom needle		Facial paralysis	1,580	66.7% cured, other 32.6% improved
Liu (161)	AP	HoKu Xiaguan (S 7)	Facial paralysis	52	67% cured and other 19% markedly improved
Wang (271)	AP		Facial paralysis	25	28% cured, 32% improv
	Laser			51	35.2% cured, 37.2% improved.
Wu (3, p. 42)	AP		Facial paralysis	234	52% cured, total effective rate 97%
Yang (295)	EAP**		Facial paralysis	180	91.5% were cured
	AP, manual			40	70% cured
Yang (298)	IAc inj.# B_{12}	Yangbai (G 14) Sibai (S 2)	Facial paralysis	300	52.7% cured and other 30% recovered basicall
Yao (301)	AP with Plum-blossom needle	Affected side	Facial paralysis	50	96% cured
Zhang (318)	AP	HoKu, Fengchi Baihui (Du 20)	Facial paralysis	280	96.8% cured
Zhang (321)	AP	HoKu, Fengchi	Facial paralysis	74	95% were cured

* AP =Acupuncture; ** EAP = Electro-acupuncture
\# IAc inj. = Intra-acupoint injection

cases of mental retardation and paralysis, acupuncture therapy was performed for more than three months. Seven children regained their intelligence equivalent to other children the same age; the mentality of another sixteen children was also improved. In another case, a child with congenital mental retardation could not count or take care of himself. After three months of acupuncture therapy, his thinking ability was greatly improved, his reasoning was good, and he could read more than six hundred Chinese words. In a survey of 558 cases of such mental retardation in China, the authors claimed that acupuncture therapy had a 20.97 percent effectiveness rate.

M. Si (232) reported 120 cases of low-intelligence children with an average age of seven years. Their IQ was below 70. They were given acupuncture therapy at the Zusanli and Sanyinjiao points or an intraacupoint injection of vitamin B12 (100–500 μg). Twenty-three percent of them showed a remarkable improvement in comprehension and speech, and their IQ was increased substantially after treatment. In another report, acupuncture therapy was used to treated forty-six low-IQ children; 96 percent showed improvement (233).

In another 128 cases of childhood retardation, auricular acupuncture or body acupuncture was given. After three months of treatment, nine children had a marked improvement in their mentality and eighty-eight had a slight improvement (251). Sixty cases of idiot children were treated with auricular paste with Vaccaria seeds, which was attached on the Shenmen point of the ear and pressed; 58 percent showed a marked improvement in their intelligence, conversation, and memory (273).

K. L. Lin and L. Y. Zhou (162) reviewed the clinical reports from Chinese hospitals on acupuncture therapy of mental retardation of children and concluded that body acupuncture, scalp acupuncture, and auricular or intraacupoint injection resulted in an improvement rate of 28–40 percent. Combination therapy, including acupuncture and intraacupoint injection, gave a greater improvement rate, up to 63–71.4 percent. The younger the age, the better the success. Usually, after three months of treatment, the child could speak more words and take care of himself in daily life and thinking ability and comprehension were greatly improved.

J. K. Li (139) reported studies on 298 cases of pediatric hypophrenia treated with the auricular acupressure method. Fifty-four percent of the children raised their IQ by one grade level, 16 percent by two grade levels and 14 percent by three grade levels. The results were very impressive. In another article published in a Chinese journal, the same author detailed the improvement of 187 pediatric hypophrenia cases as follows (138):

Acupuncture Therapy	I.Q.	Reading and Memory
Before:	25.32	28.9
After:	45.92	51.84

Table (from LI, J.K. (138)).

Patients were separated based on their symptoms, such as general appearance, slowness, studiousness, and idiocy. All were improved after the acupuncture treatment.

Anxiety and Hyperactivity

V. Lanza (132) tested the biofeedback electromyograph of twenty-four people and found that acupuncture gave a quick fall in anxiety within the first three or four sessions of treatment and then a progressive improvement through the end of therapy. Acupuncture also appeared to improve the discharge of the learning behavior.

Acupuncture was found to be quite effective in sedating the hyperactive children and promoting a quicker onset of sleepiness (186). Such an effect was confirmed by measuring the EEG pattern of the subjects. F. Z. Liu and A. D. Jin (160) reported their finding on sixty-seven cases of insomnia treated with auricular acupressure for five to six minutes and three or four times daily. Forty-four patients lost their symptoms completely and had a comfortable sleep over six hours after three to five treatments. The advantage of this technique was that the patient could do it by himself at home.

Epilepsy

Almost any type of cerebral lesion may cause epileptic seizures. Seizures are presumably due to a sudden excessive, disorderly discharge of cerebral neurons. Acupuncture is not only used as a tool to diagnose the foci of the discharge (See Chapter 22), but is also used as a therapy to treat the epileptic episode.

Convulsions can be induced by injection of penicillin into the brain tissue of animals. Many invesigators have reported that EAP was effective in reducing such epileptogenic foci in the hippocampus, theorized by regulation of the biosynthesis of preproenkephalin (PPE) in the hypocampus by an alteration in gene transcription (256).

In studies on 144 epileptic patients, K. Y. Chen, et al., (30) measured the EEG pattern before and after acupuncture treatment and found that of those patients with an abnormal EEG in the pretreatment period, 60.2 percent manifested changes after the acupuncture treatment, mainly as asynchronism (meaning a reduction or cessation of the epileptiform discharge). But in those patients with a normal EEG in the pretreated period, there was no change after the treatment. The selection of acupoint for acupuncture played an important role. While needling at the acupoints Shenmen (H 7), Taichong (Liv 3), and scalp acupuncture at *du* meridian caused a marked EEG change, needling at HoKu, Zusanli and the thoracic zone of *du* maridian caused a less pronounced change.

Acupuncture therapy and CO2 bath were used to treat 106 patients suffering from atherosclerotic dyscirculatory encephalopathy. Assessment on their EEG and REG showed that acupuncture definitely produced a positive clinical improvement and increased the blood circulation (185).

In sixty-two cases of childhood's cerebral convulsion, acupressure was applied by strong manual stimulation at the acupoint of the nasal philtrun. Ninety-one percent of the convulsions of grand mal seizure disorder subsided within thirty seconds after the treatment, but the rest did not respond to the acupressure therapy. It was claimed that acupressure is definitely superior to the medication chloraldehyde. It resulted in therapeutic efficacy within a short time and caused no sedation to the patients (209). In another fifty-one cases of neurotic disorder of epilepsy, acupuncture was combined with anticonvulsive agents and found to be highly effective (9).

Table 11-14 lists another two reports on the effects of acupuncture treatment of epilepsy.

Table 11-14. Acupuncture Therapy in Epilepsis

Source	Mode	Acupoint	Diagnosis	No. of Patients	Effectiveness %
Cheng (41)	AP* and Herbs	Neiguan (P 6) Beihui (Du 20)	Epileptic seizure	64	48% were cured, without attack for 3 years
Hsu (91)	IAc # Catgut embedding	Fengfu (Du 16)	Epilepsis	60	53% were cured and other 22% markedly improved.

* AP = Acupuncture
\# IAc = Intra-acupoint

Urination Difficulties and Enuresis

Enuresis usually occurred in children with bladder instability or inadequate neurological control, characterized by nocturnal urination, and uninhibited contraction of detrusor muscles. Mothers scolded the child about bedwetting as an abnormal behavior and solicited treatment from the acupuncturist. It has been reported that acupuncture therapy can achieve a significant result in these cases. B. Minni, et al., (193) treated twenty children with enuresis with acupuncture. Eleven had gradual elimination of their enuresis symptoms (55 percent) and seven had improvement (35 percent). Other investigators also reported satisfactory results in treating sixty-two cases with acupuncture (124). Recent study on pediatric enuresis also showed that acupuncture therapy gave a 55 percent good effective result and a 40 percent long-term success rate (21).

One hundred and eleven children suffering from enuresis, varying in age from four to fifteen years old, were treated with acupuncture. After treatment, eighty-two were cured (74.5 percent) and five failed (156). Guo (3, p. 93) treated 250 cases of childhood enuresis with acupuncture at the acupoint Sanyinjiao and obtained a 36.8 percent cure rate and 12.4 percent ineffectiveness. Acupuncture therapy was used to treat 108 cases of pediatric enuresis, in patients aged from five to nineteen years. Thirty-four percent obtained an excellent result and another 37.9 percent were improved (103). In another report, 11 cases of chronic enuresis were treated with acupuncture therapy at acupoints Zhongji (Ren 3) and Zhibian (B 54). They were completely cured (101).

Adults can also have urinary incontinence and inability to control urination. A report showed that acupuncture therapy in 58 cases produced a 69.2 percent cure rate and 36.5 percent improvement rate (137). Fifty-two women with frequent urgent urination, or dysuria, were treated with acupuncture at the acupoint Sanyinjiao. It produced a periodic increase in intraurethral pressure and induced an inhibition of the detrusor muscle and external sphincter contraction. There was a 84.6 percent improvement rate (26).

Table 11-15 lists the recent clinical reports on acupuncture treatment of urination difficulties and enuresis.

Table 11-15. Acupuncture Therapy in Patients Suffered with Urination Difficulty

Source	Mode	Acupoint	Diagnosis	No. of Patients	Effectiveness %
Guo (87)	AP*	Sanyinjiao (Sp 6) Fengchi (G 20) Ciliao (B 32)	Neurological dysuria	60	68.8% cured and other 31.7% improved
Liu (166)	EAP**	Sanyinjiao	Anuria due to infection	13	All was cured after 1-13 treatments
Po (207)	AP	Sanyinjiao	Urinary retention after lumbar injury	12	Started to have urinatio after 1-10 treatments
Lin (151)	EAP	Zusanli (S 36) Sanyinjiao	Post-labor urinary retention	20	12 of them started to urinate after 1st. treatment
Lue (179)	AP	Yingxiang (LI 20)	Post-labor urinary retention	91	69% cured after one treatment, total 92% cured after 2 treatments
Wu (281)	AP	Sanyinjiao Zusanli	Postoperative urinary retension	46	87% relieved
Yang (294)	AP	Zusanli Sanyinjiao	Post-labor urinary retention	49	All was cured after average 19 treatments
Yang (296)	AP	Shenshu (B 23)	Urinary retention	14	71.4% cured after 10-12 treatments
Zhang (317)	AP with warming needle	Mingmen (Du 4)	Uncontrolled urination in old aged	57	49.1% cured and other 43.9% improved
Huang (96)	Moxi.#	Baihue (Du 20) Fengchi	Infantile enuresis	33	64% cured after 2-4 weeks treatment
Kachan (121)	AP		Pediatric enuresis	25	68% effective
Katai (122)	AP		Pediatric enuresis	15	68% effective
Po (208)	AP	Sanyinjiao	Enuresis	62	56% were cured and other 34% improved
Song (238)	AP	Shenmai (B 62)	Enuresis	135	82% were cured

* AP = Acupuncture; ** EAP = Electro-acupuncture
# Moxi. = Moxibustion

Other Psychiatric Disease

Z. X. Shi and M. Z. Tan (230) treated 500 cases of schizophrenia with acupuncture and obtained a 55 percent cure rate and a total effectiveness rate of 88.4 percent. The patients were divided into three groups according to their diagnostic symptoms. The mania group was treated with acupuncture at the acupoint on the *du* meridian; the depressive type was acupunctured at the point along the *ren* meridian; the paranoid type was acupunctured on the spleen meridian with strength and on the gallbladder meridian weakly. There was no significant difference between groups in sex, age, or frequency of attacks. The better therapeutic result was observed in cases with a shorter duration, less than one year of the illness, and a sudden or relatively sudden onset of the disease. Nine patients who had psychiatric disorder for over ten years responded excellently to acupuncture therapy. One hundred and ninety-four patients were followed up after they were cured by acupuncture therapy. A 32.5 percent recurrence rate was observed.

In the first symposium on acupuncture held in Beijing, a team from Shenyang Hospital (2, p. 8) reported on 403 cases of schizophrenia treated by acupuncture. The cure rate was 54.4 percent and the total effectiveness rate was 88.6 percent. A report from another team (2, p. 37) showed that acupuncture therapy in eleven cases of mental depression achieved the same therapeutic effect as the tricyclic compound amitriptyline.

Shuaib, et al., (120, p. 583) treated forty psychiatric patients with EAP and obtained a good relief rate of 60–90 percent. Most symptoms such as sadness, insomnia, headache, fatigue, and tension were much improved.

V. I. Markelova, et al., (186) treated patients with neurotic depressive disorders with acupuncture and claimed that the acupuncture achieved an effective improvement of the symptoms. There was also improvement in biochemical parameters, such as 5HT levels, and urinary concentrations of NE, DA, and DOPA.

M. J. Zhang (322) treated 296 cases of hallucinations with scalp acupuncture. After ten sessions of treatment, hallucinations became less and less, finally completely disappearing.

In psychiatry, electric shock therapy (EST) was used for decades in treating manic-depressive patients. But the treatment is traumatic. The post-EST patient has to withstand stress and suffers a period of loss of memory. It creates an unshakable fear in patients and also their families after witnessing a confused disorientated period during the EST and an amnesiac period of insanity. In China EAP has been used to replace EST. Z. M. Dong (58) treated twenty cases with needling at the acupoint Renzhong (S 17) and stimulation with an electric current continuously at two- to four-second intervals until reaching a condition of tonic muscular spasm. He presented the results of acupuncture shock therapy as compared with standard EST as follows:

Treatment	No. of Cases	Cured	Failed
Electric Shock	50	38 (76%)	2 (4%)
Electric Acupuncture	20	8 (40%)	5 (25%)

Table (from Dong (58)).

In the early 1950s Xue, et al., (3, p. 33) used EAP therapy to replace the ordinary EST in the treatment of schizophrenia patients and found it to be superior. They coined the term Electric Acupuncture Shock Therapy (EAST). Sixty-eight patients with schizophrenia were studied, their ages ranging from nineteen to forty-eight years. They were divided into two groups: half were treated with EST, applied on the temporal region, with a current of 3497 joules and an average time of 3.11 seconds. The other half received EAST, with a current of 1.27 joules (less than one-thousandth of EST intensity). The acupoints Baihui (Du 20) and Renzhong (S 17) were chosen. The average treatment time was 1.87 seconds. The advantage of EAST is safety. Very few patients treated with EAST required artifical respiration, and only one needed oxygen inhalation. On EEG examination, convulsions and memory disturbance occurred more often in EST group than in the EAST group. After eight treatments, 80 percent of patients in the EST group had a memory disturbance, but only 35.7 percent in the EAST group had that problem. The time for EEG recovery to normal averaged 29.07 days for EST and 17.03 days for EAST. Two patients in the EST group still had an abnormal EEG pattern after three months, but none in the EAST group had that problem.

In terms of side effects of the therapy, fifteen patients in the EST group (44.1 percent) developed a spinal fracture, while only five cases in the EAST group (14.7 percent) had that problem.

EKG examinations and sugar tolerance tests in these patients showed no abnormalities.

Kurland (120, p. 579) used low-frequency EAP to treat three psychiatric cases. Two were suffering from manic depression and one was schizophrenic. The EAST therapy assisted in producing a significant remission in depressive symptomatology. Although it did not eradiate all disorders and did not allow complete discontinuation from the medications such as antidepressants and neuroleptic agents, the treatment was more easily adaptable to the outpatient clinic.

Vitou, et al., (120, p. 589) used the low-intensity electric stimulation (50 Hz) to treat thirty psychiatric patients at the Shenmen point of the ear. Eighty-three percent of the patients responded well to the treatment and remained completely free of drug medication use for six months. Other patients were able to reduce the dosage of drug they required.

V. D. Kochetkov, et al., (123) studied the effects of acupuncture therapy on 121 patients suffering from asthenic conditions in neurosis. They found that patients definitely were responding well to acupuncture therapy. Sixty-seven percent of the patients were improved and had a positive normal noctural sleep. The duration of sleep was lengthened, and there was an increase of their adrenal function.

Insomnia

Lee (120, p. 572) reported that fifteen out of sixteen patients with insomnia had a substantial improvement after auricular acupuncture therapy. The effect appeared almost immediately after the treatment. Eleven resumed a normal sleep pattern and were able to sleep for more than seven hours without other medications. The therapy was carried out an average of two or three times. All symptoms completely disappeared and patients remained symptom-free at three months' follow-up.

Acupuncture therapy has also been promoted to be a personalized treatment of insomnia, particularly for reharmonizing a disturbed sleep-wake cycle (198). Table 11-16 summarizes the clinical reports on acupuncture therapy in psychiatric patients.

Table 11-16. Acupuncture Therapy in Psychiatric Diseases

Source	Mode	Acupoint	Diagnosis	No. of Patients	Effectiveness %
Feng (75)	EAP *	Scalp	Schizophrenia	34	35% had their symptoms completely disappeared, other 29% markedly improved.
Sen (225)	IAc inj.# of B_{12}	Dazhu (B 11) Zusanli (S 36)	Schizophrenia	105	94% were cured
Shi (229)	AP**	Multiple	Schizophrenia	500	55% were cured; other 16.6% markedly improv[ed]
Zhang (312)	EAP	Baihui (Du 20)	Schizophrenia	69	42.1% effective, thei[r] mentality was improve[d]
Liu (157)	AP	Yongquan (K 1)	Hysteric mutism	68	97% cured after one treatment
Romoli (218)	Ear Ap		Psychosomatic disorder	50	Significantly improve[d]
Zhang (323)	AP bilateral	Yifeng (Sj 17)	Auditory hallucination	48	54% had their hallucination abolished, other 37.3% symptom relieved
Zhang (325)	Pl @ with Vaccaria seeds	Ear	Insomnia	60	60% cured and other 38% improved
Zhang (324)	AP	Baihui	Insomnia	110	62% cured and other 32% improved

* EAP = Electro-acupuncture; ** AP = Body acupuncture
# IAc inj. = Intra-acupoint injection;
@ Pl = Plaster

Pulmonary Diseases

Asthma

Bronchial asthma is prevalent in China. Its major impact lies in its ability to cripple patients, both functionally and emotionally. It is common in children, but some patients experience the onset of asthma in adult life. The Chinese herb *ma huang* has been used for thousands of years to treat both allergic and nonallergic types of asthma. It was introduced to Western medicine in the 1920s by Prof. K. K. Chen and the major ingredient, ephedrine, was isolated. Ephedrine is a potent sympathomimetic amine that produces a bronchial dilatation effect (97). But its use has limits including the development of drug tolerance and adverse effects, such as heart palpitation and elevated blood pressure.

Acupuncture has become one of the alternate remedies for asthma. It is safe and effective, especially in chronic bronchial asthma. Reports from the last decade have shown that asthma is effectively treated by several alternative acupuncture techniques. Those include the plum-blossom needle, the catgut embedding, acupoint pressing, intraacupoint injection of drug, cupping, and moxibustion. The beneficial action is partially due to promotion of immunoactivity and partially to its bronchodilating effect through stimulation of the nervous system. However, Y. M. Joshi (119) indicated that acupuncture has limited success in the treatment of acute asthma, because it is a weak bronchodilator. Nevertheless, in chronic asthma, acupuncture has an excellent prophylactic effect and can produce a modern significant improvement in pulmonary function. T. C. Medici (189) considered acupuncture as one alternative therapy for both acute and chronic allergic asthma, especially in short-term effect.

In the years 1974 to 1978, 205 cases of bronchial asthma were treated by a team from the Chinese Traditional Medical Academy (2, p. 57) with acupuncture therapy. A 22 percent cure rate and a total 82 percent effectiveness rate were reported. Another team from Shanghai Hospital (2, p. 58) reported 299 cases of asthma treated with acupuncture. A 29 percent excellent result rate and a total 70.6 percent improvement rate were obtained.

J. Q. Zang (310) treated 192 cases of bronchial asthma with acupuncture at the acupoints Kongzu (L 6) and Yuji (L10). Ninety-eight per cent of the patients had immediate relief of symptoms and 76.5 percent had a clinical remission. The effect was especially remarkable in asthma cases related to cold and allergy. N. N. Osipora, et al., (202) treated eighty-seven patients with bronchial asthma and chronic obstructive bronchitis and found that acupuncture therapy can reduce the symptoms.

In another report, ten patients with bronchial asthma, aged from eight to sixty years, were treated with EAP ten times biweekly for three minutes. The results were remarkable. Acupuncture therapy not only improved the patients' immunity and pulmonary function, but also produced a freedom from asthmatic attacks (42).

In twenty-nine chronic asthma patients acupuncture therapy was given for twelve weeks and followed up for six months. All patients were greatly improved after the treatment and remained in a stable condition, free of attacks (194).

The benefit of acupuncture therapy on asthma is not only an immediated relief of symptoms, but also a reduction in the dosage of medication. For example, acupuncture therapy was given to twelve patients with corticosteroid-dependent chronic asthma and produced a significant reduction in asthmatic attacks and the steroid dosage requirement (16). Sternfeld, et al., (244) treated nine extrinsic asthmatic patients with acupuncture therapy and found that they were able to reduce the dosage of bronchodilator and steroid medications, but there was no change in skin reactivity or in IgE level. Fifty-one cases of chronic spastic bronchitis were treated with acupuncture for three years; treatment consisted of two or three months of treatment and the two or three months of recess (235). Thirty-six patients completed their three years' treatment course and 63.8 percent of them were able to eliminate their steroid medication; 13.9 percent still took the drug, but the dosage was reduced by one-half or more. In seven cases, all other medications were no longer required.

P. A. Christensen, et al., (45) reported the results of acupuncture therapy in seventeen stable bronchial asthma patients as compared with a placebo group. The treatment lasted for eleven weeks. The acupuncture group had significant symptomatic improvement. D. Berger and D. Nolte (18) treated twelve asthma patients with acupuncture and found a significant decrease in airway resistance in nine patients (75 percent).

Wang, et al., (261) reported on acupuncture therapy in 155 cases of asthma during the years 1975–93. Forty-five patients were cured (29.6 percent), seventy-four were improved (47.7 percent), and thirty-six showed no effect. In 2,125 cases of chronic bronchitis and asthma, C. Lu, et al., (176) found that acupuncture therapy produced a remarkable effect and improvement rate. Their results are summarized in table 11-17.

Moxibustion has often been used in combination with acupuncture. J. M. Shao and Y. P. Ding (226) treated 111 cases of asthma with acupuncture and moxibustion in combination, at the acupoints Feishu (B 13) and Dazhui (Du 14). Pulmonary function was measured by electro-thoracograph before and after the treatment. They found that combined treatment gave a significant improvement in lung function and symptoms. C. P. Wu (282) treated 386 cases of pediatric asthma with moxibustion only. The age of the patients ranged from one to eighteen years, and some had suffered from the disease for over seventeen years. The acupoints Dazhui, Feishu, and Yongquan (K 1) were chosen. The results are summarized in table 11-18.

K. P. Fung, et al., (78) treated nineteen children who had exercise-induced asthma with acupuncture therapy and concluded that the treatment provided a good protective effect against asthmatic attacks.

However, there is some doubt about the effectiveness of acupuncture therapy in the treatment of asthma. A team from UCLA (248) studied twenty-five cases of moderate to severe asthma, treated them with acupuncture, as compared with placebo (sham acupuncture). The course of treatment was twice per week for four weeks. They failed to show any significant effect in either group in terms of symptoms, medication use, or lung function measurements. Only two subjects demonstrated a significant favorable response to the real acupuncture therapy, but they failed to show any short-term or long-term beneficial effect. O. K. W. Chow, et al., (43) reported on sixteen cases of exercise-induced asthma treated with auricular acupuncture over lung loci, as compared with sham needle over lumbago loci. They found no significant change in baseline forced expiratory volume or the vital capacity, suggesting that acupuncture did not alter basal bronchomotor tone in these patients.

A very interesting therapeutic technique for asthma has been described by N. L. Tang (247). He treated 1,500 cases of chronic bronchitis and asthma with a cross-embedding technique of xenogeneic fat from the acupoint Tanzhong (Ren 17) of patient A to the acupoint Yuji (L 10) of patient B, or vice versa. After one month of such cross embedding from two different acupoints, 652 patients showed a significant improvement or cure (42 percent), and 7.7 percent did not show any effect.

Table 11-19 summarizes other clinical data on acupuncture treatment of asthmatic patients.

Acupuncture is also a useful alternative approach to the treatment of allergy and homeopathy, especially in the treatment of allergic asthma. In one study, 143 patients suffering from type I allergy, including allergic asthma, allergic rhinitis, and chronic urticaria, were treated with acupuncture. The patients responded better to acupuncture therapy than desensitization therapy (131).

Table 11-17. Acupuncture Therapy of Bronchitis and Asthma

Diagnosis	No. of	Cured		Improved		Failed
	Cases	No.	%	No.	%	
Chronic Bronchitis	702	158	22.5	541	77	3
Asthma	1,423	141	9.9	1,274	89.5	8
Total	2,125	299	14.0	1,815	85.4	11

(From Lu et al. (176))

Table 11-18. Effectiveness of Acupuncture Therapy on Asthmatic Children Related to Their Age

Age (Yrs.)	No. of	Effectiveness					
	Patients	Cured		Improved		Failed	
		No.	%	No.	%	No.	%
Under 5	96	39	40	48	50	9	9
6-12	152	53	38	39	25.6	15	10
13-18	138	55	40	70	51	13	9.4
Total	386	147	38	157	41	38	10

(From Wu (282))

Table 11-19. Acupuncture Therapy in Asthma and Other Respiratory Diseases

Source	Mode	Acupoint	Diagnosis	No. of Patient	Effectiveness %
Chu (48)	AP* and IAc inj.# of Herb extract	Tianzhu (B 10)	Bronchial asthma	1,113	9.3% were cured; 68% improved; 2% failed
Academy Tradit. Med. (2, p. 57)	AP	Feishu (B 13)	Asthma	205	22% clinically cured; effective rate 82%
Yea (2, p. 58)	AP and Moxi. @		Asthma	299	29% excellent result; total effective rate 70.6%
Peng (3, p.51)	AP		Asthma	30	85.7% symptomatic relieved, and 5 cases had an elevation of cAMP
Shao (3, p. 50)	AP	Zusanli (S 36) Feishu	Asthma	111	43.2% effective
Chondkury (42)	AP		Asthma	10	Free of attack and improvement of all symptoms and pulmonary functions
Osipor (202)	AP		Asthma	87	Effectively improved
Wang (261)	AP		Asthma	155	29.6% cured; other 47.7% improved
Zang (310)	AP	Kongzu (L 6) Yuji (L 10)	Asthma	192	76.2% clinically remission
Zwolfer (338)	AP		Adult asthma	17	Over 70% showed significantly improved
Chen (32)	IAc inj. of Herb extract	Zusanli Feishu	Pediatric asthma	63	40% markedly effective; and other 44% improved
Wu (282)	AP		Pediatric asthma	386	38% clinically cured; other 40.7% improved
Wu (286)	AP	Dazhui (Du 14) Feishu	Pediatric asthma	386	39.4% were cured;other 51% improved

Table 11-19. (continued)

Source	Mode	Acupoint	Diagnosis	No. of Patients	Effectiveness %
Lu (176)	AP	Multiple	Chronic bronchitis & asthma	2,125	44% were cured; total effective rate 85.4%
Moi (196)	Em.** with Catgut	Danzhong (Du 17)	Chronic bronchitis & asthma	100	87% effective
Tang (247)	Cr.Bed.##		Chronic bronchitis & asthma	1,500	42% improved
Slivinski (235)	AP		Spastic bronchitis	51	63.8% improved, patie[illegible] stopped their sterol administration
Yang (299)	PL*** with Vaccaria seeds	HoKu (LI 4) Dachangshu (B 25)	Pediatric respiratory diseases	104	46.8% cured and other 50.5% improved
Zhang (315)	PL	Ear	Pediatric respiratory diseases	370	61% cured and other 27.6% markedly improv[illegible]

* AP = Acupuncture
\# IAc. inj. = Intra-acupoint injection
@ Moxi. = Moxibustion
** EM = Acupoint embedding with Catgut
\## Cr. Bed. Cross bedding of acupoint's fat from one point to other
*** Pl. = Plaster

Hansen (120, p. 670) described a two-year experience on the use of acupuncture therapy in the treatment of patients whose illnesses had not responded to conventional Western medicine approaches. He found that acute and chronic respiratory tract infections, such as the common cold, chronic bronchitis, chronic sinuitis, chronic lingual tonsillitis, and nonspecific laryngitis responded to acupuncture therapy with surprisingly good results. Cough and congestion were decreased, breathing was improved, and there was a marked sense of general improvement. Also, he stated that intractabale hiccup responded well to acupuncture therapy. One patient suffering from constant hiccups for ten days after open heart surgery had not responded to any conventional approaches. He was treated with acupuncture. The hiccups stopped within fifteen minutes. In a second case, a child with cerebral palsy had been overwhelmed with hiccups for forty-eight hours and had not responded to any medication but responded to acupuncture within twenty minutes.

Lau, et al., (120 p. 688) treated twenty-two subjects with allergic rhinitis with acupuncture. After a series of six treatments, eleven (50 percent) were virtually symptom-free. Eight patients (36 percent) had a marked reduction in symptoms. Three (14 percent) showed no improvement. Laboratory tests showed a significant decrease in blood eosinophils and a reduction in plasma IgE level to 64 percent of baseline in patients who completed the treatment and to 76 percent level at two months' follow-up.

Whooping Cough

L. M. Zhang found that acupuncture therapy is very effective in treating pediatric whooping cough (316). In this report, 120 patients aged three months to seven years received acupuncture once a day for five days and were compared to a control group consisting of thirty- patients treated with antibiotics and Chinese herbs for five days. The acupuncture group had a remarkable effect as shown below:

Table of Treatment Outcome, Acupuncture vs. Medication.

Treatment	No. of Cases	Cured	Failed
Acupuncture group	120	89	3
Medication group (antibiotics + chinese herbs)	38	1	28

Three hundred and ten children suffering from pertussis were treated with acupuncture at Dazhui (Du 14) and Feishu (B 13) points and cupping for five minutes. After three treatments 72.5 percent were cured, and after four treatments all were cured (279).

Chronic Obstructive Pulmonary Disease

Twenty-four patients suffering from disabling breathlessness due to chronic obstructive pulmonary disease were divided into two groups. Half were treated with acupuncture and the other half with placebo (sham acupuncture). After three weeks of treatment, the acupuncture group had a significant benefit in terms of breathlessness and six-minute walking distance. There was no objective change in lung function in either group (116).

Other Infectious Diseases

Epidemic Encephalitis

During the years 1970–89, a total of 500 cases of epidemic encephalitis B were treated in a Chinese hospital (219). Three hundred and forty-eight people received acupuncture therapy. The duration of the ailment ranged from fifteen days to one year. Some patients suffered a type of paralysis and were treated with auricular acupuncture and scalp acupuncture. A cure rate of 52.8 percent was obtained. G. Z. Luo (182) reviewed 910 cases of encephalopathy treated with scalp acupuncture techniques in which 150 cases (16 percent) were basically cured, 370 (40.6 percent) were markedly improved, and 390 (42.9 percent) did not show any beneficial effect.

Q. F. Cheng reported on forty-three cases of encephalitis while he was practicing in Africa. The patients had not responded to any medical treatment and were given acupuncture therapy at the Fengchi and HoKu points. Thirty-five of them were cured (87.4 percent) (39).

Hepatitis

The Hubei Hospital in China (2, p. 41) reported 212 cases of icteric viral hepatitis treated with auricular acupuncture and the supplemental medications, glucuronic acid, and vitamins B and C. After an average of 14.2 days of treatment the patients recovered from the illness and were symptom-free. The SGPT level decreased to a normal range. Another team from Chengdu Hospital (2, p. 43) reported 68 cases of viral hepatitis treated with body acupuncture at the acupoints HoKu and Sanyinjiao. Sixty patients (88 percent) were clinically cured. A follow-up of 46 cases in twenty-six months showed no relapse. Two hundred and three cases of acute toxic hepatitis were treated with auricular acupuncture. Ninety percent of them had a satisfactory result (158).

Acupuncture therapy has been used to treat chronic hepatitis B infection. After three months of treatment 18.2 percent of patients showed a marked effectiveness and another 20.4 percent showed improvement (77). In another study in eighty-two hepatitis B carriers, acupuncture therapy attenuated the plasma levels of IgG and IgA, with little effect on IgM level (35).

Skin Infections

Acupuncture has been used to treat sixty cases of skin infection with furuncles that had not responded well or were resistant to antibiotic therapy. Fifty-seven of them (95 percent) were completely cured (258).

Herpes Zoster

Postherpetic neuralgia is especially serious in elderly people. In twenty-nine such cases treated with acupuncture, H. C. Dung (65) found no significant improvement in patients over sixty-five years old, but in young patients, especially those who had been sick less than six months, a better symptomatic relief was obtained. Similar conclusions have been reported by other investigators treating herpes zoster with EAP techniques (23).

Acute Epidemic Parotidis

In a seven-year period, Long, et al., (174) treated 262 patients suffering with epidemic parotidis involving one or both sides, with acupuncture or medication. The patients had the infection from about two days, with fever, headache and anoxia, swelling of the gland(s), and intense pain. Of the 192 patients treated with auricular acupuncture, 119 were cured (61.9 percent) and 5 failed. In another 170 cases treated with medication, only 26 were cured (15.3 percent).

Gonorrhea

One hundred and eleven cases of gonococcal arthritis were treated with acupuncture therapy at the Zusanli point. Seventy-four patients were cured (63.8 percent) after three courses of treatment (268). S. J. Wang (269) reported his experience on the use of acupuncture in treating 405 cases of nongonorrheal urethritis while practicing medicine in East Africa. The patients received an average of three courses of treatment at the acupoints Taichong (Liv 3) and Sanyinjiao (Sp 6). A cure rate of 64.4 percent, an improvement rate of 21 percent, and a failing rate of 14 percent were observed.

Leprosy

EAP has been used effectively in the treatment of leprosy. When given at the correct acupoint, it can stimulate the paralyzed muscles of the patient and prevent disuse atrophy. It also serves as a more effective method to get physicial therapeutic improvement and healing of early deformities. Acupuncture also relieves pain in leprosy patients (107).

Prostatitis

Twenty-five cases of chronic incurable prostatitis were treated with EAP and magnetic plaster. A total effectiveness rate of 72 percent was obtained. Some associated symptoms, such as constipation, diarrhea, and lumbago, were also improved after the treatment (82). In fifteen cases of incurable chronic prostatitis, EAP was given weekly. Excellent clinical efficacy was demonstrated in 10 cases and moderate efficiency in 5 cases (221). In another 100 cases of chronic prostatitis, acupuncture therapy was curative in 46 (178). Seventeen patients suffering from chronic prostatitislike syndrome and refractory to conventional medical treatment were treated with EAP with low frequency. The overall efficacy rate for long-term treatment reached 100 percent. Patients either were completely withdrawn from previous medication or reduce the dosage of the drug taken (102).

Acquired Immune Deficiency Syndrome

AIDS is still a major problem faced by Western nations because of the lack of a specific curative medicine or an effective vaccine to eradicate the virus (HIV). There have not been many cases of AIDS reported in China. So neither the government nor the medical profession has made much of an effort to find a cure for this disease. However, it has been claimed that acupuncture can increase body immunity and may indirectly be of benefit in AIDS treatment. N. Rabinowitz (213) reported 200 cases of AIDS and AIDS-related complex treated with acupuncture. He stated that although acupuncture therapy is not a cure, it was beneficial to patients on a physiological, emotional, and spiritual level and had a significant prophylactive success.

While practicing in Thailand, Si reported five cases of AIDS treated with acupuncture with a plum-blossom needle and moxibustion combination. The patients also suffered from herpes zoster over the chest and face. After fourteen treatments, scars were healed and pain was relieved, but the patients remained HIV positive (234).

Lithiasis

Acupuncture therapy has been claimed to promote relaxation of the sphincter muscle. Therefore, it could be helpful in treating lithiasis. In a report from Wendeng Hospital in China (2, p. 5), a total of 592 cases of cholelithiasis were treated with acupuncture. The acupoints Qimai (SJ 18) and Riyue (G 24) were chosen, and other therapies, such as antishock and fluid therapy, were given concomitantly. Three hundred and sixty patients (69 percent) had their gallstones expelled within one to five treatments. In seventy-three patients serving as controls and receiving medication therapy, only fifteen (20.5 percent) had expulsion of the stones. Zhou, et al., (25, p. 588) reported 522 cases of cholelithiasis treated with EAP plus a dose of $MgSO_4$ once a day. Seventy-eight percent of the patients had their stone expelled in the feces and sixteen patients had no effect; among them, six died.

In another report, 365 cases of cholelithiasis were treated with acupressure over the ear points (57). The treatment was remarkably effective; after thirty to forty-five treatments, 81.9 percent of the cases showed total stone expulsion, and a short-term cure was obtained in 19.7 percent of them. W. S. Gon and E. H. Shem (85) reported on fifty-six cases of biliary colic due to acute choleangitis, cholecystitis, or cholelithiasis. Acupuncture therapy produced symptomatic relief and pain suppression within 3.64 minutes in twenty-nine patients (57.1 percent). Another group of patients was treated with atropine and analgesics that proved to be inferior and took a longer time (average 10.9 minutes) to produce similar pain relief.

M. P. Wang (266) treated 454 cases of urolithiasis with auricular acupuncture and body acupuncture at the acupoint Sanyinjiao. Ninety-two percent were cured. The stones were expelled automatically after a while and the patients were symptom-free. Eleven patients did not obtain any benefit from the treatment.

In forty-eight cases of urolithiasis, uretero-renal colic was immediately relieved by acupuncture therapy and local anesthetic block at the acupoint Jianyu (LI 15) (1 percent lidocaine solution was injected into the acupoint) (223). Some patients had recurrence of pain, but it was much milder than before treatment. In another report, acupuncture therapy effectively relieved renal colic, better than medications (134).

Table 11-20 summarizes other clinical data on acupuncture therapy of lithiasis.

Overweight and Obesity

Ovverweight and obesity are mainly a dietary problem occurring in Western countries, being uncommon in China. H. C. Dung (62) has summed up his four years of practice in an acupuncture clinic in San Antonio, Texas. Among 3,464 patients, 6.64 percent (more females than males) came in for weight reduction. In China it is rare to see a fat woman or man on the street or in a clinic

Table 11-20. Acupuncture Therapy in Lithiasis

Source	Mode	Acupoint	Diagnosis	No. of Patients	Effectiveness %
Dong (57)	Pl * with Vaccaria seeds	Ear	Cholelithiasis	365	81.9% have stone expelled
Li (146)	AP**	Weizhong (B 40) Zusanli (S 36)	Renal lithiasis	25	88% stone expelled
	Medication			27	only 26% had stone expelled
Du (60)	AP with bristle-like needle	Sanyinjiao (Sp 6)	Urinary lithiasis	32	62.5% had their stone expelled
Wang (265)	AP or Ear AP	Sanyinjiao Shenshu (B 23)	Urinary colic and Lithiasis	454	92% had their stone expelled and symptoms disappeared

* Pl = Plaster
** AP = Body Acupuncture

seeking weight reduction treatment, except for other medical reasons or under the advice of a physician. Z. P. Lei reported his experience in treating forty-two cases of obesity, in which the weight ranged from eighty to eighty-two kilograms (This would be considered practically a normal body weight by Western standards!) Acupuncture therapy was performed at the acupoints Liangqiu (S 34) and Gongsun (Sp 4) once every three days and electically stimulated for twenty minutes. Ten sessions constituted one course. After three courses of treatment an average weight reduction of seven and one-half kilograms was obtained (135).

In their studies on forty-four cases of obesity, Z. C. Liu et al., (172) found that a combination therapy of acupuncture and moxibustion provided a significant effect, decreasing both body weight and blood sugar. Their results are presented in table 11-21.

The mechanism of action of acupuncture in reducing obesity is not completely understood. Some investigators believe acupuncture can stimulate hypothalamic centers, sending a signal to the gastrointestinal tract and reducing absorption and appetite. It has also been shown that acupuncture can lower the high 5HT and histamine content in obese patients. X. Liu, et al., (168) suggested that acupuncture can enhance the functioning of the sympathetic adrenal system and the hypothalamic-pituitary-adrenal system. Dung suggested that the weight-reducing effect of acupuncture is mediated through vagal stimulation (63). He and his coworker also reported that weight reduction was not effectively obtained by auricular acupuncture technique. However, in an early report, Soong (120, p. 685) treated twenty-one obese patients with auricular acupuncture therapy for two to six weeks. The patients ranged in age from twenty-seven to fifty-nine years and achieved a weight loss of two to sixteen pounds at the end of the treatment. All experienced a decrease in appetite to varying degrees.

A. K. Alkaysi, et al., (5) reported a five-year experience with auricular EAP treatment in fifty obese patients. An average weight loss of five and one-half kilograms per month was obtained after the treatment. Other problems, such as hypertension and hyperglycemia, were also improved.

Studies in sixty-two children with constitutional exogenic obesity have shown that EAP had a beneficial effect on various pathogenetic components of the disease. There was a reduction in the body mass and fatty tissue content, an increase in the performance abilities, recovery of normal cardiovascular function, and normalization of serum lipids (81).

H. Q. Qu (212) studied the effects of acupuncture therapy on fifty-two obese individuals and found that it can significantly decrease the body weight (from average 74.68±12.45 Kg down to 67.97 ±11.23 Kg) and increase both plasma corticosterone and aldosterone concentrations, with little change in triglyceride and cholesterol levels. In another study, X. P. Ma (184) reported that an acupuncture and moxibustion combination therapy in thirty-one obese individuals produced a satisfactory effect by reducing body weight and abdominal fat.

Recently, Chinese acupuncturists used a modified technique, namely auricular plaster containing Vaccaria seeds, applied on the Shenmen point of the ear, and obtained a good therapeutic result. The advantage of the technique is that patients can be taught to do it themselves; this is especially valuable in patients with needle phobias. Qi applied this technique to 959 obese people; 59.4 percent lost more than six kilograms. In 342 cases in which the auricular plaster technique in combination with body acupuncture was used, 68.7 percent of the patients had a significant weight loss. After treatment, the blood sugar level of the patients was lowered and the corticosterone and T3 levels were increased (211).

Table 11-21. Effectiveness of Acupuncture and Moxibustion Therapy on Obese Individuals

Parameter:	Before Treatment	After Treatment
Body Weight (Kg)	76.66 ± 10.03	71.83 ± 9.66
Abdominal Fat (thickness mm)	40.18 ± 7.3	35.39 ± 8.46
Blood sugar (mg/dl)	138.96± 27.7	117.32± 27.0
Adrenaline conc. (ng/ml)	16.82 ± 2.79	19.41 ± 4.90
Cortisol conc. (μg/ml)	10.26 ±2.17	12.99 ± 3.99

(From Liu et al. (172))

Bone and Joint Diseases

Acupuncture therapy has been found to be effective in treating osteoarthritis deformans and rheumatoid arthritis. Arichi, et al., (8) treated their patients with acupuncture on the normal side, and with a flexion-extension exercise and massage on the affected side. A remarkable cure rate was achieved. However, such method of therapy treatment showed less effective in postcerebral hemorrhage or thrombotic knee mobility disorders or rheumatic arthritis. Acupuncture therapy was successible in the treatment of snapping finger.

S. Zarski, et al., (311) reported their experience in treating lumbar discopathy with acupuncture or with epidural steroid-xylocaine block and found that the later was the most effective, producing a better a relief than acupuncture in all cases.

A microacupuncture technique was used in the treatment of eight-seven patients with neurodystrophic syndromes of cervical osteochondriosis, including brachioclavicular periarthrosis, brachial epicondylitis, and styloiditis. The effectiveness rate was 1.5 to 2 times better and the effect occurred faster than with drug therapy (84). In another report, acupuncture was used to treat patients suffering from osteochondrosis of the spine combined with ischemic heart disease. A remarkable effect involving relieving of the pathological reflex reaction, normalization of cardiac rhythm, and improvement in coronary circulation in 89.2 percent was observed (53).

Forty cases of osetoarthritis were treated with acupuncture. It was found that the pain, motor function, and periarticular edema were greatly improved after the treatment (204).

Thirty-two patients suffering from osteoarthritis were treated with EAP (2 Hz) at the acupoints Sanjian (LI 3), Feng Chi (G 20), Dazhui (Du 14), and Baihui (Du 20) bilaterally. After several treatments, the chronic nociceptive pain was alleviated significantly. Pretreatment with diazepam or naloxone can reduce such effect but not completely block it (68). The result is summarized in table 11-22.

Table 11-22. Effectivenss of Electro-acupuncture Therapy on Osteoarthritis

No. of Patients	Pre-administered Drug		Affective Score	Sensory Score
32	none	Before	2.6 ± 0.9	2.1 ± 0.8
		After	1.7 ±1.7	1.5 ± 1.1
32	Diazepam	Bef.	2.5 ±0.5	1.7 ± 0.7
		Aft.	2.0 ± 1.5	1.6 ± 1.1
32	Naloxone	Bef.	2.5 ±1.3	1.9 ± 0.9
		Aft.	2.2 ± 1.2	1.5 ± 0.9

(From Eriksson et al. (68))

H. H. Buelow, et al., (20) treated forty-two cases of osteoarthritic knee with acupuncture at acupoints HoKu and Zusanli. Patients averaging sixty-nine years of age received 6 treatments. The success rate varied from 50 to 70 percent, depending upon the duration of the disease. In general, the less chronic cases responded well to acupuncture therapy and received the best long-term effect. Several patients were further improved at follow-up observation, even without further treatment.

Forty-two patients suffering from chronic cervical osteoarthritis were treated with acupuncture and compared with a group treated with diazepam or placebo. The acupuncture group had higher improvment rate (44, 180, 250). Some clinicians consider acupuncture an alternative treatment for this disease, because of its lack of adverse effects (118).

Studies on eighteen patients with osteoarthritis of the knee have shown that after acupuncture treatment the pO_2 of the synovial fluid was increased significantly, with no change in pH, pCO2, or base. This indicates that acupuncture could increase blood flow to the knee and stimulate metabolism and replacement of gases in the synovial fluid (1).

Acupuncture therapy was also used to treat 113 patients suffering from a strain of the intrapatellar fat pad accompanied in some cases by traumatic arthritis of the knee and malacia of the patella. A 100 percent cure rate was observed, with marked alleviation of all symptoms (86).

Arthritis and Systemic Lupus Erythematosis

Rheumatoid arthritis is a chronic inflammation of the synovial lining of the joint, subsequently causing edema, exudation, and cellular infiltration, due to the synovial hypervascularity. In traditional Chinese medicine it is called "wind and wet disease." The cause of the disease is not completely understood. Acupuncture therapy has been applied for centuries. X. Y. Kong (125) reported fifty-nine cases of acute rheumatism treated with acupuncture at the acupoints Dazhui (Du 14) and Sanyinjiao (Sp 6) and found that thirty-four patients (73.9 percent) were cured, nine (19.6 percent) improved, and only three were failures.

In his report, X. H. Jai (108) divided patients suffering from rheumatoid arthritis into two groups. One group was treated with stick needle acupuncture and the others with EAP. The acupoints Quchi (LI 11) and Yanglingquan (G 34) were needled once a day, ten treatments to a course. After a one-week rest the treatment was repeated. The results are summarized in table 11-23.

Table 11-23. Acupuncture and Electro-acupuncture Therapy on Rheumatic Arthritis

Type of Treatment	No. of Cases	Cured	Improved	Failed
Acupuncture	286	83 (29%)	184 (71.8%)	19
Electro-acupuncture	134	32 (33.9%)	88 (65.7%)	14

(From Jai (108))

Yao, et al., (302) compared acupuncture therapy with herbal medication in the treatment of gouty arthritis and found that acupuncture therapy gave a superior result, as shown in Table 11-24:

Table 11-24. Acupuncture and Herbal Therapy on Arthritis

Type of Treatment	No. of Cases	Result		
		Markedly Improved	Moderately Improved	No Effect
Acupuncture	61	48 (78.7%)	11 (18%)	2
Herbal	40	10 (20.8%)	15 (31.2%)	23

(From Yao et al. (302))

Sixty-three cases of bursitis were treated with either scalp acupuncture or body acupuncture. Thirty-three to 38 percent of the patients were cured and imflammation subsided (288). In another report, fifty-four cases of bursitis were treated with acupuncture at the acupoints Feng Chi and Zusanli. Thirty-nine patients were cured (72.2 percent), one failed, and the others were slightly improved (329). Seventy-one patients with gonarthrosis underwent acupuncture therapy or twenty-one days of spa treatment. Both treatments were equally effective and gave a 67.3 percent improvement rate (109). Acupuncture therapy was recommended especially for cases with severe painful decompensation, in which it was superior to nonsteroidal antiinflammatory drug therapy, or cases with significant knee edema, or cases in which the use of balneotherapy must be restricted, such as in elderly patients or patients with cardiovascular diseases.

S. M. Li, et al., (145) reported twenty-three cases of gouty arthritis treated with acupuncture using the pricking blood technique. A 100 percent cure rate was obtained, the plasma level of uric acid decreased, and the urinary excretion of uric acid increased after the treatment.

Table 11-25 summarizes the other clinical reports on arthritis treated with acupuncture therapy.

Systemic lupus erythematosis (SLE) is an autoimmune disease, resulting from the elaboration of antibodies to native (one's own) DNA and nuclear proteins. Active SLE involves the joints, skin, kidney, and heart. Although there was no specific description of this disease in traditional Chinese medicine, practitioners apparently treated it symptomatic to relieve suffering, without knowing the mechanism. Ginseng is a useful remedy because of its stimulating effect on the pituitary adrenal axis (97, p. 33), but it is an expensive herb and its exact dosage has not been determined. For rural populations, acupuncture became more practical and useful when patients did not respond well to other medications.

S. F. Feng, et al., (73) treated twenty-five cases of SLE with acupuncture. Ten patients did not receive any corticosterone therapy, and another fifteen patients, including twelve with the nephrotic syndrome, had corticosterone therapy for three months and failed to obtain relief. After several acupuncture treatments, there was considerable improvement in symptoms in all patients. The laboratory findings showed a definite immunological change.

Table 11-25. Acupuncture Therapy in Arthristis

Source	Mode	Acupoint	Diagnosis	No. of Patients	Effectiveness %
Liu (170)	AP * with warmed needle or IAc inj #	Zusanli (S 36) Sanyinjiao (Sp 6)	Rheumatic arthritis	54	78% markedly effective and other 17% improved
Liu (169)	AP with warmed needle or IAc inj.		Rheum. arthritis	54	100% effective by changing the cellular and humoral immunity.
Ji (110)	AP	Multiple	Rheumatic arthritis, bursitis, sciatic neuralgia	200	67% clinically cured; symptom-free
Wang (267)	AP	Ququan (Liv 8)	Arthritis	80	94.1% basically cured
Lin (152)	AP	HoKu (LI 4) Fengchi (G 20)	Mandibular arthritis	40	88% cured
Wang (263)	AP	Dazhui (Du 14) Quchi (LI 11) Zusanli	Gonorrheal arthritis	116	64% cured and other 11% improved
Yen (305)	AP	HoKu, Ququan	Gouty arthritis	61	78.7% markedly effective
	Medication			48	20.8% markedly effective
Zhou (331)	AP	Chengshan (B 57) HoKu	Bursitis	60	82% were cured

* AP = Acupuncture
# IAc inj. = Intra-acupoint injection

Metabolic and Other Diseases

Diabetes Mellitus

Diabetes mellitus is quite common in China. Herbal medicine is commonly used. The best-known herb is ginseng. It is effective but expensive. In the Chin Dynasty, ginseng was considered to be a royal property, not readily available for the common people. Acupuncture therapy was then tried and claimed to be helpful. In the late 1970s, Chang (3, p. 28) reported success in the treatment of twenty-four cases of diabetes mellitus by acupuncture therapy and recorded a 45.8 percent effectiveness rate. In 1991, C. F. Chu (46) treated 246 cases with acupuncture at the acupoint Zusanli bilaterally once a day for a month. The blood sugar of the patients fell to a normal level. Another 136 cases serving as controls were treated with sham acupuncture and only with dietary management. The results are shown in table 11-26.

Table 11-26. Effect of Acupuncture Therapy on Diabetes Mellitus

Type of Treatment	No. of Cases	Blood Sugar (mg/dl)	
		Before	After
Control (sham acupuncture)	136	364.3 ±38.5	334.5 ±52.2
Acupuncture	246	383.1 ±50.8	117.4 ± 30.6

(From Chu (46))

A. Szczudlik and A. Lypka studied ten healthy volunteer subjects receiving acupuncture treatment. All showed a significant slow-term decrease in insulin concentration (245). Studies on 40 healthy individuals also showed that acupuncture can significantly suppress the hyperglycemia and cortisol response induced by surgical stress (82).

Table 11-27 summarizes the other clinical reports on acupuncture effects in the treatment of diabetes mellitus.

Hypoglycemia

In a case of hypoglycemia reported by G. Chen (27), a thirty-two-year-old male had functional hypoglycemic symptoms, the glucose level was 25 mg/dl and was unresponsive to dietary control for two years. Ten sessions of acupuncture therapy were given. The hypoglycemic symptoms disappeared the fifth day after treatment and the patient was able to shift to a normal diet and had a normal glucose tolerance test.

Table 11-27. Acupuncture Therapy in Diabetes Mellitus

Source	Mode	Acupoint	Diagnosis	No. of Patients	Effectiveness %
Fung (79)	AP*	Qihai (Ren 6)	Insulin-independent diabetes	309	71.2% markedly effective
Chen (29)	AP	Pishu (B 20) Zusanli (S 36)	Diabetes	26	Blood sugar was down from 300-500 mg/dl to 130 mg/dl; and blood insulin was up
Liu (167)	AP	Ear	Diabetes	86	40.7% were cured and other 32.6% markedly improved

* AP = Acupuncture

Thirty-one patients who had suffered from reactive hypoglycemia for one to five years had common symptoms including headache, cold sweating, vertigo, tremors, and depression. They responded favorably to acupuncture therapy. After one to three weeks of treatment, the depression, fatigue, and other symptoms disappeared and it was possible to discontinue all other medications. All but two were able to take normal food without any discomfort (28). The author concluded that a dysautonomia was probably the cause of this hypoglycemia and acupuncture therapy could correct the dysfunction.

Hyperthyroidism

J. S. He, et al., (89) reported 136 patients with hyperthyroidism who could not tolerate the side effects of antithyroid agents and came to the acupuncture clinic for treatment. They received the acupuncture at the Neiguan (P 6), Zusanli, and Sanyinjiao points once a day for thirty minutes. After fifty treatments, 39 percent of the patients became symptom-free and 43 percent were greatly improved. Their plasma level of T4 was reduced from 212.6±5.99 to 145.4±4.63 ng/ml, and the T3 level decreased from 5.63±0.18 to 3.24±0.16 ng/ml.

Bladder Instability

Twenty patients with lower urinary tract symptoms or sensory urgency were treated with acupuncture. Seventy-seven percent were symptomatically cured, but urodynamic assessment revealed no consistent change. The instability was abolished in one case. In patients with diurnal symptoms associated with idiopathic bladder instability, acupuncture offered an effective therapy (206).

The Kidney and Urinary Excretion

Nakamura, et al., (199) tested the effects of acupuncture on the urinary excretion of water and sodium in thirteen healthy volunteers. The acupoint Shenshu (B 23) was chosen for needling because it was used traditionally for kidney diseases; each treatment lasted fifteen minutes. All subjects had a remarkable increase in urinary flow and sodium excretion, as high as three times the pretreatment value. Blood pressure and pulse rate were not changed. Plasma renin activity (PRA) and plasma concentrations of aldosterone, catecholamines, DOPA, and urinary kallikrein (UK) were not significantly affected. However, atrial natriuretic peptide (ANP) concentration was signfificantly increased, from 85.97 ± 23.7 pg/ml to 151.6 ±45.1 pg/ml.

Studies in 102 cases of pyelonephritis treated with acupuncture showed that 60 percent of patients had a positive response to treatment. Acupuncture not only promoted earlier recovery or remission, but also reduced the required dose of chemotherapeutic agents (52).

In animal experiments, Lin, et al., (150) induced an increase in urine flow and urinary sodium excretion by acupuncture and found that the effect disappeared after bilateral cervical vagotomy or bilateral renal nerves denervation.

Postirradiation Edema

Acupuncture therapy has been used to treat edema of the arms and legs induced by radiation therapy and multimodality therapy in breast and cervical cancer patients (15). Studies in 141 patients with the postirradiation edema showed that acupuncture therapy effectively improved lymph flow in 122 patients and there was a normalization of hemostasis. The best result was observed in Stages I and II of edema.

Acupuncture therapy was also used to treat postirradiation edema in the upper limbs of thirty-six cancer patients (129). It effectively decreased edematous fluid by 22–37 percent.

References

1. Aida, S. J. Journal of Japanese Asso. Physical Medicine Balneology and Climatol. 55:191, 1992.
2. All China Society of Acupuncture and Moxibustion: National Symposium of Acupuncture and Acupuncture Anesthesia. Beijing: 1979.
3. All China Society of Acupuncture and Moxibustion: Second National Symposium of Acupuncture and Moxibustion and Acupuncture Anesthesia. Beijing: People Health Publisher, 1984.
4. Akhmelov, T. I., et al. Vrachcbnol Delo 0(8):100, 1991.
5. Alkaysi, A. K., et al. American Journal of Acupuncture 19:323, 1991.
6. Ande, J. Journal of Traditional Chinese Medicine 7:141, 1987.
7. Anshelevich, Y. V., et al. Ter. Arkh. 57:42, 1985. (4a) Anshelevich, Y. V., et al. Klin. Med. (Moscow) 66:54, 1988.

8. Arichi, S., et al. American Journal of Chinese Medicine 11:146, 1983; 11:143, 1983; 11:137, 1983.
9. Aviridova, E. I., and N. I. Oleimikov. ZH. Nevropatol. Psikhiatr. IM S.S. Korsakova 84:1381, 1984.
10. Ballegaard, S., et al. Journal of Internal Medicine 229:357, 1991.
11. Ballegaard, S., et at. Acta Med. Scand. 220:307, 1986.
12. Ballegaard, S., et al. Acupuncture Electro-Ther. Res. 18:103, 1993.
13. Bao, Y. X., et al. Chinese Medical Journal 95:824, 1982.
14. Bao, X. Y., et al. Shanghai Journal of Acupuncture and Moxibustion 8(2):1, 1989.
15. Bardychev, M. S., et al. Vopr. Onkol. 34:319, 1988.
16. Batra Y. K. et al. American Journal of Acupuncture 14:261, 1986.
17. Bei, S. Y., et al. Journal of Chinese Acupuncture and Moxibustion 8(4):16, 1989.
18. Berger, D., and D. Nolte from F. F. Kao, eds. Recent Advances in Acupuncture Research, Garden City, NY: Institute for Advance Research in Asian Science and Medicine, 1979, p. 680.
19. Berns, A. V., et al. Fiziologiya Cheloreka 19:36, 1993.
20. Buelow H. H., et al. American Journal of Chinese Medicine 20:17, 1992.
21. Caione, P., et al. Minerva-Pediatr. 46:437, 1994.
22. Cao, Q. S., et al. Journal of Traditional Chinese Medicine (in english) 1:83, 1981.
23. Ceghlan, C. Journal of Cent, Afr. J. Med. 38:466, 1992.
24. Chan, C., and G. H. Chai. Journal of Chinese Acupuncture and Moxibustion 14(2):53, 1994.
25. Chang, H. T., ed. Acupuncture and Moxibustion Research. Beijing: Science Publishing Company, 1986.
26. Chang, P. L. Journal of Urology 140:563, 1986.
27. Chen, G. American Journal of Acupuncture 11:131, 1983.
28. Chen, G. American Journal of Acupuncture 15:105, 1987.
29. Chen, J. F., and J. Wei. Journal of Traditional Chinese Medicine (in English) 5(2):79, 1985.
30. Chen, K. Y., et al. Journal of Traditional Chinese Medicine 3:121, 1984.
31. Chen, S. C., and C. X. Liu. Journal of Chinese Acupuncture and Moxibustion 13(5):41, 1993.
32. Chen, S. J. Shanghai Journal of Acupuncture and Moxibustion 13(2):61, 1994.
33. Chen, S. Y. Jiangsu Journal of Traditional Chinese Medicine 15:224, 1994.
34. Chen, S. X., et al. Journal of Traditional Chinese Medicine 3:113, 1983.
35. Chen, W. H., et al. Journal of Chinese Acupuncture and Moxibustion 13(2):33, 1993.
36. Chen, W. J., and J. P. Doyle. American Journal of Acupuncture 15:305, 1987.
37. Chen, Y. H., et al. Shanghai Journal of Acupuncture and Moxibustion 12(1):12, 1993.
38. Chen, Y. H., et al. Shanghai Journal of Acupuncture and Moxibustion 12(1):12, 1993.
39. Cheng, Q. F. Journal of Chinese Acupuncture and Moxibustion 14(1):37, 1994.
40. Cheng, Y. M. and Y. A. Fang. Acupuncture Electro-Ther. Res. 15:9, 1990.
41. Cheng, Y. M., et al. New Journal of Traditional Chinese Medicine 26(1):38,1994.
42. Chondkury, L. Y., and D. J. O. Ffoulkes-Chzabbe, Alternative Medicine 3:127, 1989.
43. Chow, O. K. W., et al. Lung 161:321, 1983.
44. Christensen, B. V., et al. Ugestr.-Laeger 155:4007, 1993.
45. Christensen, P. A., et al. Allergy 39:379, 1984.
46. Chu, C. F. Journal of Chinese Acupuncture and Moxibustion 11 (1):5, 1991.
47. Chu, F. S., et al. Journal of Chinese Acupuncture and Moxibustion 11(3):19, 1991.
48. Chu, G. S. Shanghai Journal of Acupuncture and Moxibustion 12(2):61, 1993.
49. Chu, P. C. and M. M. Hsu. Journal of Chinese Acupuncture and Moxibustion 13(1):33, 1993.
50. Cui, J. C. Journal of Chinese Acupuncture and Moxibustion 14(2):17, 1994.
51. Dancim, A., and E. Dancim. American Journal of Acupuncture 13:247, 1985.
52. Darenkov, A. F., et al. Urologiya i Nefrologiya 0(2):10, 1993.
53. Davydov, O. V. Klin. Medicine 65:98, 1987.
54. Debrecein, L. and L. Dean. Acupuncture Electro-Ther. Res. 13:105, 1988,
55. Deng, X. C. Shanghai Journal of Acupuncture and Moxibustion 13(1):11, 1994.
56. Ding, S., et al. Journal of Japanese Assoc. Physical Medicine Balneoli and Climat. 56:95, 1993.
57. Dong, S. R., et al. Journal of Traditional Chinese Medicine 6:1, 1986.
58. Dong, Z. M. Journal of Chinese Acupuncture and Moxibustion 11 (6):15, 1991.
59. Dovgeyallo, O. G., et al. Ter. Arkh. 59:16, 1987.
60. Du, L. Tianjin Journal of Traditional Chinese Medicine (2):10, 1993.
61. Dundee, J. W. and C. M. McMillan. Acup-Elect.-Ther. Res. 15:211, 1990.
62. Dung, H. C. Chinese Medical Journal 98:855, 1988.
63. Dung, H. C. American Journal of Acupuncture 14:249, 1986.
64. Dung, H. C. American Journal of Acupuncture 14:117, 1986.
65. Dung, H. C. American Journal of Acupuncture 15:5, 1987.
66. Duo, L. J. Nephron 47:179, 1987.
67. Emelyanento, I. V. Vrach. Delo 0:98, 1991.

68. Eriksson, S. V., et al. American Journal of Chinese Medicine 19:1, 1991.
69. Fan, W. P., and P. C. Fan. Journal of Chinese Acupuncture and Moxibustion 11(2):15, 1991.
70. Fan, Y. A., et al. Shanghai Journal of Acupuncture and Moxibustion 8(4):1, 1989.
71. Fan, Y. L. and C. C. Zhang. Chinese Medical Journal 96:491, 1983.
72. Fam, S. J. Journal of Traditional Chinese Medicine 25(0)32, 1993.
73. Feng, S. F., et al. Chinese Medical Journal 93:71, 1988.
74. Feng, X. Q., et al. Beijing Journal of Traditional Chinese Medicine February (1):37, 1993.
75. Feng, X. G., et al. Beijing Journal of Traditional Chinese Medicine April(2):36, 1994.
76. Fon, Y. H., et al. Journal of Chinese Acupuncture and Moxibustion 11(5):1, 1991.
77. Fu, N. L. Journal of Chinese Acupuncture and Moxibustion 14(2):9, 1994.
78. Fung, K. P., et al. Lancet 2:1419, 1986.
79. Fung, M. S., et al. Journal of Traditional Chinese Medicine (in Chinese) 35(1):25, 1994.
80. Ga, S., et al. Journal of Chinese Acupuncture and Moxibustion 13(1):11, 1993.
81. Gadzhiew, A. A., et al. Problemy Endokrinologii 39(3):21, 1993.
82. Galoic-Krleza, R. Lijec-Vjesn. 113(9):327, 1991.
83. Gao, Z. W., et al. Journal of Traditional Chinese Medicine 7:185, 1987.
84. Goadenko, V. S., et al. ZH. Nevropatol. Psikhiatr. IM S.S. Korsakova 89:45, 1989.
85. Gon, W. S. and E. H. Shem. Journal of Traditional Chinese Medicine (in Chinese) 34(11):660, 1993.
86. Guo, X. Journal of Traditional Chinese Medicine (in English) 13:294, 1993.
87. Guo, W.P., et al. Journal of Chinese Acupuncture and Moxibustion 13(4):22, 1993.
88. Harada, K and Y. Yamata. Jpn. J. of Clin. Urol. 38:967, 1984.
89. He, J. S., et al. Shangahi Journal of Acupuncture and Moxibustion 13(2):54, 1994.
90. Hong, Y., et al. Journal of Chinese Acupuncture and Moxibustion 13(5):1, 1993.
91. Hsu, F., et al. Journal of Chinese Acupuncture and Moxibustion 13(6):25, 1993.
92. Hsu, Y. C., et al. Shanghai Journal of Acupuncture and Moxibustion 8(4):16, 1989.
93. Hu, E.W. and S. J. Lu. New Journal of Traditional Chinese Medicine 25(2):28, 1993.
94. Hu, H. H., et al. Neuroepidemology 12(2):106,1993.
95. Huang, C. H. Journal of Chinese Acupuncture and Moxibustion 13(2): 17, 1993.
96. Huang, J. M., et al. Journal of Traditional Chinese Medicine (in Chinese) 34(5):293, 1993.
97. Huang, K. C. Pharmacology of Chinese Herbs CRC Press, Florida 1993, p. 229.
98. Huang, M. Journal of Chinese Acupuncture and Moxibustion 13(3):21, 1993.
99. Huang, M. Journal of Chinese Acupuncture and Moxibustion 13(2): 21, 1993.
100. Huo, J. S. Journal of Traditional Chinese Medicine 8:195, 1988.
101. Hwang, Y. C., and E. M. Jenkins. American Journal of Vet. Res. 49:1641, 1988.
102. Ikeuchi, T., and H. Iguchi. Acta Urologica Japonia 40(7):587,1994.
103. Ionescii-Tirgoviste, C. et al. American Journal of Acupuncture 11:119, 1983.
104. Itaya, K., et al. Acupuncture Electro-Ther. Res. 12:45, 1987.
105. Ja, H. J., et al. Shanghai Journal of Acupuncture and Moxibustion 12(4):148, 1993.
106. Ja, K. T., et al. Journal of Chinese Acupuncture and Moxibustion 11(4): 3, 1991.
107. Jagirdan, P. C. American Journal of Acupuncture 14:155, 1956.
108. Jai, X. H. Journal of Chinese Acupuncture and Moxibustion 11(3):31, 1991.
109. Jezek, J. Balneol. Bohem. 16:1190, 1987.
110. Ji, X. P. Journal of Traditional Chinese Medicine (in Chinese) 34(1):151, 1993,
111. Jian, Y. C., et al. Journal of Chinese Acupuncture and Moxibustion 11 (4):9, 1991.
112. Jiang, Y. C., et al. Journal of Chinese Acupuncture and Moxibustion 13(4):1, 1993.
113. Jin, D. L. Journal of Chinese Acupuncture and Moxibustion 10(2): 21, 1990.
114. Jin, R., et al. Journal of Chinese Acupuncture and Moxibustion 13(1):11, 1993.
115. Jin, S. M., et al. Journal of Chinese Acupuncture and Moxibustion 11 (4):3, 1991.
116. Jobst, K., et al. Lancet 2:1416, 1986.
117. Johanssan, K., et al. Neurology 43:2189, 1993.
118. Jones, A., and M. Doherty. British Journal of Clin. Pharm. 33:357, 1992.
119. Joshi, Y. M. Journal of AsSociety Physicians India 40:327, 1992.
120. Kao, F. F., and J. J. Kao. Recent Advances in Acupuncture Research. Garden City, NY: Institute for Advanced Research in Asian Science and Medicine, 1979.
121. Kachan, A. T., et al. Rh. Neuropatol. Psikhiatr. Im S S Korsakova 93(5):40, 1993.
122. Katai, S., and K. Nishigyou. Jpn. Assoc. Physical. Medicine Balneology and Climatology 54:178, 1991.
123. Kochetkov, V. D., et al. ZH Nevropatol. Psikhiatr. I M S S Korsakora 88:102, 1988.
124. Komissarov, V. I., and E. E. Tretyokora, ZH Nevropatol. Psikhiatr. I M S S Korsakora 90:44, 1990.
125. Kong, Y. Y. Journal of Chinese Acupuncture and Moxibustion 13(2):3, 1993.
126. Kravtosova, T. I., et al. Vopr-Kurortol-Fizioter-Leh-Fiz-Kult (1):22, 1994.
127. Kravtosova, T. I., et al. Zh. Neuropatol. Psikhiatr. Im S.S. Korsakova 93(6):50, 1993.

128. Kum, C. W., et al. Journal of Chinese Acupuncture and Moxibustion 11(2):13, 1991.
129. Kuzmina, E. G. and A. A. Deytyareva, Medical Radiology 32:42, 1987.
130. Kurosaka, H., et al. Gastroenterol. Endosci. 31:35, 1989.
131. Lai, X. Journal of Traditional Chinese Medicine 13(4):243, 1993.
132. Lanza, U. Acupuncture Electro-Ther. Res. 11:53, 1986.
133. Le, J. K. Journal of Chinese Acupuncture and Moxibustion 11(1):13, 1991.
134. Lee, Y. H., et al. Journal of Urology. 147:16, 1992.
135. Lei, Z. P. Journal of Traditional Chinese Medicine 8:125, 1988.
136. Li, C. H. Journal of Chinese Acupuncture and Moxibustion 13(3):36, 1993.
137. Li, C. M., and Y. H. Zhey. Journal of Chinese Acupuncture and Moxibustion 13(1):15, 1993.
138. Li, J. K. Shanghai Journal of Acupuncture and Moxibustion 8(3):10, 1989.
139. Li, J. K. Journal of Chinese Acupuncture and Moxibustion 10(4):3, 1990.
140. Li, J. T., and Y. F. Gong. Shanghai Journal of Acupuncture and Moxibustion 12(4):154, 1993.
141. Li, J. T., and S. I. Yang. Tianjin Journal of Traditional Chinese Medicine (6):25, 1993.
142. Li, K. Y. Journal of Chinese Acupuncture and Moxibustion 10 (3):1, 1990.
143. Li, L. S. Journal of Chinese Acupuncture and Moxibustion 13(1):21, 1993.
144. Li, P. Journal of Traditional Chinese Medicine 5:211, 1985.
145. Li, S. M., et al. Journal of Chinese Acupuncture and Moxibustion 13(4):11, 1993.
146. Li, T. H., and J. H. Hsu. Journal of Chinese Acupuncture and Moxibustion 13(2):13, 1993.
147. Li, T. F., et al. Journal of Chinese Acupuncture and Moxibustion 11(3):5, 1991.
148. Li, Y., et al. American Journal of Gastroenterol. 87:1372, 1992.
149. Liang, D., and Y. Zhao, Journal of Traditional Chinese Medicine 14:110, 1994.
150. Liang, L. M. Journal of Chinese Acupuncture and Moxibustion 11(5):47, 1991.
151. Lin, J. S., et al. New Journal of Traditional Chinese Medicine 26(2):34, 1994.
152. Lin, L. New Journal of Traditional Chinese Medicine 26(4):35, 1994,
153. Lin, M. Z., et al. Acta Physiol. Sinica 38:332, 1986.
154. Lin, T. L., and L. Y. Zhou. Journal of Chinese Acupuncture and Moxibustion 12(2):48, 1992.
155. Lin, Y. C. Journal of Traditional Chinese Medicine 28:288, 1987.
156. Liu, E. S., and G. Shen. Journal of Chinese Acupuncture and Moxibustion 10(3): 19, 1990.
157. Liu, G. Journal of Traditional Chinese Medicine (in English) 1(2):143,1981.
158. Liu, H. S., et al. Journal of Chinese Acupuncture and Moxibustion 11(3): 9, 1991.
159. Liu, C. M., et al. Journal of Chinese Acupuncture and Moxibustion 10(6): 13, 1990.
160. Liu, F. Z., and A. D. Jin. Journal of Traditional Chinese Medicine (in Chinese) 28:213, 1987.
161. Liu, J. H. Jiangsu Journal of Traditional Chinese Medicine 15(2):76,1994.
162. Liu, K. L., and L. Y. Zhou. Journal of Chinese Acupuncture and Moxibustion 13(2):48, 1993.
163. Liu, K. S. Journal of Chinese Acupuncture and Moxibustion 13(6):23, 1993.
164. Liu, M. H., et al. New Journal of Traditional Chinese Medicine 26(2):32, 1994.
165. Liu, M. P., and L. Liu. Journal of Chinese Acupuncture and Moxibustion 11(6): 23, 1991.
166. Liu, S. H., et al. Journal of Chinese Acupuncture and Moxibustion 13(1):7, 1993.
167. Liu, S. K. Journal of Chinese Acupuncture and Moxibustion 13(3):40, 1993.
168. Liu, X., et al. Journal of Traditional Chinese Medicine 13(3):174, 1993.
169. Liu, X. L., et al. Journal of Chinese Acupuncture and Moxibustion 14(2):1, 1994.
170. Liu, X. L. Journal of Chinese Acupuncture and Moxibustion 13(3):5, 1993.
171. Liu, Y. C., and T. Z. Guo. Journal of Chinese Acupuncture and Moxibustion 14(1): 16, 1994.
172. Liu, Z. C., et al. Shanghai Journal of Acupuncture and Moxibustion 8(1):4, 1989.
173. Lo, G. C., and M. F. Yang. Journal of Chinese Acupuncture and Moxibustion 13(4):26, 1993.
174. Long, M. J., et al. Journal of Chinese Acupuncture and Moxibustion 11(6):19,1991.
175. Lovacky, S., et al. American Journal of Acupuncture 18:105, 1990.
176. Lu, C., et al. Journal of Chinese Acupuncture and Moxibustion 11(1):1, 1991.
177. Lu, W. Journal of Traditional Chinese Medicine 14:180, 1994.
178. Lu, Y. N., et al. Journal of Chinese Acupuncture and Moxibustion 13(6):1, 1993.
179. Lue, Y. Z. New Journal of Traditional Chinese Medicine 25(4):31, 1993.
180. Lundeberg, T., et al. Pain Clinic. 4:155, 1991.
181. Luo, C. C. Journal of Chinese Acupuncture and Moxibustion 11(4):8, 1991.
182. Luo, G. Z. Journal of Chinese Acupuncture and Moxibustion 10(4):5, 1990.
183. Luo, G. S. Journal of Chinese Acupuncture and Moxibustion 13(6):21, 1993.
184. Ma, X. P. Shanghai Journal of Acupuncture and Moxibustion 12(2):56, 1993.
185. Manucharyan, G. G., et al. Zh. Neuropatologii I. Psikhiatric M. S S Korsakova 92:60, 1992.
186. Markelova, V. I., et al. ZH Nevropatol. Psikhiatr. I M. S S Korsakova 86:1708, 1986.
187. Matsurmoto, K., et al. American Journal of Acupuncture 18:359, 1990.

188. McMillan, C., et al. British Journal of Cancer. 64:971, 1991.
189. Medici, T. C. Schwerzerische Med. Wochenschr. Supplem. 0(62):39, 1994.
190. Mew, S., et al. Journal of Chinese Acupuncture and Moxibustion 13(5):37, 1993.
191. Meng, C. D., et al. Journal of Chinese Acupuncture and Moxibustion 13(4):9, 1993.
192. Milanov, I. American Journal of Acupuncture 19:107, 1991.
193. Minni, B., et al. Acupuncture Electro-Ther. Res. 15:19, 1990.
194. Mitchell, P. and J. Elisabeth. American Journal of Acupuncture 17:5, 1989.
195. Mitrovskaya, V. N. and N. N. Loshkareva. ZH Nevropatol. Psikhiatr. I M. SS Korsakova 91:16, 1991.
196. Moi, T. P. Journal of Chinese Acupuncture and Moxibustion 13(5):13, 1993.
197. Monaenkov, A. M., et al. American Journal of Acupuncture 12:313, 1984.
198. Montakab, H., and G. Laugel. Schwerzerische Medicine Wochenschr. Supplem. 0(62):49, 1994.
199. Nakamura K., et al. J. Med. Soc. Toho Univ. 35:54, 1988.
200. Noguchi, E., and T. Sato. J. Jpn. Assoc. Phys. Med. Balneol. Climatol. 51:88, 1988.
201. Nosalinia, A., et al. Digestive Surg. 3:243, 1986.
202. Osipora, N. N., et al. ZH Nevropatol. Psikhiatr. IM SS Korsakova 0:89, 1990.
203. Ouyang, S., et al. Acta Physiol. Sinica 35:34, 1983.
204. Pacini, D., et al. Acta Anesthesiol. Ital. 36:129,1985.
205. Pei, J. L., and S. Yun. Journal of Chinese Acupuncture and Moxibustion 13(5):25, 1993.
206. Philip, T., et al. British Journal of Urology 61:490, 1988.
207. Po, K. P. Journal of Chinese Acupuncture and Moxibustion 14(1):5, 1994.
208. Po, S. G. Journal of Traditional Chinese Medicine (in Chinese) 34(1):26, 1993.
209. Pothmann, R., and G. Schmitz. Alternative Medicine 1:63, 1985.
210. Qi, L. Y., et al. Journal of Traditional Chinese Medicine 8:161, 1988.
211. Qi, L. Z. Shanghai Journal of Traditional Chinese Medicine April(4):15, 1994.
212. Qu, H. Q. Journal of Chinese Acupuncture and Moxibustion 14(1):1, 1994.
213. Rabinowitz, N. American Journal of Acupuncture 15:35, 1987.
214. Radzievskii, S. A., et al. Journal of Chinese Medicine 17:111, 1989.
215. Radzievskii, S. A., et al. Kardiologiya 27:66, 1987.
216. Raut, C. American Journal of Acupuncture 12:245, 1984.
217. Richter A., et al. Finnish Heart Journal 12:175, 1991.
218. Romoli, M., and A. Giommi. Acupuncture Elect-Ther. Res. 18:185, 1993.
219. Sam, F. S. Journal of Chinese Acupuncture and Moxibustion 11(3):7, 1991.
220. Satoh, S., and Y. Yamata, Nishinihon. J. Urol. 50: 456, 1988.
221. Saku, K., et al. Clinical Cardiology 16:415, 1993.
222. Sato, A., et al. Neuroscience Research 18:53, 1993.
223. Seguchi, T., et al. J. Clin. Urol. 42:319, 1988.
224. Semenova, K. A., and V. I. Dotsuko. ZH Nevropatol. Psikhiatr. I M SS Korsakova 88:32, 1988.
225. Sen, Y. L. Shanghai Journal of Acupuncture and Moxibustion 13(1):16, 1994.
226. Shao, J. M., and Y. P. Ding. Journal of Traditional Chinese Medicine 5:23, 1985.
227. Shi, C. L. Guangdon Medical Journal 14(3):149, 1993.
228. Shi, Y., and Z. Y. Song. Journal of Traditional Chinese Medicine (in Chinese) 34(1):34, 1994.
229. Shi, Z. X., and M. Z. Tan. Journal of Traditional Chinese Medicine (in English) 6:99, 1986.
230. Shi, Z. X., and M. Z. Tan. Journal of Traditional Chinese Medicine 6:99, 1986.
231. Shu, H. P. Journal of Chinese Acupuncture and Moxibustion 10(3):7, 1990.
232. Si, M., et al. Shanghai Journal of Acupuncture and Moxibustion 13(2):58, 1994.
233. Si, P. P., et al. Shanghai Journal of Acupuncture and Moxibustion 13(2):60, 1994.
234. Si, Y. Z. Shanghai Journal of Acupuncture and Moxibustion 12(3):119, 1993.
235. Sliwinski, J., and R. Ratusiewicz. Acupuncture Electro-Ther. Res. 9:203, 1985.
236. Smith, M. O. and N. Rabinowitz. American Journal of Acupuncture 14:143, 1986.
237. Sodipo, J., American Journal of Chinese Medicine 21:85, 1993.
238. Song, B. Z., and Y. Wang. Journal of Traditional Chinese Medicine 5:27, 1985.
239. Song, L. L. Shanghai Journal of Acupuncture and Moxibustion 12(2):93, 1993.
240. Steinberger, A. American Journal of Chinese Medicine 14:175, 1986.
241. Sternfeld, M., et al. American Journal of Acupuncture 14:127, 1986.
242. Sternfeld, M., et al. American Journal of Acupuncture 15:149, 1987.
243. Sternfeld, M., et al. American Journal of Acupuncture 17:119, 1989.
244. Sternfeld, M., et al. American Journal of Chinese Medicine 17:129, 1989.
245. Szczudlik, A., and A. Lypka. Acupuncture Electro-Ther. Res. 9:1, 1984.
246. Takahashi, T. Japan Anesthesiol. 34:1258, 1985.
247. Tang, N. L. Journal of Chinese Acupuncture and Moxibustion 11(2):1, 1991.
248. Tashkin, D. P., et al. Journal of Allergy Clin. Immol. 76:855, 1985.

249. Thieman, T. G., in Kao F.F. and J. J. Kao, eds. Recent Advances in Acupuncture Research. Garden City, NY: Institute for Advanced Research in Asian Science and Medicine, 1979, p. 341.
250. Thomas, M., et al. American Journal of Chinese Medicine 19:95, 1991.
251. Tian, L. T., et al. Journal of Traditional Chinese Medicine (in Chinese) 34(10):600, 1993.
252. Tian, S. D., et al. Journal of Chinese Acupuncture and Moxibustion 11(4):15, 1991.
253. Tongas, G., et al. Digestive Disease and Science. 37:1576, 1992.
254. Tsuei, W. M. Journal of Chinese Acupuncture and Moxibustion 11(2):50, 1991.
255. Vasilenko, A. M., et al. Fiziol. Cheli 12:940, 1986.
256. Wang, B. E., et al. Acupuncture Electro-Ther. Res. 19:129, 1994.
257. Wang, C., and C. H. Guo. Shanghai Journal of Acupuncture and Moxibustion 13(2):63,1994.
258. Wang, C. H., et al. Tianjin Journal of Traditional Chinese Medicine 15(5):221, 1994.
259. Wang, C. D., et al. Journal of Chinese Acupuncture and Moxibustion 13(4):9, 1993.
260. Wang, C. S., et al. Journal of Chinese Acupuncture and Moxibustion 11(3):1, 1991.
261. Wang, C. Y., et al. Journal of Chinese Acupuncture and Moxibustion 13(1):17, 1993.
262. Wang, G. H. Journal of Chinese Acupuncture and Moxibustion 13(1): 18, 1993.
263. Wang, K. Journal of Traditional Chinese Medicine (in Chinese) 34(12):728, 1993.
264. Wang, L. P. American Journal of Acupuncture 14:217, 1986.
265. Wang, M. C. Shanghai Journal of Acupuncture and Moxibustion 12(2):66, 1993.
266. Wang, M. P. Shanghai Journal of Acupuncture and Moxibustion 12(2):66, 1993.
267. Wang, S. F., and Z. H. Zhang. Journal of Chinese Acupuncture and Moxibustion 14(1):46, 1994.
268. Wang, S. Journal of Chinese Acupuncture and Moxibustion 13(1):5, 1993.
269. Wang, S. Journal of Chinese Acupuncture and Moxibustion 11(5):7, 1991.
270. Wang, W. Z., and W. Z. Lin. Journal of Traditional Chinese Medicine 7:238, 1987.
271. Wang, Y. P., and M. Y. Hsu. Shanghai Journal of Acupuncture and Moxibustion 10(4):13, 1991.
272. Wang, Y. T., and H. An. Journal of Chinese Acupuncture and Moxibustion 10(3):21, 1990.
273. Wen, S. H. Beijing Journal of Traditional Chinese Medicine February (1):34, 1993.
274. Weng, S. Y., and Z. F. Yin. Shanghai Journal of Acupuncture and Moxibustion 12(4):143, 1993.
275. Wong, C. C., and H. C. Huang. Journal of Chinese Acupuncture and Moxibustion 11(5):11, 1991.
276. Wong, C. Journal of Chinese Acupuncture and Moxibustion 13(5): 11, 1993.
277. Wong, K. C., et al. Journal of Chinese Acupuncture and Moxibustion 13(6):4, 1993.
278. Wong, H. Z. Journal of Chinese Acupuncture and Moxibustion 11(6):1, 1991.
279. Wong, Y. L., and Y. S. Tan. Journal of Chinese Acupuncture and Moxibustion 13(5):21, 1993.
280. Wu, C. Journal of Chinese Acupuncture and Moxibustion 10(5):1, 1990.
281. Wu, C. K. New Journal of Traditional Chinese Medicine 25(4):32, 1993.
282. Wu, C. P. Journal of Chinese Acupuncture and Moxibustion 13(4):5, 1993.
283. Wu, D. Z. American Journal of Acupuncture 16:113, 1988.
284. Wu, H. J., and H. P. Chen. Journal of Chinese Acupuncture and Moxibustion 14(2): 51, 1993.
285. Wu, J. J. Journal of Chinese Acupuncture and Moxibustion 13(3): 16, 1993.
286. Wu, S. P. Journal of Chinese Acupuncture and Moxibustion 13(4):5, 1993.
287. Wu, S. F., and Y. C. Ky. Journal of Chinese Acupuncture and Moxibustion 11(2):11, 1991.
288. Wu, S. T. Shanghai Journal of Acupuncture and Moxibustion 12(1):30, 1993.
289. Wu, Y. Y. Shanghai Journal of Acupuncture and Moxibustion 12(1):25, 1993.
290. Xiang, L. M., and H. Yan. Shanghai Journal of Acupuncture and Moxibustion 12(4):150,1993.
291. Xiao, Y. F., et al. Acta Physiol. Sinica 35 :257, 1983.
292. Xue, C. C. Chinese Medical Journal 98:669, 1985.
293. Yang, C. H., and Y. C. Jin. Shanghai Journal of Acupuncture and Moxibustion 12(3):104, 1993.
294. Yang, D. L. Journal of Traditional Chinese Medicine 5(1):26, 1985.
295. Yang, E. W. Journal of Chinese Acupuncture and Moxibustion 10(3):18, 1990.
296. Yang, L. F. Shanghai Journal of Acupuncture and Moxibustion 12(1):33, 1993.
297. Yang, L. H., and C. Y. Huang. Jiangsu Journal of Traditional Chinese Medicine 15(1):27, 1994.
298. Yang, Y. C., et al. Journal of Traditional Chinese Medicine 3(1):41, 1983.
299. Yang, S. H., et al. Journal of Chinese Acupuncture and Moxibustion 14(2):4, 1994.
300. Yang, Y. M., et al. New Journal of Traditional Chinese Medicine 25(11):33, 1993.
301. Yao, F. Y., and L. Y. Wang. Shanghai Journal of Acupuncture and Moxibustion 12(2):74, 1993.
302. Yao, Z. H., et al. Journal of Traditional Chinese Medicine 4:97, 1984.
303. Yao, Z. L., and C. Z. Yang. Shanghai Journal of Acupuncture and Moxibustion 8(1):12, 1989.
304. Yazawa K. J. Jpn. Assoc. Phys. Med. Balneol. Clinatol. 48:183, 1985.
305. Yen, K. T., et al. Journal of Chinese Acupuncture and Moxibustion 13(1):8, 1993.
306. Yu, Y. Y. Shanghai Journal of Acupuncture and Moxibustion 12(2):54, 1993.
307. Yuan, C. J. Journal of Traditional Chinese Medicine 25(10):33, 1993.

308. Yuan, Q. Journal of Chinese Acupuncture and Moxibustion 14 (1):6, 1994.
309. Yuan, Y. M., et al. Journal of Traditional Chinese Medicine 7:235, 1987.
310. Zang, J. Q. Journal of Traditional Chinese Medicine 10:89, 1990.
311. Zarski, S., et al. Reumatolog. (Warsaw) 25:8, 1987.
312. Zhang, B., et al. Journal of Chinese Acupuncture and Moxibustion 14(1):17, 1994.
313. Zhang, C. F. Shanghai Journal of Acupuncture and Moxibustion 12(3):106, 1993.
314. Zhang, H. L., et al. Journal of Traditional Chinese Medicine 3:259, 1983.
315. Zhang, L. F. Journal of Chinese Acupuncture and Moxibustion 14(1):36, 1994.
316. Zhang, L. M. Shanghai Journal of Acupuncture and Moxibustion 12(1):28, 1993.
317. Zhang, L. S. Journal of Chinese Acupuncture and Moxibustion 13(5):3, 1993.
318. Zhang, L. Y. New Journal of Traditional Chinese Medicine 25(3):33, 1993.
319. Zhang, M., and J. C. Cheng. Journal of Chinese Acupuncture and Moxibustion 13(6):28, 1993.
320. Zhang, M., and S. C. Chen. Journal of Chinese Acupuncture and Moxibustion 11(1):45, 1991.
321. Zhang, M. Z., and H. Li. New Journal of Traditional Chinese Medicine 26(4):31, 1994.
322. Zhang, M. J. Journal of Traditional Chinese Medicine 8:153, 1988.
323. Zhang, P. G., and X. G. Zhu. Journal of Chinese Acupuncture and Moxibustion 13(3):9,1993.
324. Zhang, P. M. Shanghai Journal of Acupuncture and Moxibustion 13(2):64, 1994.
325. Zhang, X. F. Journal of Chinese Acupuncture and Moxibustion 13(6):17, 1993.
326. Zhang, S. Z. New Journal of Traditional Chinese Medicine 26(3):33, 1994.
327. Zhang, Y. Journal of Chinese Acupuncture and Moxibustion 13(4):15, 1993.
328. Zhang, Y. C., and J. F. Zhang. Journal of Chinese Acupuncture and Moxibustion 13(4):16, 1993.
329. Zhang, Y. S. Shanghai Journal of Acupuncture and Moxibustion 12(1):31, 1993.
330. Zhou, C. F., and F. Zhang. Journal of Chinese Acupuncture and Moxibustion 13(3):3, 1993.
331. Zhou, C. S. Shanghai Journal of Acupuncture and Moxibustion 12(1):48, 1993.
332. Zhou, C. S., et al. Journal of Chinese Acupuncture and Moxibustion 13(6):19, 1993.
333. Zhou, E. P., and S. F. Li. Journal of Chinese Acupuncture and Moxibustion 13(1):38, 1993.
334. Zhou, K. F., et al. New Journal of Traditional Chinese Medicine 26(2):33, 1994.
335. Zhou, L., and Wm. Y. Chey. Life Science 34:2233, 1984.
336. Zhou, R. X., et al. Shanghai Journal of Acupuncture and Moxibustion 12(2):62, 1993.
337. Zhou, Y., et al. Journal of Traditional Chinese Medicine (in English) 13(4):277, 1993.
338. Zwolfer, W., et al. American Journal of Chinese Medicine 21:113, 1993.

12
Acupuncture in Ophthalmology

Ophthalmology was not a separate speciality in traditional Chinese medicine. The sense organs, including the eye, are not listed as parts of Zhan-Fu (organs and viscerals) and no meridian is branched into any one of them. Chinese medical literature on the treatment of eye diseases is scarce, and little was listed in the ancient classics. The applications of acupuncture in eye illness usually involved eye symptoms in conjunction with other diseases. Examples included visual disturbances related to headache or migraine headache, and trigeminal neuralgia, a sort of functional ophthalmological disturbance. Acupuncture therapy targeting the major pathological conditions would also benefit vision disturbances.

In patients with functional opthalmological disturbances undergoing acupuncture treatment for an average of seven sessions, it has been reported that 34 percent were free of complaints after the treatment and another 53 percent were greatly improved (22).

Chinese schoolchildren were taught the acupoints around the eye socket and instructed to massage them daily as an exercise for eye fitness (23).

Since acupuncture anesthesia was introduced in China in the late 1950s, this technique has also been successfully applied to ophthalmological surgery. H. Masula, et al., (14) reported on twenty-four patients undergoing eye surgery under acupuncture anesthesia who required much less of the analgesic agent, fentanyl (about 25 percent of the regular dose) than the group operated on with other anesthetic techniques. H. Ogata, et al., (17) reported successful results with acupuncture anesthesia in cataract operations.

Wang (1, p. 214) operated on patients with glaucoma under acupuncture anesthesia and obtained a 91 percent success rate. Zusanli was selected as the main acupoint.

Retinitis and Retinopathy

A team from Zhejiang University Hospital (1, p. 102, 21) studied 600 cases of exudative central chorioretinopathy under the treatment of acupuncture. A special acupoint, Xiang-Yang Yao, located between the largest laryngeal cartilage and the sternocleidomastoid muscle and approximately one finger lateral to the thyroid was selected. The right Xiang-Yang Yao was needled for right eye disease and the left Yao for left eye disease. Treatment was performed once a day and lasted for fifteen to twenty minutes. In seven years of observations on 600 patients receiving an average one to four courses of treatment (ten days as a course), 46.2 percent were cured with resolution of all symptoms and recovery of vision to 1.0 in the International Vision Index. Inflammation subsided and the Fovea Centralis reflex reappeared. Another 309 patients (51.5 percent) were improved and only fourteen failed to respond (2.34 percent). In 167 cases followed up for one year, seventy-one patients maintained in normal condition.

Li (1, p. 101) reported on 403 patients suffering from chronic central angioretinopathy who were treated with acupuncture at the acupoint Meichong (B 3). Sixty-one percent recovered to a normal condition, 29.6 percent showed improvement, and only 2.3 percent failed. One hundred and twenty-three patients suffering from recurrent retinal hemorrhage were treated with acupuncture at the acupoint Feng Chi (G 20). The short-term cure rate was 26.8 percent and the long-term rate was 77.3 percent. There was a 12.6 percent failing rate (1, p. 103). Wang, et al., (2, p. 5) reported the successful treatment of 116 cases of central retinitis with acupuncture therapy over the years 1976–83. Ninety-six patients were cured (82.7 percent). Their vision was improved from a pretreatment index of 0.51 ±0.122 increased to 0.86 ± 0.14.

F. C. Wong, et al., (26) reported on the use of acupuncture in the treatment of ninety-two patients suffering from hemorrhage of eye base and other ophthalmological disorders. A total of 150 eyes were treated at the acupoint Feng Chi. In 38 of the eyes there was complete recovery from the illness; of 52 eyes with peripheral retinal inflammation, 17 were cured (32.7 percent); of 36 eyes with retina embolism, 14 were cured; and of 6 eyes with optic nerve inflammation 1 was cured (16.7 percent). In other cases there was partial recovery, and 27 eyes did not respond to the treatment.

P. Q. Li (11) reported on 972 cases of central angiospastic retinopathy treated with acupuncture. Of 861 chronically affected eyes in 533 patients, 66 percent showed remarkable improvement and a total of 97 percent had at least some improvement in their vision.

S. Dabov, et al., (6) used acupuncture in fifty patients suffering from retinitis pigmentosa, myopia, glaucoma, or optic nerve atrophy. Acupuncture was performed bilaterally at the acupoints Yangbai (G 14) Cheng Qi (S 1), and YinTang (Extra 2), which are in the close proximity to the eye. All patients showed a subjective improvement in visual baseline value. Three glaucoma patients had a decrease in intraocular pressure, by tonometric measurements.

Surveying clinical experience over seven years, C. Y. Chen (4) reported on the treatment of 162 cases of central retinitis (total 233 eyes) with acupuncture in combination with Qi Gong technique. (See Chapter 23.) He claimed he could concentrate his body force (or Qi) into his finger and transmit this force by pointing to needles inserted at two acupoints, one of which was Zusanli and the other the eyeball. The needle remained at each point for five or six minutes. Of the 233 eyes, 163 were cured (70 percent). Vision was restored to normal. There were three failures; the others were slightly improved.

Disorders of the Optic Nerve

In forty-six patients (a total of eighty-two eyes) suffering from optic nerve disorders treated with acupuncture (8), a total effectiveness rate of 76.9 percent was obtained. Of fifty-six eyes with optic neuritis, 60.7 percent were markedly improved and in 16.1 percent there was no effect. Of twenty-six eyes with optic atrophy, only sixteen (61.5 percent) showed moderate improvement; in ten there was no effect. It appears that the duration of the diseases did not have any influence on the response to therapy.

A recent report by Wong (26) described forty-eight cases of optic nerve atrophy treated with acupuncture at the acupoints Qiuhou (Extra 7) and Feng Chi, once daily for twelve days. Fifteen patients had marked improvement, twenty-five moderate improvement, and there were seven failures.

C. M. Shi (21) reported twenty-four cases of optic nerve atrophy treated with acupuncture at the acupoint Feng Chi three times per week. After twelve treatments the effectiveness rate was 62.5 percent.

Congenital Color Blindness

Probably the most surprising claim about acupuncture is the report by Chen, et al., (2, p. 47) that it produced a remarkable reversal of congenital color blindness. Ninety red-green color blind subjects were treated with acupuncture at the acupoints Zusanli and Sanyinjiao. The control group received a sham acupuncture. In the acupuncture group fifteen were cured: they were able to acurately distinguish colors they could not do previously. Among the other seventy-three subjects, who were followed for six months with continued treatment, color vision was much improved. In the control group, no patient was improved during the same observation period.

Strabismus

Gao (2, p. 48) reported 100 cases of strabismus treated with acupuncture at the acupoints Feng Chi and Taichong (Liv 3) for inward strabismus or at the acupoints HoKu and Jingming (B 1) for outward strabismus. Treatments were given every other day for a total of three to forty sessions. Sixty-five patients fully recovered, seven failed, and the others had some improvement.

Sixty-six patients, aged three to twelve years, underwent surgery to correct strabismus under the acupuncture anesthesia. Bilateral needling was applied at the acupoint Neiguan (P 6) and produced very satisfactory results (9).

In 167 cases of paralytic squint (175 eyes) treated with acupuncture, Z. Zheng, et al., (33) reported that short term cure rate in 33.6 percent, marked improvement in 26.6 percent, and failure in 12 percent. The researchers stated that if the squint was less than twenty degrees and the duration of the disorder was less than one month, then, the acupuncture therapy was associated with a good prognosis. In patients followed up for two and one-half years, the total cure rate was 34 percent to 67 percent.

Myopia

M. Liang (12) reviewed the clinical application of acupuncture therapy in eye diseases over the last forty years in China. Totally, in 1,100 cases of myopia treated with acupuncture, a 90 percent effectiveness rate was observed.

Yan (2, p. 277) treated sixty youngsters with myopia with acupuncture at the acupoints HoKu and Taichong once a day for fifteen days. After resting for a couple of days, a second treatment session could be performed. Among 109 treated eyes, the diopter was decreased by more than 0.75 D.S. after the treatment, indicating that acupuncture not only improved accommodation, but also influenced the diopteric power of the eyes. The visual acuity of the patients was increased; of the treated eyes 23 percent returned to normal.

In another report, 150 cases of myopia (a total of 267 eyes) were treated with magnetic blunt needle and manual massage at the acupoints HoKu, Feng Chi, and Sishencong (Extra 6). Totally, 201 eyes were cured (73.5 percent), and the rest were improved (3).

Table 12-1. Acupuncture Therapy in Ophthalmological Diseases

Source	Mode	Acupoint	Diagnosis	No. of Patients	Effectiveness %
Chu (5)	AP-pr.* with Vaccaria seeds	Ear	Myopia	326 (488 eyes)	20.9% were cured and other 74.6% improved
Li (10)	AP** and IAc inj.#	Jingming (B 1) Qiuhou (Extra 7)	Myopia	332 (652 eyes)	26% were cured and other 48% improved
Liu (13)	AP	Jingming Chengguang (B 6)	Myopia	150 (278 eyes)	11% were cured and other 25% markedly improved
Pasmanik (18)	AP		Amblyopia	52 (75 eyes)	More effective than the group treated with pleoptics technique
Deng (7)	AP	Ear	Acute conjunctivitis	64	100% were cured after 5½ days treatment
Yang (29)	AP	Zusanli (S 36) Sanyinjiao (Sp 6) Fengchi (G 20)	Optic nerve myelitis	28	21 of them were cured
Wang (25)	AP	Jianli (Ren 11) Yintang (Extra 2)	Optic nerve atrophy	110 (164 eyes)	11% were cured and other 35% improved
Wong (27)	AP	Jingming Sizhukong (Sj 23)	Ophthalmo-plegia	120	75% markedly effective after 1-30 treatments
Wu (28)	AP	Tianzhu (B 10) Fengchi	Endocrine ophthalmo-pathy	40	23% completely recovered 13% markedly improved
Yin (32)	AP	Shousanli (LI 10) Zusanli Sanyinjiao	Eye lip ptosis	30	87% were cured
Zhong (34)	AP with Plum-blossom needle		Squint eyes	182 eyes	31% functional cures; visual acuity restored.

* AP-pr. = Acupressure with plaster
** AP = Acupuncture
# IAc. inj. = Intra-acupoint injection

Other Eye Disorders

In 1,617 young subjects suffering from hypometropia, 359 cases (22.2 percent) were cured with acupuncture, with vision returning to 1.0 or above, 296 cases (18.2 percent) did not show any effect, and the others were improved (19).

A. Nishida, et al., (16) reported several cases of asthenopia due to working with video display terminals. Patients were treated with EAP for fifteen minutes with low frequency applied bilaterally at the acupoints Tai Yang (Extra) and Zanshu (B 2). A significant improvement was obtained.

Acupuncture therapy was found to be very effective in treating occipital neuralgia. Forty-three patients suffering from asthenopia with ocular pain and headache received acupuncture treatment with or without massage. All symptoms were effectively relieved (15).

K. Yazawa (30) reported thirty cases of subacute myelo-optico-neuropathy treated with acupuncture over three years. A highly successful result was obtained in 77.3 percent of the patients.

Acupuncture therapy seems to be ineffective in Graves' ophthalmopathy (20).

Table 12-1 lists additional clinical data on the treatment of ophthamological diseases by acupuncture therapy.

References

1. All China Society of Acupuncture and Moxibustion. First National Symposium on Acupuncture and Moxibustion and Acupuncture Anesthesia. Beijing: 1979.
2. All China Society of Acupuncture and Moxibustion. Second National Symposium on Acupuncture, Moxibustion and Acupuncture Anesthesia. Beijing: People Health Publisher, 1984.
3. Chao, S. M., et al. Journal of Chinese Acupuncture and Moxibustion 10(4): 15, 1990.
4. Chen, C. Y. Journal of Chinese Acupuncture and Moxibustion 11(6): 9, 1991.
5. Chu, S. P. Journal of Chinese Acupuncture and Moxibustion 13(2):19, 1993.
6. Dabov, S., et al. Acupuncture Electro-Ther. Res. 10:793, 1985.
7. Deng, S. F. Journal of Traditional Chinese Medicine (in English) 5:263, 1985.
8. Huang, S. Y., and Y. C. Zeng. Journal of Traditional Chinese Medicine 5:187, 1985.
9. Lewis, I. H., et al. British Journal of Anesthet. 67:23, 1991.
10. Li, K. Z., et al. Journal of Chinese Acupuncture and Moxibustion 13(6):9, 1993.
11. Li, P. Q. Chinese Medical Journal 98:343, 1985.
12. Liang, L. M. Journal of Chinese Acupuncture and Moxibustion 11(5):47, 1991.
13. Liu, C. Y., and T. M. Wang. Journal of Chinese Acupuncture and Moxibustion 14(1):35, 1994.
14. Masula, H., et al. Acupuncture Electro-Ther. Res. 11:259, 1986.
15. Nakagawa, S., and M. Takake Jpn. J. of Clin. Ophthalmol. 42:1130, 1988.
16. Nishida, A., et al. Jpn. J. of Clin. Ophthalm. 42:712, 1988.
17. Ogata, H., et al. American Journal of Chinese Medicine 11:130, 1983.
18. Pasmanik, E. D., and T. R. Nizovtseva. Vestn-Oftalmol. 109:6, 1993.
19. Po, C. C. Journal of Chinese Acupuncture and Moxibustion 10(2):1, 1990.
20. Rogvi-Hansen, B., et al. Acta Endocrinol. 174:143, 1991.
21. Shi, C. M. Chinese Acupuncture and Moxibustion. Tianjin: Science and Tecbology Publisher, 1991 p. 646.
22. Sold-Darseff, J., and W. Leydhecker. Klin. Monatschr. Augenheilkd. 189:169, 1986.
23. Spoerel, W. E. American Journal of Chinese Medicine 10:70, 1982.
24. Wang, S. H. Journal of Chinese Acupuncture and Moxibustion 13(2): 5, 1993.
25. Wang, X. F., and X. Y. Jiang. Journal of Chinese Acupuncture and Moxibustion 13(6):9, 1993.
26. Wong, F. C., et al. Journal of Chinese Acupuncture and Moxibustion 10(1):11, 1990.
27. Wong, L. Z., et al. Journal of Chinese Acupuncture and Moxibustion 13(5):7, 1993.
28. Wu, Z. S., et al. Journal of Traditional Chinese Medicine 5(1):19, 1985.
29. Yang, Y. C., and G. L. Zhang. Journal of Chinese Acupuncture and Moxibustion 14(2):13, 1994.
30. Yazawa, K. J. Jpn. Assoc. Phy. Med. Balneol. Climatol. 48:267, 1985.
31. Yi, L. M., et al., from Chang, H., ed. Acupuncture and Moxibustion and Acupuncture Anthesthesia. Beijing: Anesthesia Research Science Publisher, 1986. p. 652.
32. Yin, Z. C. New Journal of Traditional Chinese Medicine 25(3):32, 1993.
33. Zheng, J. Z., et al. Journal of Traditional Chinese Medicine 4:177, 1984.
34. Zhong, M. Q. Journal of Traditional Chinese Medicine 4(1):7, 1984.

13
Acupuncture in Otolaryngology

Following President Nixon's visit to China in 1972, many American medical professionals went to China to explore the mysterious acupuncture therapy. Prof. J. J. Bonica was one who led a delegation to investigate acupuncture. He published a report based on his personal observations and information from other visiting physicians and scientists (3). Besides its use in anesthesia and pain relief, he emphasized the use of acupuncture in the treatment of deafness, on which it has been applied in China since 1968, the most intriguing and exciting application of acupuncture. Reports from some clinics have claimed an improvement rate up to 80 percent in the treatment of childhood deafness. But Bonica, himself an anesthesiologist and scientist, was skeptical of such claims, because the clinical assessment of patients before the treatment frequently was incomplete.

After a visit to China to observe the treatment of deaf mutism by acupuncture, which is performed in several hospitals, S. Rosen applied the technique in forty cases of pediatric deafness and concluded that it failed to produce any consistent improvement (17).

Q. Liu, et al., (12) reviewed their twenty-year experience with acupuncture treatment of sensorineural deafness and deaf mutism. In the vast majority, acupuncture did not exert a beneficial effect. They specifically stated that acupuncture should not be used, especially in deaf mutism. During the years 1971–72, 204 students from a Chinese deaf-mute school were treated by acupuncture. Not a single case had a beneficial effect. In the years 1972–73, 157 deaf-mute students were treated with acupuncture under the supervision of an American otologist. Again no improvement was observed.

However, several subsequent publications claimed that acupuncture is effective in the treatment of toxic deafness. Whether the reported cases had a functional and not anatomical hearing loss is unclear. Basically, there is no scientific explanation of the mechanism by which acupuncture may improve hearing. D. X. Ja (6) reviewed the use of acupuncture therapy in the treatment of otolaryngological diseases in the last ten years. In 109 cases of toxic deafness due to drug intoxication (aminoglycoside antibiotics were the major cause) acupuncture therapy produced a cure rate of 83.9–94 percent. The patients' hearing returned to 15 decibels or above. By comparison, a group treated with medications had an effectiveness rate of 74 percent.

Hanson (8, p.670) reported on 100 patients with neurosensory hearing loss, 50 treated with EAP and 50 with manual acupuncture. Audiograms revealed that a ten decibel or more improvement in speech frequencies in ten cases. At the end of the treatment, one-third of the patients were significantly improved and did not require the use of any hearing aid, one-third slightly improved, and the rest had no response to treatment.

In 125 cases of deafness, including 12 due to congenital defects and 110 due to drug intoxication, acupuncture therapy was applied at the acupoints Tinggong (SI 19) and Renying (S 9) once a day for twenty-six days as a treatment course. Twenty-seven patients (21.6 percent) were cured and 19 (15.2 percent) were improved (25).

In another sixty-nine patients suffering with toxic deafness for up to twelve years treated with acupuncture therapy at the HoKu, Feng Chi, and Ermen (SI 21) acupoints. There was a remarkable improvement in hearing in forty-six cases (24).

EAP was used to treat 180 cases of deafness (in 300 affected ears) at the acupoints Tinggong and Ermen; 190 of the affected ears were cured (26).

Kao, et al., (8, p. 603) reported 6 cases of sensorineural deafness treated with acupuncture. The patients were examined thoroughly by X ray, biochemical, and physiological tests before and after treatment. The efficiency of acupuncture therapy was judged by the improvements in speech discrimination. It was concluded that acupuncture therapy produced some beneficial effect.

In a ten-year period, Yang treated 87 cases of auditory deafness (a total of 137 ears) by EAP plus intraacupoint injection of vitamin B12 at the acupoint Xiaguan (S 7). Thirty-five of the ears (28 percent) were markedly improved (23).

In the United States, Peng (8, p. 599) performed acupuncture therapy in 10 cases of sensorineural deafness. The age ranged from thirty-six to eighty-four years and the duration of deafness was five to thirty-one years. After four to fourteen treatments, six patients were cured or remarkably improved, three were moderately improved, and two had no effect.

A team from the Jilan Medical University Hospital (7) devised a transtympanic technique to study the amplitude of voltage changes in the internal ear by electrical stimulation of a needle inserted into the tympanum. Based on these measurements and electrocochleaograms, they were able to determine whether the acupuncture therapy would be beneficial in cases of deafness. In a total of 129 deafness cases, EAP was applied every other day for ten minutes. A course consisted of ten treatments. Thirty-four cases (24 percent) showed an improvement, and 98 (76 percent) failed to improve. Among the improved cases, there was an increase of more than ten-decibal power in speech discrimination.

In the first national symposium on acupuncture, held in Beijing in 1979, a team from Shanghai Hospital reported 34 cases of deafness treated with acupuncture. Eleven patients (36.9 percent) were improved. Five of 20 deaf mutism cases were improved by acupuncture (1, p. 108).

Wang, et al., (1, p. 106) measured the auditory cochlear potentials of fifty-three patients (a total of sixty affected ears). Acupuncture therapy was given at the acupoint Tinggong (SI 19). Eleven ears (18.3 percent) showed an increase in cochlear activity, but 78.4 percent had no significant change. In 41 cases the promontorium tympani cavity was needled; 20.7 percent of the affected ears showed an increase in cochlear activity.

Studies on the effect of acupuncture on hearing in deaf patients have shown that the effectiveness of the therapy depended upon the degree of deafness. Xu, et al., (2, p. 49) treated 50 cases of toxic deafness due to streptomycin with acupuncture at the acupoints Tinggong and Ermen. Twenty-one patients whose hearing was between five and fifteen decibels were markedly improved after the treatment, but twenty-nine patients whose hearing was below 5 decibels showed no improvement.

In studies on a group of normal male volunteers, T. J. Liao, et al., (11) found that acupuncture stimulation can promote middle-latency auditory-evoked potentials. This could explain the beneficial effect of acupuncture therapy in some cases of deafness.

Other Auditory Disturbances

Acupuncture therapy has been shown to be effective in the treatment of vestibular disturbances (16). V. F. Filatov, et al., (5) reported eighty-five patients with vestibular dysfunction treated with acupuncture. A prolonged remission was obtained in twenty-three of thirty patients with Meniere's disease, twenty of thirty-seven patients with cervical osteochondriosis, nine of eleven patients with vestibulopathies, and seven of these patients suffering with vestibulopathies due to a complication after middle ear surgery.

S. Nilsson, et al., (15) treated fifty-six patients with continuous severe tinnitis. Three patients reported an improvement lasting for at least eighteen days without recurrence, indicating a possible long-term effect. Seventeen patients (31 percent) reported a transient intensity reduction lasting for hours or days.

Other reports also showed that Meniere's disease responded well to acupuncture therapy. Thirty-four patients who were nonresponsive to medical treatment were transferred to the acupuncture clinic. After a couple of acupuncture treatments the vertigo resolved and the central hearing threshold became stable and returned to normal (20).

T. Nagahama of Japan developed a new technique employing acupuncture and lidocaine injected into an acupoint for the treatment of tinnitus (14). N. J. Marks (13) reported that acupuncture treatment of tinnitus resuslted in a beneficial effect in 35 percent of the patients, but there was no difference in response between the acupuncture group and the placebo group.

G. G. Bubnova, et al., (4) reported that acupuncture therapy can restore auditory function in children with otitis media.

One hundred and twenty-five active-duty flying pilots suffering from aero-otitis media were treated with acupuncture on the acupoints Ermen (SI 21) and Tinghui (G 2). Fifty-six percent were cured and another 15 percent showed marked improvement (21).

Acupuncture anesthesia has been used in China in tonsillectomy and laryngoectomy with reported success. (See chapter 9.) A. Kusuma, et al., from Indonesia Hospital used a combination acupuncture and "Sluder-Guillotene Gauze pressure" technique in thirty tonsillectomy cases with excellent results (10).

Acupuncture therapy has also has used successfully in the treatment of acute tonsillitis. In fifty cases in which acupuncture was performed bilaterally at the acupoint Shousanli (LI 10), twenty-three patients (46 percent) were cured after one treatment, and the other twenty-four (48 percent) were cured after another one or two treatments (22).

Sixteen patients suffering from phonasthenia (due to emotional stress) and showing some polymorphic neurotic manifestations (hypochondriac or depressive) were treated with acupuncture. All were improved and had normal sleep. Laryngeal muscle pain was relieved, and voice quality was improved (18).

Fourteen patients with unilateral paralysis of the recurrent laryngeal nerve were treated with acupuncture in combination with medications. Excellent results were obtained. Eleven patients recovered within two or three weeks after the treatment, and the other·three recovered after two or three months (9).

Meyer (8, p. 553) reported two cases of peripheral nerve paralysis of the larynx treated with acupuncture. After four months' treatment their voices had returned to normal. One case with facial paralysis was completely healed after two months.

Acupuncture therapy was also found to be effective and painless in the treatment of vasomotor and allergic rhinitis in children (19).

References

1. All China Society of Acupuncture and Moxibustion: First National Symposium on Acupuncture and Moxibustion and Acupuncture Anesthesia. Beijing: 1979.
2. All China Society of Acupuncture and Moxibustion: Second National Symposium on Acupuncture and Moxibustion and Acupuncture Anesthesia. Beijing: People Health Press, 1984.
3. Bonica, J. J. JAMA 228:1544, 1974.
4. Bubnova, G. G., et al. Vestn. Otorinolaringol. 0(5):58, 1988.
5. Filatov, V. F., et al. Vestn. Otorinolaringol. 0:14, 1988.
6. Ja, D. Y. Journal of Chinese Acupuncture and Moxibustion 11(4):16, 1991.
7. Jilin Med. Univ. Team: from Chang, H. T., ed. Acupuncture Moxibustion and Acupuncture, Beijing: Anesthesia Research Science Publisher, 1984, p. 656.
8. Kao, F. F., and J. J. Research Advances in Acupuncture Research, Garden City, NY: Institute for Advanced Research in Asian Science and Medicine, 1979.
9. Karnova, O. Y. Vestn. Otorinolarinogol. 0:41, 1989.
10. Kusuma, A., et al. Alternative Medicine 1:69, 1985.
11. Liao, T. J., et al., Tohoku Journal of Exp. Med. 170:103, 1993.
12. Liu, Q., et al. Chinese Medical Journal of 95:21, 1982.
13. Marks, N. J., et al. J. Laryngol. Otol. 98:1103, 1984.
14. Nagahama, T. Otol. Fukuoka 32:206, 1986.
15. Nilsson, S., et al. Scad. Audiology 21:245, 1992.
16. Paskar, N.D. Vestn. Otorinolaringol. 0(6):20, 1985.
17. Rosen, S. Laryngoscope, December 1974, p. 1.
18. Salivon, L. G. Vestn. Otorinolaringol. 0:23, 1988.
19. Shevrygin, B. V., and E. P. Karpora. Vestn. Otorinolaringol. 0:21, 1988.
20. Steinberger, A., and M. Pansini. American Journal of Chinese Medicine 11:102, 1983.
21. Tian, Z. M. Journal of Traditional Chinese Medicine 5(4):259, 1985.
22. Wong, C. H. Shanghai Journal of Acupuncture and Moxibustion 12(1):46, 1993.
23. Yang, S. C. Shanghai Journal of Acupuncture and Moxibustion 12(4):158, 1993.
24. Zhang, W. P. Journal of Chinese Acupuncture and Moxibustion 10(3):16, 1990.
25. Zhang, X. Y. Journal of Chinese Acupuncture and Moxibustion 11(4):16, 1991.
26. Zhou, S. H., and C. H. Wang. Journal of Chinese Acupuncture and Moxibustion 1(4):9, 1990.

14

Acupuncture in Dermatology

Chinese traditional medicine strongly believes that the skin is communicated with the internal organs (Zhan-Fu) through the meridian channels and that some stubborn skin diseases that cannot be cured by topical therapy on the affected area could be treated at the cause of the origin, namely by the way of the affected meridian channel, to reach the responsive Zhan-Fu.

For more than twenty years D. C. Li and his colleagues have theorized about this phenomenon by connecting various dermatological diseases with the meridian distribution. They reported ninety-three cases of dermatitis, including scleroderma, neurodermatitis, eczema, seborrhea sicca, psoriasis, and purpura (17). With photographic illustrations they demonstrated that the spread of the dermatitis tended to follow the route of the twelve pairs of meridians. Patients were treated with acupuncture therapy or intraacupoint injection of Chinese herbs. Excellent results were observed. Usually itching was graduately reduced and inflammation resolved. The skin became normal after two or four weeks of treatment.

L. P. Chao (3) summarized ten years' experience in acupuncture therapy in the treatment of dermatitis at his clinic and others. Cures were reported in seventeen of thirty-four cases of chronic urticaria (50 percent); sixty-two of 80 cases of acne (77.5 percent); 8 of 46 cases of flat wart (17.4 percent); and 108 of 283 cases of chloasma (38.3 percent). Of 227 cases of leukoderma, only 11 cases (4.8 percent) were cured. Five hundred cases of psoriasis received longer acupuncture treatment over three months, and 56.6 percent were cured. Of thirty cases of pruritis, 25 were cured (83.3 percent) after acupuncture therapy.F. W. Chan reported 600 cases of psoriasis treated with acupuncture (2). Some patients had had the disease for more than forty years. Three hundred and sixteen were in a progressive active stage and 104 were in a regressive stage. Treatment involved use of a three-edged needle at the acupoints Ganshu (B 18) and Pishu (B 20) and electrical stimulation at a frequency of 26/minute. A total of 370 patients were been cured (61.7 percent), and another 148 were significantly improved.

Auricular acupuncture was used to treat 78 patients suffering from eczema. High effectiveness rates were obtained (1).

S. J. Liao reported on the use of acupuncture therapy in 4 cases of contact dermatitis due to poison ivy. After one treatment, the itching subsided within a few hours. In one severe case, the symptom subsided two days after the treatment. The skin lesions of all patients were dried up in four days. Acupuncture therapy involved an antiinflammatory action, possibly caused by a release of ACTH and/or corticosteroids (21).

Acupuncture therapy has also been used to treat senile dermatitis and vascular dermatitis at the acupoints of Baihui (Du 20) and Qiangjian (Du 18) in combination with intraacupoint injection of acetyl-glutaminate. K. Chen, et al., (5) reported that 7 of 17 cases of senile dermatitis were improved and 9 of 21 cases of vascular dermatitits were improved.

Forty-one cases of neurodermatitis were treated with acupuncture, employing a plum-blossom

Table 14-1. Acupuncture Therapy in Dermatology

Source	Mode	Acupoint	Diagnosis	No. of Patient	Effectiveness %
Liao (18)	EM*	Quchi (LI 11) Zhigou (SJ 6) Sanyinjiao (Sp 6)	Psoriasis	348	83.6% were cured after 3 months treatment
Liao (19)	AP**	Dazhui (Du 14)	Psoriasis	61	49% completely clear; 23% had 2/3 clear; 13% had 1/3 of skin lesion clear
Liang (22)	AP with 3-edged needle	Dazhui Feishu (B 13)	Psoriasis	158	50.6% were cured and other 22.7% markedly improved.
Lu (27)	AP	Quchi Xuehai (Sp 10)	Psoriasis	26	62% were cured, follow up for 2 yrs, no recurrence
Wang (34)	AP	Lingtai (Du 10)	Neurotic dermatitis & psoriasis	1,000	60% were cured and other 20% improved
Chen (6)	AP	Dazhui Lingtai	Neurotic dermatitis	68	78% were cured
Li (16)	AP	Near the affected area	Neurotic dermatitis	56	73.2% were cured
Wang (33)	AP	Ear	Neurotic dermatitis	69	86% were cured, follow up for 3 months, no recurrence
Rosled (31)	AP		Atrophic dermatitis and acne	4	excellent result, all was cured
Lin (25)	AP	Zusanli (S 36) Quchi Feishu	Eczema	46	87% were cured,other 9% improved
Lin (24)	IAc inj.# of own blood	Quchi Zusanli	Chronic urticaria	38	76.2% were cured and other 16% markedly improved
Chen (5)	IAc inj. of peni-cillin	Quchi Xuehai	Urticaria	36	64% were cured
Zhang (40)	AP with Plum-blossom needle	Quchi	Urticaria	52	83% were cured

Table 14-1. (continued)

Source	Mode	Acupoint	Diagnosis	No. of Patients	Effectiveness %
Zhou (41)	Pl@ with Vaccaria seeds	Ear	Urticaria	121	29% were cured and other 34% markedly improved
Chiang (8)	AP	HoKu (LI 4) Taichong (Liv 3)	Verruca plana	46	57% were cured and other 34.8% improved
Lin (23)	IAc inj. with own blood	Quchi, Xuehai	Verruca plana	36	92% were cured
Wang (35)	AP		Verruca	186	All disappeared after 7-14 treatments
Ding (11)	AP and Cu##	Dazhui	Acne	50	54% were cured, other 42% markedly improved
Yang (37)	Pl with Vaccaria seeds	Ear	Acne	106	91.5% were cured
Yi (38)	AP with 3-edged needle	Zusanli, HoKu Sanyinjiao	Acne	68	28% were cured, other 35% markedly improved
Zhan (39)	IAc inj. of own blood	Zusanli Feishu	Acne	256	83% were cured
Dai (10)	AP	Zusanli, HoKu Sanyinjiao	Choasma	63	21 of them completely cured, 90% pigment was disappeared
Liao (20)	AP		Herpes simplex Herpes genitalis	2 3	All showed a marked reduction of episode
Long (26)	IAc inj. of B_{12}	Beihui (Du 20) Fengchi (G 20)	Baldhead	180	64% had hair reappearance in their head

* EM = Embedding with Catgut; ** AP = Acupuncture
# IAc inj. = Intra-acupoint injection
Cu = Cupping @ Pl = Plaster

needle (37). A 97.6 percent short-term success rate was obtained. Sixteen cases were followed up for a year and had a satisfactory long-term effect at the acupoint where the needle was applied and at the area along both sides of the spinal column.

T. Lundeberg, et al., (28) experimentally induced itching in 10 healthy people by injecting histamine subcutaneously and treated the subjects with manual acupuncture or EAP (2 Hz or 80 Hz) at the affected site for five minutes. Both manual acupuncture and EAP significantly decreased itching intensity, suggesting that acupuncture should be an effective remedy for the treatment of pruritis.

Six patients suffering from uremic pruritis were treated with acupuncture (13). Drastic improvement was observed. In another group of patients serving as controls, electrical stimulation was applied without acupuncture. No beneficial effect was observed.

Seven patients with warts, including anogenital and cluster warts, unresponsive to conventional therapy were treated with both acupuncture and moxibustion. After several treatments, all warts had disappeared and no recurrence was observed (4).

M. Masda, et al., (30) treated 4 cases of progressive systemic sclerosis with EAP, once or twice a week, with low frequency. There was remarkable improvement in the imflammatory reaction and the sense of well-being of the patients. The authors also reported a forty-seven-month-old girl suffering from scleroderma and hyperpigmentation who was treated with low-frequency EAP once a week for twenty to thirty months. The needle was inserted at the far edge of the longer axis of the linear scleroderma lesion. There was definite improvement in the cutaneous sclerosis, hyperpigmentation and perilesional alopecia.

EAP employing a plum-blossom needle was used in 186 cases of alopecia (14). One hundred and forty-six patients (78.6 percent) were cured, and another thirty-six were improved (19 percent).

Four patients with skin ganglia were treated with acupuncture. Six to eight needles were inserted around the peripheral region of the ganglion. After a single treatment, the ganglion was completely eliminated within approximately three weeks (12).

Twenty cases of polytrichosis were treated with acupuncture at the acupoint Zusanli for twenty minutes every other day. After fifteen sessions the density of hair growth and the length of hair were greatly reduced (36).

H. H. Lao (15) reported on the effects of acupuncture therapy in mycosis fungoides. After an average of eighty sessions of treatment the skin lesions completely resolved.

While in Kuwait, F. S. Chu (9) treated 357 cases of pemphigus ortheoarthropathy with acupuncture, achieving a cure in 62 cases (17.3 percent). Two hundred and twenty-nine patients showed improvement (63.7 percent), and sixty-eight failed to respond (18.9 percent).

Table 14-1 summarizes the other clinical data on the effectiveness of acupuncture therapy in the treatment of various dermatological problems.

References

1. Bukharovich, M. N., and V. A. Bocharov. Vestn. Dermatol. Veneral. 0(7): 59, 1988.
2. Chan, F. W., et al. Journal of Chinese Acupuncture and Moxibustion 11(2):3, 1991.
3. Chao, L. P. Journal of Chinese Acupuncture and Moxibustion 10(6):41, 1990.
4. Chen, G. S. American Journal of Acupuncture 15:221, 1987.
5. Chen, K. Shanghai Journal of Acupuncture and Moxibustion 13(2):70, 1993.
6. Chen, S. L. New Journal of Traditional Chinese Medicine 25(8):30, 1993,
7. Chen, Y. M., et al. Journal of Chinese Acupuncture and Moxibustion 11(4):20, 1991.
8. Chiang, W. Y., and J. L. Hu. Journal of Chinese Acupuncture and Moxibustion 13(2): 11, 1993.

9. Chu, F. S. Journal of Chinese Acupuncture and Moxibustion 10(4):13, 1990.
10. Dai, Y. Y., et al. Shanghai Journal of Acupuncture and Moxibustion 12(4):151, 1993.
11. Ding, L. N. Journal of Traditional Chinese Medicine 5(2):128, 1985.
12. Dung, H. C. Alternative Medicine 1:371, 1985/86.
13. Duo, L. Journal of Nephron 47:179, 1987.
14. Kuo, S. H. Journal of Chinese Acupuncture and Moxibustion 11(1):17, 1991.
15. Lao, H. H. American Journal of Acupuncture 16:221, 1988.
16. Li, C. M. Tianjin Journal of Traditional Chinese Medicine (6):24, 1993.
17. Li, D. C., from Chang, H. T., ed. Acupuncture, Moxibustion and Acupuncture Anesthesia. Beijing: Anesthesia Research Science Publisher, 1986, p. 528.
18. Liao, J. F. Journal of Chinese Acupuncture and Moxibustion 13(6):15, 1993.
19. Liao, S. J., and T. A. Liao. Acupuncture-Electro-Ther. Res. 17:195, 1992.
20. Liao, S. L., and T. A. Liao. Acupuncture Electro-Ther. Res. 16:135, 1991.
21. Liao, S. J. Acupuncture Electro-Ther. Res. 13:31, 1988.
22. Liang, H. Z. Journal of Chinese Acupuncture and Moxibustion 14(2):23, 1994.
23. Lin, L. Shanghai Journal of Acupuncture and Moxibustion 13(2):71, 1994.
24. Lin, N. Journal of Chinese Acupuncture and Moxibustion 14(2): 19, 1994.
25. Lin, P. Journal of Chinese Acupuncture and Moxibustion 13(4):4, 1993.
26. Long, T. F. New Journal of Traditional Chinese Medicine 26(4):37, 1994.
27. Lu, M. C. Journal of Chinese Acupuncture and Moxibustion 13(4):7, 1993.
28. Lundeberg, T., et al. British Journal of Dermatology. 117:771, 1987.
29. Masda, M., et al. Nishinihon Journal of Dermatology 49:270, 1987.
30. Masda M., et al. Journal of Dermatology (Tokyo) 15: 133, 1988.
31. Rosled, P. American Journal of Acupuncture 20:34, 1992.
32. Wang, J. Y., and Y. L. Pan. Journal of Chinese Acupuncture and Moxibustion 213(2):22, 1993.
33. Wang, M. H., and T. S. Yor. New Journal of Traditional Chinese Medicine 25(8):31, 1993.
34. Wang, S. L., et al. Tianjin Journal of Traditional Chinese Medicine (6):24, 1993.
35. Wang, X. F. Journal of Chinese Acupuncture and Moxibustion 13(3):18, 1993.
36. Wu, J. S., and S. A. Choi. Journal of Traditional Chinese Medicine 29:26, 1988.
37. Yang, S. P. Journal of Chinese Acupuncture and Moxibustion 14(1):26, 1994.
38. Yi, Z. Y. Shanghai Journal of Acupuncture and Moxibustion 13(2):72, 1994.
39. Zhan, S. Z., and C.F. Lu. Shanghai Journal of Acupuncture and Moxibustion 12(4):151, 1993.
40. Zhang, H. P. Shanghai Journal of Acupuncture and Moxibustion 13(2):69, 1994.
41. Zhou, P. Z., and L. M. Li. Journal of Chinese Acupuncture and Moxibustion 13(1):27, 1993.

15

Acupuncture in Dentistry and Oral Surgery

In the early nineteenth century, French physicians initiated the use of electrical stimulation as a painkilling remedy, especially for toothache and dental extraction. Actually, thousands of years ago the travelling practitioners in China had used acupuncture in markets and bazaars for dental extractions. They placed teeth, broken and unbroken, in front of their desk to advertise their experience. By the early 1970s, acupuncture therapy had become widely used in all Chinese dental clinics, especially for relief of dental pain. It was also used in rural areas as a substitute for opium smoking, which was often seen prior to the 1949 revolution.

Recently W. P. Chen and C. K. Hsu (5) reported on their eighteen years' experience dated from 1971 to 1989 in the use of acupuncture anesthesia for dental extractions. They selected the HoKu point (LI 4) as the acupoint. The needle was manually vibrated 180–200 times per minute for a period of three to five minutes. Of 1,153 cases, 429 (37.2 percent) showed an excellent results, 543 (47.1 percent) had good results, and 33 (2.9 percent) failed.

Z. Q. Gu, et al., (9) reported their ten -year experience in dental extraction under acupuncture anesthesia. The acupoint Xiaguan (S 7) was chosen. Totally 315 cases were done and excellent results were achieved in 60–86.7 percent, averaging 80.1 percent.

D. E. Bresler (4) applied EAP (180 Hz) at the acupoint HoKu for thirty minutes in the extraction of an abscessed second molar tooth and obtained a good result. There was no pain or bleeding. The analgesic effect persisted for nearly twelve hours following removal of the needle. He pointed out that such a long lasting analgesic effect is certainly not a counterirritant effect.

T. J. Kitade performed dental extraction in fifty-six patients under acupuncture anesthesia; eighteen patients also received an injection of DPA, a peptidase inhibitor, to slow the metabolism of opioid peptides. (See chapter 6.) The anesthetic effect was better in the group receiving DPA and acupuncture than in the group receiving acupuncture only. Eight patients showed excellent results, six had good results, and three failed (12).

The major advantages of acupuncture anesthesia over local anesthesia in dentistry are numerous, including the lack of toxicity, allergic reaction, and systemic reactions. Acupuncture can affect an extensive anatomic area and does not disturb local tissues, thus promoting faster postoperative healing. Furthermore, it is inexpensive and an ideal procedure for rural practices (19).

S. Sun (21) surveyed the clinical data from Chinese medical records and suggested that acupuncture therapy is the preferred treatment for dental patients who had suffered myocardial infarction. It was much safer than other anesthetic agents.

H. Ishi, et al., (11) performed oral surgery under acupuncture anesthesia during the years 1977–82 and obtained a 43-percent effectiveness rate in dental extractions. Seventy percent of the patients had pain relief; 6 percent had some complications after extractions.

It was reported that oral surgery was performed under acupuncture anesthesia in eighty patients with tongue carcinoma without any difficulty. Seventy-seven patients were followed up for seven years. The primary lesion disappeared in 95 percent of the patients (22).

In surgical operations in 117 cases of sinusitis under acupuncture anesthesia it was reported that sixty-two patients (53 percent) had no pain and went through the surgical procedure without any difficulty (15).

W. Y. Fu (7) treated 121 patients with chronic periodontitis with a three-edged needle acupuncture at the Sibai (S 2) and Xiaguan (S 7) points. Thirty-five patients (29 percent) were cured and sixty-nine (57 percent) showed marked improvement.

S. W. Odell proposed acupuncture as a reprogramming therapy in dentistry as well as in medicine, to control habits and stress, and as a substitute for hypnosis (20).

A. Ekblem, et al., (6) removed the mandibular third molar tooth in 50 patients and administered either preoperative or postoperative acupuncture therapy to determine whether acupuncture could produce analgesic effects. The results were compared with those in 60 other patients who were operated on under general anesthesia. The results were disappointing. Patients in the acupuncture group suffered more pain with acupuncture therapy and required large amounts of analgesic agents to relieve pain.

Another report has also shown the failure of acupuncture anesthesia in oral surgery. Twenty-eight patients were operated on under acupuncture to remove an impacted third molar. Only 2 patients tolerated the acupuncture procedure; both had severe pain at the end of the operation (10).

However, J. A. Gershman and P. O. Wikstrom (8) reported successful use of acupuncture anesthesia in the extraction of two lower molar teeth. M. H. M. Lee, et al., (14) performed twenty cases of dental surgery under acupuncture anesthesia, which was successful in sixty cases.

Acupuncture has also been used in other oral problems. EAP therapy has been used in the treatment of xerostomia in patients with Sjoegren's syndrome; reportedly the procedure could induce increase local blood flow and salivation (2, 3).

T. List and associates (16, 17, 18) used acupuncture therapy in patients suffering from craniomandibular disorders and who had had pain for at least six months. There was a significant short-term improvement, which was as good as obtained with the occluded spinal therapy and far better than that obtained with placebo. The researchers stated that acupuncture therapy also had other beneficial effects, such as a relaxed feeling and improvement of sleep. The majority of patients were satisfied with the therapy because there were no serious adverse effects.

A. Kozma (13) discussed the use of acupuncture in the prevention and treatment of general toxic accidents in dental practice. He reported a total of nine cases of drug accidents treated with acupuncture. Good results were obtained. The treatment was simple and well accepted by the patients. They recovered from the toxic symptoms faster than with other classical therapeutic methods.

References

1. Anderson, S. A., and E. Holmgren. Brain Res. 63:393, 1973.
2. Blom, M., et al. Oral Surgery, Oral Med., Oral Path. 73:292, 1992.
3. Blom, M., et al. Journal of Oral Rehabilitation 20:541, 1993.
4. Bresler, D. E., from Jenerik, H. P., ed. Proceedings NIH Acupuncture Res. Conf. DHEW 74-165. 1973, p. 68.
5. Chen, W. P., and C. K. Hsu. Journal of Chinese Acupuncture and Moxibustion 11(2):33, 1993.
6. Ekblem, A., et al. Pain 44:741, 1991.
7. Fu, W. Y. Journal of Chinese Acupuncture and Moxibustion 13(2):9, 1993.
8. Gershmann, J. A., and P. O. Wikstrom. Swed. Dent. J. 8:225, 1984.

9. Gu, Z. Q., et al. from All China Society of Acupuncture and Moxibustion. Second National Symposium on Acupuncture and Moxibustion and Acupuncture Anesthesia. Beijing: People Health Publisher, 1984. p. 175.
10. Hansson, P., et al. Oral Surg. Oral. Medicine Oral Pathol. 64:283, 1984.
11. Ishi, H., et al. Yokohoma Medical Journal 38:847, 1987.
12. Kitade, T. J. Osaka Med. Colleg. 45:28, 1987.
13. Kozma, A. Rev. Chir. Oncol. Radiol. ORL Oftolmol. Stomatol. Ser. Stomatol. 33:197, 1986.
14. Lee, M. H. M., et al. from Jenerick, H. P., ed. NIH Acupuncture Research Conf. DHEW 74-165, 1973, p. 76.
15. Lin, C. Y. Journal of Chinese Acupuncture and Moxibustion 13(2):8, 1993.
16. List, T., et al. Journal of Orofacial Pain 7:275, 1993.
17. List, T., and M. Helkino. Acta Odontologia Scand. 50:375, 1992.
18. List, T., and M. Helkino. Cranio 10:318, 1992.
19. Lu, D. D., and G. P. Lu. Compendium 14:182, 1993.
20. Odell, S. W. American Journal of Acupuncture 14:151, 1986.
21. Sun, S. Journal tradit. Chin. Med. (in Engl.) 11:15, 1991.
22. Wang, S. C. Chinese Medical Journal 97:131, 1984.

16

Acupuncture in Drug Abuse, Smoking, and Alcoholism

Smoking and drinking are two social problems often seen in the United States. Not long ago, smoke-filled rooms were the places where political and business king makers made important deals. In modern days people gradually became aware that both smoking and excessive drinking are health hazards. Back in 1840 the British started the Opium War with China. Opium addiction was a treacherous disease in China until it was gradually eradicated after 1950. The Chinese picked up the cigarette smoking habit from the West and considered it a privilege for well-to-do people. At home, they served cigarettes instead of tea. In business, they bribed others with cigarettes. According to a recent report, of the 1.2 billion Chinese people 300 million, mainly males, smoke one to three packs of cigarettes a day. Almost 70 percent of the adult males in China are smokers, but only 8 percent of the females smoke, compared with 26 percent in the United States. Lung cancer morbidity and mortality rates are rising steadfastly in large Chinese cities. For example, in Shanghai, the mortality due to lung cancer has increased from 30.8 deaths per 100,000 population in 1964 to 61.9 deaths per 100,000 in 1985. The mortality rate due to coronary heart disease is also rising, mainly due to smoking (33).

The Chinese government and people have often overlooked the long-term effects of smoking, focusing instead only on the short-term economic consequences. It took more than a century for the Chinese to get rid of opium. A cigarette war would be an extreme method to get rid of cigarette smoking. At present, very few people voluntarily go to hospitals or clinics for treatment to stop smoking, unless strongly advised to do so by their doctor.

Nicotine, the major active ingredient in tobacco, can cause addiction. However, the craving for cigarettes is not as severe as that for opium in addicted people. Many people have tried but found it difficult to stop smoking. The acupuncture therapy has been introduced in the last ten years in the treatment of smoking withdrawal and is claimed to be effective. H. C. Dung surveyed his practice in his acupuncture clinic in San Antonio, Texas, from the years 1981 to 1984 (9). He reported that in his clinic, acupuncture therapy was mainly for the treatment of three major types of problems: pain, smoking, and overweight. There were 3,464 patients who received acupuncture treatments, 639 of the treatment (18.4 percent) for smoking withdrawal. Male and female patients were about equal in number. In Dung's own evaluation, the individuals sought the acupuncture treatment of their own free will and returned back to the clinic steadily for the treatment. The undiminished number coming back for treatment indicates that patients accepted the treatment favorably. As he argued, if the treatment were ineffective, the number of patients returning to the clinic would be reduced, but visits to his clinic actually did not decline.

Recently M. Tsuai and I. P. Chiang (31) reviewed sixty-four publications in Chinese journals dealing with smoking withdrawal treatment. Totally 15,000 patients received acupuncture treatment. The effectiveness rate was 84 percent. No adverse effects were being reported with the treatment.

In follow-up studies it was noted that the effectiveness rate gradually decreased with time, indicating that some individuals were not cured and took up smoking again.

In a European study of 996 smokers the effectiveness of acupuncture therapy in smoking withdrawal was comparable to that of medication (7).

J. L. Schwartz (25) treated thirteen patients undergoing smoking withdrawal with acupuncture and followed them up for six months. The median effectiveness rate was 25 percent. It was concluded that acupuncture therapy did not promote a complete cessation of smoking as others had claimed. In a recent article he argued that the use of acupuncture therapy as a method for quitting smoking is not warranted (26).

In contrast to such negative results, some investigators have found a beneficial effect of acupuncture therapy for smoking withdrawal. Q. S. Li, et al., (21) treated twenty-eight heavy smokers with auricular acupuncture. After several sessions the subjects developed greater sensitivity to sour and sweet tastes. Their elevated plasma level of the LEK-like substance during smoking graduately fell to a normal concentration equal to that of nonsmokers.

Kusumi (17) treated 518 chronic smokers with auricular acupuncture therapy and microelectric stimulation. Three hundred and eight patients (59.5 percent) stopped smoking completely and eighty-four (16.2 percent) reduced the number of cigarattes smoked; 126 patients (24.3 percent) did not respond to the treatment.

In another report on 100 cigarette smokers treated with auricular acupuncture at the Shenmen point of the ear, thirty were rated to completely withdraw from smoking while fifteen had no beneficial effect. The remainder were improved with a reduction in the number of cigarettes they smoked (13).

Data from a Chinese tobacco detoxification clinic showed that auricular acupuncture therapy had an effectiveness rate of 60 percent in 488 individuals; 30 percent of those people who effectively stopped smoking remained symptom-free for six months to one year. In contrast, individuals treated with medication had less successful results (17).

J. L. Olms reported a three-year experience in treating 2,282 cases of cigarette smoking by acupuncture and laser irradiation. The effectiveness rate reached 90 percent (24).

J. A. Cottraux, et al., (8) divided 558 cigarette smokers into three groups; one was treated with acupuncture, one with behavior therapy, and the third with placebo. Individuals receiving acupuncture therapy had a significantly greater withdrawal rate from smoking than those in the placebo group at the end of two therapeutic courses. (Generally, seven sessions constituted a course.) At the end of nine to twelve months, the acupuncture group had a statistically significant greater number who stopped smoking than the behavioral therapy group.

Auricular acupuncture therapy was used in the treatment of 95 smokers (19). Patients receiving acupuncture reduced their cigarette smoking much more rapidly than those in a behavioral therapy group. Treatment with a combination of acupuncture and behavioral therapy produced a much high effectiveness rate in both the short and long term.

While in Africa, F. L. Wang treated 254 cigarette smokers with acupuncture therapy (32). The acupoints Zusanli and HoKu were chosen and electrical stimulation was applied for thirty minutes. One hundred and sixty-nine patients (66.5 percent) completely withdrew from smoking. Among those individuals, seventy-one of them needed only one treatment and the rest required two to five treatments. Seventy-seven smokers (30.3 percent) reduced their daily number of cigarettes by 50–80 percent. The treatment was ineffective in only eight subjects, who continued to smoke at the pretreated level.

In one study, 108 cigarette smokers were treated with either auricular acupuncture or body acupuncture with Zusanli as the acupoint. There was no difference between the two groups in term

Y. A. Feng, et al., (11) divided 150 cigarette smokers into two groups. One group received acupuncture treatment at the acupoint Zusanli and the other received acupuncture at random nonacupoints; 70 percent of those receiving specific acupuncture had given up smoking at the end of treatment, while only 11 percent of those in the nonspecific group had quit smoking.

Other clinical trials of acupuncture therapy on cigarette smoking are summarized in table 16-1.

Table 16-1. Acupuncture Therapy for Cigarette Smokers

Source	Mode	Acupoint	Diagnosis	No. of Patients	Effectiveness %
Wu (34)	AP* and Ear AP	Baihui (Du 20)	Heavy cigarette smoking	210	90.9% stopped their smoking completely after 1-3 courses of treatment
Yin (36)	AP and Ear AP	Zusanli (S 36) Lieque (L 7) Yangxi (LI 5)	Heavy cigarette smoking	61	55.7 % completely stopped to smoke; 30% reduced more than 2/3 of smoking/day

* AP = Acupuncture

The opium smoking habit in China was completely eradicated after 1950, but in the cities of the United States and Europe heroin addiction is still a major problem. Since acupuncture can increase opioid peptide levels in the brain (see chapter 6) and the opiate antagonist naloxone can provoke abstinence symptoms similar to those of opium withdrawal, the question has been asked whether acupuncture would be effective in the treatment of morphine or heroin addiction. M. M. P. Yang and J. S. L. Kwok answered this question in experiments on morphine-addicted rats (35). They found that EAP was the most effective method to reduce morphine withdrawal symptoms. The result with acupuncture was better than with herbal medication or opioid peptide treatment. In 119 addicted rats treated with EAP, the effectiveness rate was 50.9 percent, compared to 6.3 percent in a control group treated with saline.

Acupuncture therapy for acute drug withdrawal in humans was first developed in Hong Kong in 1972. The results were very promising. At present, over 175 acupuncture chemical dependency programs are in operation in the United States and there are dozens more elsewhere in the world. A. G. Brumbaugh has advocated acupuncture for relief of classic symptoms during acute and postacute withdrawal (3). He mentioned the experience of the Santa Barbara, California, Substance Abuse Treatment Program, where "the use of acupuncture treatment is particularly promising in homeless shelters where alcohol and drug treatment is often resisted due to unmanageability of withdrawal symptoms. Acupuncture therapy gave a 90 percent success rate of program completion and aftercare placement rate."

Acupuncture therapy is also superior to other detoxification methods with medication in the treatment of drug abuse in prenatal women. In these cases, it can reduce the risk for abrupt withdrawal, which can be damaging to the mother and fetus. Acupuncture also reduces the possible teratogenic effects of the abused drugs or the detoxification agents on the fetus.

A. Lewenberg (20) reported on the treatment of opium addicts with auricular acupuncture or self-administered TENS. In addition, the patients received antidepressants and Clonidine. The results were excellent. The individuals withdrew from opium within three weeks or less after treatment. Of 106 patients, 56 needed 4 or more treatments. Thirty-three of the 56 subjects stopped smoking opium or reduced the dosage to a minimum level.

F. A. Alling, et al., (1) reviewed the use of cranial electrostimulation (CES) to alleviate the opiate withdrawal symptoms. Electrical stimulation was applied to the skin over the cranium. No conclusive benefit could be shown. Some subjects achieved more benefit from these treatments than from methadone therapy, but others did not.

M. Smith and R. A. Kleenat described the results of acupuncture therapy in 250 cases of drug abuse and alcoholism in New York and Minnesota (27). Ninety percent of the patients obtained relief from the acute withdrawal symptoms. Agitated patients felt the beneficial effects even while the needle was still in place. It was surprising to observe that the patients substantially reduced their consumption of the drug. They craved more frequent acupuncture treatments, especially chronic alcoholics who were previously considered "untreatable." EAP was the primary form of therapy, since it was simple and could be applied to several patients simultaneously in a lounge setting. Such group treatment in a hall can intensify the confidence of the new patients, in a manner analogous to AA meetings!

In a Pakistan clinic, Struaib (15, p. 509) treated nineteen drug abuse cases with EAP. Withdrawal symptoms, especially in opium abusers, were effectively controlled within thirty minutes after the treatment. All patients were symptom-free by six to eight days after the treatment. The efficacy of acupuncture therapy was highly praised.

Wen, et al., (15, p. 514) reported that plasma ACTH and corticosterone concentrations were usually high in drug addicts (about 42 and 32 percent higher, respectively, than normal control values), but cAMP levels were lower. Forty drug addicts who had been addicted to opium for two to twenty-seven years received EAP (125 Hz) for three to five minutes, continued over many sessions. Their ACTH and corticosterone levels were significantly decreased (17 percent for ACTH and 15 percent for corticosterone) and they achieved a good clinical result. In normal non-addicted subjects, acupuncture produced no change in ACTH or corticosterone level.

In another report, fifty heroin users were treated with EAP; forty-one responded well to the treatment. The withdrawal symptoms disappeared within one half hour after the treatment. Injection of naloxone in some subjects caused recurrence of the abstinent symptoms, suggesting that acupuncture therapy provides symptomatic relief but does not cure the addiction. The report also showed that older patients had a better response to EAP therapy (15, p. 520).

D. S. Lipton, et al., (22) reported that acupuncture therapy decreased the severity of cocaine withdrawal symptoms and reduced cocaine/crack craving and consumption. Urine analyses were performed in 150 acupuncture-treated patients and in a group receiving placebo. Patients who received acupuncture treatment for one month had lower urinary content of cocaine and its metabolite(s) than the placebo group. Figure 16-1 illustrates the effects of acupuncture therapy on crack-cocaine patients in comparison with the placebo group. Similar results were reported at the 1991 NIDA meeting held in the United States (23).

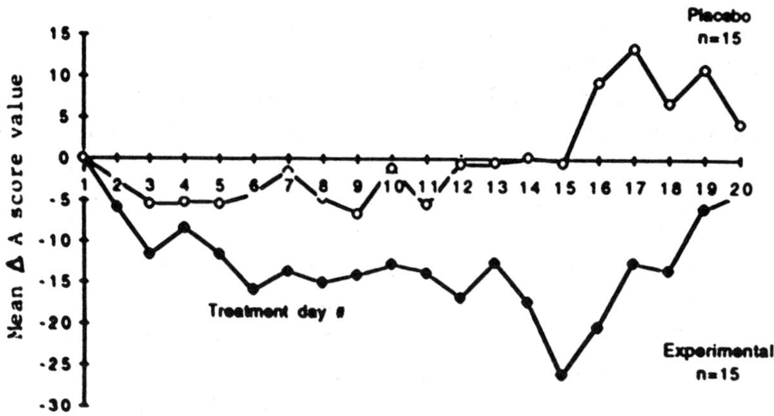

Figure 16-1. Effect of Acupuncture Therapy on Crack-Cocaine Patients as Evaluated by the Urine Specimen Analysis of Cocaine Metabolite(s) Level

o: patients received sham acupuncture

•: patients received acupuncture for 5 days

(From Lipton et al. (22)

Alcoholism is not only a social problem, but also a serious psychiatric and medical problem. In Russia, drinking is a common phenomenon for relieving boredom in daily life. However, this problem is rare in China. Chinese consider alcohol a medicine and use it to preserve the potency of herbs and serve it before meals as an appetizer or at bedtime to induce sleep. The life-style of the Chinese working class, which works more than twelve hours a day, does not include the habit of having Irish coffee for breakfast, three-martini lunches, or cocktails before dinner. Therefore, drinking problems are almost unheard of in China, except a few rare cases. Very seldom is a drunk seen sleeping on a street corner as in New York City. Consequently, clinical reports on the use of acupuncture in the treatment of alcoholics are rare. C. T. Sun, et al., (28) studied the effects of acupuncture therapy on 310 alcoholics and found that it was quite effective. The patients had been drinking for periods of three to forty years. Their average daily consumption of alcohol (45 percent, or 90 proof) was 550 milliliters. Two hundred and thirty-eight subjects were cured by acupuncture (76.8 percent). At a three-month follow-up none had touched the bottle again. In thirty-four individuals there was no effect. The remaining thirty-eight subjects were improved but resumed drinking after the treatment.

E. A. Gerasimor (12) treated alcoholic patients who also had pulmonary tuberculosis disease with a combination of acupuncture and hypnosis. After the treatment the patients were able to stop taking all antialcoholic medicines. The treatment also accelerated the disappearance of the somatovegetative and neurological symptoms of abstinence within two to five days.

In another report, thirty-five patients with alcoholism and depression were treated with acupuncture (6). The alcoholic symptoms disappeared completely by the end of therapy. The EEG interhemispheric asymmetry in these patients could be used for diagnosis, prevention, and prophylaxis (15).

M. Bullock, et al., (4, 5) reported the treatment of fifty-four hard-core alcoholics with acupuncture therapy. Patients were divided into two groups; one was treated with acupuncture at exact acupoints and the other at random nonacupoints. The majority of patients receiving specific acupuncture expressed the feeling that it had a definite impact on their desire to drink. They had fewer drinking episodes than the group receiving acupuncture at nonacupoints.

F. Facchinetti, et al., (10) found that acupuncture therapy in alcoholic addicts elevated plasma ß-endorphin levels to 128 percent of the pretreatment levels, suggesting this as a possible explanation of the effectiveness of acupuncture mechanism in the treatment of alcoholism.

D. M. Tabeeva reported that magnetic acupuncture therapy is highly effective in the treatment of alcoholism (30). Auricular and body acupuncture were both used in twenty-four male alcoholic patients for twelve or thirteen sesssions. It was found that parasympathetic activity was enhanced at the end of treatment. It was also claimed that acupuncture exerted a stablizing effect in those patients (29).

In their recent review, V. Brewington, et al., (2) concluded that research findings from several areas have provided evidence supporting the role of acupuncture as an aid in treatment of abuses including opiate, heroin, and cocaine abuses and alcoholism.

References

1. Alling, F. A., et al. Journal of Substance Abuse Treatment 7:173, 1990.
2. Brewington, V., et al. Journal of Substance Abuse Treatment 11(4):289, 1994.
3. Brumbaugh, A. G. Journal of Substance Abuse Treatment 10:35, 1993.
4. Bullock, M., et al. Alcohol Clin. Exp. Res. 11:292, 1987.
5. Bullock, M. L., et al. American Journal of Acupuncture 15:313, 1987.
6. Cherkezova, M., and S. Totera. ZH Nevropatol. Psikhiatr. IM S S Korsakova 91:83, 1991.
7. Clavel, F., and C. Paoletti. Rev. Epidemiol. Sante Publique 38:133, 1990.
8. Cottraux, J. A., et al. Behav. Res. Ther. 21:417, 1987.
9. Dung, H. C. Chinese Medical Journal 98:835, 1985.
10. Facchinetti, F., et al. Subst. Alcohol Actions and Misuse 5:281, 1984/85.
11. Fang, Y. A., et al. from All China Society of Acupuncture and Moxibustion: Second National Symposium on Acupuncture and Moxibustion and Acupuncture Anesthesia. Beijing: People Health Publisher, 1984 p. 95.
12. Gerasimor, E. A. Probl. Tuberk. 0(12):59, 1989.
13. Hsu, X. M., et al. Journal of Chinese Acupuncture and Moxibustion 10(2):22, 1990.
14. Johansson, K. Vardfacket 17(6):26, 1993.
15. Kao, F. F., and J. J. Kao eds. Recent Advances in Acupuncture Research. Garden City, NY: Institute for Advanced Research in Asian Science and Medicine, 1979.
16. Koehma, A., et al. ZH Nevropatol. Psikhiatr. IM S S Korsakova 91:88, 1991.
17. Kusumi, Y. T. American Journal of Acupuncture 14:325, 1986.
18. Labeau, B., et al. Rev. Med. Interne 7:471, 1986.
19. Leung, J. P. Psychologia 34:177, 1991.
20. Lewenberg, A. Adv. Ther. 2:143, 1985.
21. Li, Q. S., et al. Journal of Traditional Chinese Medicine 7:243, 1987.
22. Lipton, D. S., et al. Journal of Substance Abuse Treatment 11:205, 1994.
23. McHellan, A. T., et al. Journal of Substance Abuse Treatment 10:569, 1993.
24. Ohms, Journal of American Acupuncture 12:339, 1984,
25. Schwartz, J. L. American Journal of Acupuncture 16:135, 1988.
26. Schwartz, J. L. Med. Clin. North America 70:451, 1992.
27. Smith, M., and R. A. Kleenat. Alcoholism 23:25, 1987.
28. Sun, C. T., et al. Journal of Traditional Chinese Medicine 28(3):215, 1987.
29. Tabeeva, D. M. ZH Nevropatol. Psikhiatr. IM S S Korsakova 88:33, 1988.
30. Tabeeva, D. M. Ter. Arkh. 61:104, 1989.
31. Tsuai, M., and I. P. Chiang. Journal of Traditional Chinese Medicine 34 (4):243, 1993.
32. Wang, F. L. Journal of Chinese Acupuncture and Moxibustion 11(3):33, 1991.
33. Wang, X. Z. Chinese Medical Journal 101(5):371, 1988.

34. Wu, Y. R. Journal of Traditional Chinese Medicine 1:65, 1981.
35. Yang, M. M. P. and J. S. L. Kwok. American Journal of Chinese Medicine 14:46, 1986.
36. Yin, X. C. Journal of Traditional Chinese Medicine (in Chinese) 34(11):679, 1993.
37. Zhang, C. Journal of Chinese Acupuncture and Moxibustion 10(5):23, 1990.

17
Acupuncture in Impotence

Impotence is the failure to achieve an erection, ejaculation, or both. Males with sexual dysfunction usually complain of loss of libido, inability to initiate or maintain an erection, difficulty in ejaculating or premature ejaculation, or inability to achieve an orgasm. Impotence may be primary or secondary testicular hormonal failure, but the majority of cases are psychogenic. In ancient Chinese feudal society, impotence was a common symptom of the rich and royal families, because of their practice of polygamy, overindulgence in sex, and excessive use of alcohol or opium. In the poor, excessive masturbation was also a major cause of impotence. According to Chinese traditional medicine, this could lead to a decline of the Mingman (the spiritual gate or the juice's fire) and exhaustion of the kidney's (as the Chinese call the testes) essence.

The common symptomatic remedy for impotence is an aphrodisiac. In Chinese herbal medicine, many agents are listed for rejuvenation and stimulation of the reproductive system. Ginseng (*Panax ginseng*) is considered to be the best for revitalization and rejuvenation in exhausted men. But in the old dynasties, ginseng was reserved for royalty and the rich because of its rarity and expense. Thus many substitutes are on the market, including Wu Ja Pei, a species from Panax, Wu Wei Zi, the *Schisandra chinesis,* and rhino horn (4). The effectiveness of these herbs has not been defined or proven. But to the rural people, especially the illiterate farmers and laborers, travelling practitioners on street corners have advertised acupuncture as a remedy for impotence for centuries.

However, the application of acupuncture therapy for impotence was not described explicitly in the ancient Chinese texts and the effectiveness was never documented. Only recently have articles appeared in several Chinese acupuncture journals indicating its usefulness in the treatment of impotence and ejaculation difficulties and complaints of asthenia of the penis and weakness in erection.

The selection of acupoints is varied, depending on the preference of the acupuncturist, and there are no specific guidelines to follow. Usually acupoints along the ren meridian or the one close to the penis are selected. The success of acupuncture is age-dependent; in general, the younger the individual, the better the results.

Recent clinical reports demonstrated that acupuncture therapy could help to correct the sexual dysfunction either by electric stimulation or by intraacupoint injection of vitamin B1. The acupoints Zusanli and Sanyinjiao were chosen as the main acupoints (7). In 160 impotent individuals who were treated with acupuncture therapy, 85 were cured (53.1 percent), 67 improved (41.8 percent), and 8 failed. The total effectiveness rate was 95 percent. In another 106 cases of sexual difficulties, 66 patients had penile asthenia. The acupoints Zhongji (Ren 3), Guanyuan (Ren 4), and Sanyinjiao were alternately needled and electrically stimulated for fifteen minutes once a day for twenty sessions. All 66 subjects were cured.

C. Z. Wu, et al., (10) reported on the treatment of 100 impotent males with acupuncture. The subjects were twenty-four to fifty-three years old. The acupoints Jugu (LI 16) and Ciliao (B 32) were needled and stimulated for ten minutes every two to three days. A course consisted of ten treatments. Among the 100 patients, 63 were cured, 13 had no response, and the rest were improved.

In another report, ninety-one impotent males were treated with acupuncture at the acupoints Sanyinjiao (Sp 6) and Guanyuan. The needle was twisted slightly until it reached the perineum or the root of the penis which was then electrically stimulated for ten to twenty minutes. The procedure was performed once every other day. A course consisted of ten sessions. After three to five days of rest, a second course could be started if needed. Among the ninety-one men treated, sixty-seven were cured (73.6 percent) and 7 failed (2).

Two hundred and fifty-eight impotent individuals, twenty to forty years old, were treated with acupuncture at the acupoint Guanyuan for thirty minutes every other day. After twelve sessions, eighty-seven of the subjects were cured (33.7 percent), fourteen failed and the rest were improved (13).

Y. H. Tan, et al., (9) reported seventy-five impotent males, aged twenty-two to sixty-five years, who were treated with acupuncture at the acupoints Zhonglushu (B 29) and Huiyang (B 35). After ten to twelve treatments, forty-nine were cured (65.3 percent), five had failed, and the rest were improved. The younger the patient, the better the results.

In 106 cases of impotence, S. L. Ho (3) reported that acupuncture therapy was very effective in treating the sexual dysfunction. Fifty-two of 100 patients were cured, but the acupuncture was less effective in cases of impotence due to organic injury. In 6 such cases, only 1 patient was cured.

Wu reported 12 cases of impotence treated with acupuncture at the Zusanli point. Eight patients were cured (66.7 percent). After the treatment, penile erection could be maintained for one-half hour and the patient could again enjoy sexual activity. Only one subject failed to respond to the treatment (10). L. S. Yamen, et al., (12) reported 29 cases of psychogenic impotency treated with acupuncture. Twenty patients demonstrated successful erection following a varying number of treatments.

In cases of ejaculation difficulty, acupuncture therapy also exerts some beneficial effect. Q. Zhang, et al., (15) treated eighty-two males who complained of difficulty in ejaculation during sexual intercourse. Their ages ranged from twenty-five to thirty-nine years. The acupoints Qugu (Ren 2) and Yinlians (Liv 11) were chosen. After ten treatments, seventy patients reported that their ejaculation had returned to normal; only twelve failed to respond to the treatment.

Seventy cases of functionally defective ejaculation were treated with acupuncture at the acupoint Sanyinjiao. The age of the individuals was twenty-five to forty-one years. At the end of ten treatments sixty-five patients were cured (92.8 percent) (1).

H. D. Xue (11) compared the effectiveness of acupuncture therapy and herbal medication (his own Chinese herbal recipe) in 100 cases of defective ejaculation. His results were as follows:

Effect of Acupuncture on Defective Ejaculation in Men

Treatment	Acupoint	No. of Subjects	Cured		Failed
			No.	%	No.
Acupuncture Gr.	Sanyinjiao (Sp 6)	60	55	91.6	5
Medication Gr. (chinese herbs)		40	5	12.5	35

(From Xue (11))

Recently, G. Z. Qin (6) reviewed the effectiveness of acupuncture in 6,036 cases of men's diseases, which were published in nineteen Chinese journals over the last ten years. Totally, 1,614 impotence cases were treated. An average of 77.1 percent of the patients had a beneficial response; penile erection could be maintained and patients enjoyed their sex life afterward. Some patients received an intraacupoint injection of vitamin B12 at the acupoint Zusanli or Shenshu (B 23). Ninety-three percent of these patients were cured, which was better than the results obtained with EAP therapy or moxibustion. In 581 cases of ejaculation difficulties, acupuncture was applied at the Sanyinjiao point; 86 percent of the patients were cured. Of 160 individuals suffering from oligospermia, after acupuncture treatment 78 percent were improved and were subsequently able to father a child. Fifty patients with spermatorrhea, who received an injection of 0.25 percent procaine solution into the acupoint Xialiao (B 34), were completely cured. Based on the data published in nine journals, acupuncture therapy had a 63.2 percent cure rate in 850 cases of chronic prostatitis.

Table 17-1 summarizes recent clinical data on the acupuncture therapy of impotence and ejaculation difficulties.

Table 17-1. Acupuncture Therapy in Men's Diseases

Source	Mode	Acupoint	Diagnosis	No. of Patients	Effectiveness %
Ho (3)	AP * and EAP**	Baihui (Du 20) Zusanli (S 36) Sanyinjiao (Sp 6)	Impotence	106	52% were cured; other 16% effective
Lei (5)	AP	Sanyinjiao Mingmen (Du 4)	Impotence	28	64% were cured and 18% effective
	IAc inj.# of strychnine and glucose			48	85% were cured
Tan (8)	AP and Ear AP	Baihui	Impotence	15	67% were cured
Zhang (16)	IAc. inj of Muscone	Sanyinjiao	Ejaculation difficulty	12	50% were cured

* AP = Acupuncture
** EAP = Electro-acupuncture
\# IAc. inj. = Intra-acupoint injection

References

1. Chen, E. J. Journal of Chinese Acupuncture and Moxibustion 10(2): 19, 1990.
2. Fu, C. K., et al. Journal of Chinese Acupuncture and Moxibustion 11(2):27, 1991.
3. Ho, S. L. Shanghai Journal of Acupuncture and Moxibustion 12(2): 68, 1993.
4. Huang, K. C. The Pharmacology of Chinese Herbs. Boca Raton, FL: CRC Press 1993 pp. 31 and 201.
5. Lei, S. P. Shanghai Journal of Acupuncture and Moxibustion 13(10:14, 1994.
6. Qin, G. Z. Journal of Chinese Acupuncture and Moxibustion 13(6):40, 1993.
7. Shi, S. M., ed. Chinese Acupuncture and Moxibustion Miracle. Tiajin: Tianjin Technology and Translation Publisher, 1992, p. 233.
8. Tan, E. Shanghai Journal of Acupuncture and Moxibustion 12(2):67, 1993.
9. Tan, Y. H., et al. Journal of Chinese Acupuncture and Moxibustion 11(6): 11, 1991.
10. Wu, C. Z., et al. Journal of Traditional Chinese Medicine (in Chinese) 29:214, 1988.
11. Xue, H. D. Journal of Chinese Acupuncture and Moxibustion 10(4):17, 1990.
12. Yamen, L. S., et al. European Urology 26:53, 1994.
13. Yin, L. K., and S. L. An. Journal of Chinese Acupuncture and Moxibustion 11(5):15, 1991.
14. Yu, K. C. Shanghai Journal of Acupuncture and Moxibustion 10 (2):23, 1991.
15. Zhang, Q., et al., All China Society of Acupuncture and Moxibustion: Second National Symposium on Acupuncture and Moxibustion and Acupuncture Anesthesia. Beijing: People Health Publisher, 1984, p. 70.
16. Zhang, W. L. New Journal of Traditional Chinese Medicine 26(2):35, 1994.

18

Acupuncture Therapy on Immunity, Allergy, and Hypersensitivity

The human immune system contains the dual limbs, T cells, and B cells. Through the differentiated B cells, the immunoglobins are produced, which play a role in mediating the humoral arm of the immune response. It has been claimed that acupuncture can exert many effects to relieve allergy and hypersensitivity and improve body immunity. It also has been postulated that acupuncture may act through the central nervous system, via the hypothalamic pituitary axis, or that it may directly stimulate the B-lymphocytes, including bone marrow stem cells, to increase immunoglobulin production or release, or both. Although the mechanism of acupuncture on body immunity is still much in debate, it appears clear that acupuncture can produce a therapeutically beneficial change in immunoreactivity.

In animal experiments, T. Lundeberg, et al., (16) found that acupuncture can enhance the plaque-forming cells (PFC) in nonimmunized mice. The enhancement did not occur if the mice were preinjected with a specific antibody and complement and was abolished by propranolol, a ß-adrenergic antagonist. They suggested that acupuncture can modulate the immune system through activation of the sutonomic nervous system.

Bilateral acupuncture or EAP in rats can cause a pronounced change of the immunomodulating activity and a reduction in adrenal gland weight (19). J. C. Zhao and W. Q. Lin demonstrated that EAP can promote T-lymphocyte transformation through stimulation of endogenous opioid peptide production; naloxone can reverse the effect (25). They postulated that the effect is due to promotion of anabolism in T-lymphocytes including DNA synthesis. Acupuncture accelerates the rate of α-naphthylacetate esterase (ANAE) reaction, which suggests that the immunity induced by acupuncture is probably influenced by the central cathecholaminergic neuron (26).

Chu and Affronti (10, p. 388) studied the effects of acupuncture in rabbits and guinea pigs and found that it can elevate antibody titers by two to eight times by increasing the activity of reticuloendothelial cells and prolong the presence of the antibody in the circulation by reducing its rate of degradation. The effect involves both the anatomical, physiological, and biochemical properties of enzymes and cells.

In experiments with dogs, EAP caused a significant increase in total erythrocyte count and white cell count, especially neutrophils (17).

However, controversial results have also been reported. T. Kudo, et al., (14) performed acupuncture on twenty-four healthy mongrel dogs at the acupoint Zusanli bilaterally for thirty minutes each day. There was a depression of immunological response, mainly decreases in T-lymphocytes and immunoglobulins.

M. M. P. Yang, et al., (24) analyzed salivary IgA levels in seventy healthy volunteers before and after a thirty-minute acupuncture therapy. They found the IgA concentration significantly increased with acupuncture in subjects whose pretreatment level was low and fell in those whose pretreatment level was high. When acupuncture therapy was continued for two weeks, the average salivary IgA level increased by 20 percent in all cases. However, the IgG concentrations in serum and gingival sulcus fluid were decreased at the end of the thirty-minute acupuncture treatment. However, with chronic acupuncture (seven- to ten- day sessions), the IgG concentration was significantly increased in both serum and gingival sulcus fluid. Table 18-1 summarizes the acute effects of acupuncture therapy on salivary IgA concentration in saliva. Table 18-2 summarizes the chronic effects of acupuncture on IgA and IgG concentration

Table 18-1. Effect of Acupuncture Therapy on Saliva Concentration of IgA of Volunteers

Voltunteers:		Saliva IgA Concentration (mg/dl)	
		Control Group	Acupuncture Group
A. With low IgA	Initial	7.7 ±0.76 (18)*	7.8 ± 0.64 (12)
	30. min.	7.7 ±0.74	10.0 ± 2.2
	24 hr.later	7.9 ± 0.74	12.7 ± 1.64
B. With High IgA	Initial	14.6 ±0.58 (6)	16.6 ± 2.38 (6)
	30. min.	12.8 ±1.34	10.4 ± 1.54
	24 hr.later	13.6 ±1.02	10.6 ± 2.06

* Mean ± S.D. (no. of individuals)

(From Yang et al. (24))

Table 18-2. Chronic Effect of Acupuncture Therapy on IgA and IgG Concentration in Volunteers

Days of Treatment	IgA Conc.in Saliva (mg/dl)		IgG Conc. in Serum ng./dl)		IgG Conc. in Gingival Sulcus Fluid (μg in 3 minutes)	
	Before	After	Before	After	Before	After
7-10 days	10.7± 0.66 (10)*	11.3±0.75	13.6±0.91 (7)	16.6±1.78	0.5±0.05 (9)	0.91±0.11
24 days	9.3±0.52 (6)	11.4±0.51	12.8±0.69 (8)	12.0±0.72	0.56±0.06 (9)	0.58±0.05

* Mean ± S.D. (no. of individuals)

(From Yang et al. (24))

W. H. Chen, et al., (3) reported significant elevations in serum IgA and IgG levels in their patients after acupuncture therapy, but there was less effect on serum IgM levels. Serum IgA was increased from a pretreatment level of 2.1 mg/100 ml to a posttreatment level of 7.56 mg/100 ml, and serum IgG increased from 6.67 mg/100 ml initially to 81.12 mg/100 ml after treatment.

J. Han reported forty-nine individuals in the Beijing area who had a senile deficiency syndrome and were treated with acupuncture at the Guanyuan (Ren 4) and Sanyinjiao acupoints. After thirty treatments, the patients were significantly improved. Their plasma levels of immune factors, such as IgA, IgG, and IgM, were increased to the normal level (9).

Yan, et al., (23) reported that EAP can modulate immune functions, as assayed by the T-lymphocyte proliferation response, and that the effect can be enhanced by microinjection of leucine-enkephalin (LEK) into the CNS striatum and inhibited by naloxone. They postulated that the EAP effect on cellular immune function is mediated through an action in the CNS striatum, either as a neurotransmitter or as a neuromodulator. T. Kashara, et al., (11) found a similar result in mice; EAP suppressed a delayed-type hypersensitivity reaction and the effect could be blocked by naloxone.

Acupuncture therapy causes not only an elevation of certain immunoglobulin levels, but also an elevation in circulating interferon levels. T. F. Chin, et al., (6) studied thirty-two healthy volunteers receiving acupuncture at the acupoint HoKu bilaterally for twenty minutes. The average plasma α-interferon concentration elevated at 323.2 I U/ml twenty-four hours after acupuncture and 167.6 I U/ml at forty-eight hours but had decreased to 23 I U/ml or less by ninety-six hours. The α-interferon level in the control group (acupuncture at random nonacupoints) remained below 23 I U/ml throughout the experiment.

Acupuncture can also affect the white blood cell count. Brown, et al., (10, p. 372) studied the effect of acupuncture therapy on the white blood cells in twelve healthy males and found that EAP provokes a greater increase in white cell count than manual acupuncture, especially at the site where the needle is inserted. The white cell count was increased regardless of whether the needle was inserted at acupoints or nonacupoints. The increase was transient and gradually returned to the initial value at the end of acupuncture. This response is probably a sign of local irritation rather than an effect mediated through the meridian channel or a central action.

Studies in mice have shown that EAP or moxibustion can increase phagocytic activity and splenic white cell count significantly (18). J. H. Chao, et al., (1) showed that acupuncture at the acupoint Zusanli markedly increased the leucocyte count in rabbits. The leucocyte count was increased to 166 percent of the initial value three hours after the treatment; the neutrophil count was increased by 51.7 percent, and the lymphocyte transformation was increased by 46 percent. B. Gong, et al., (8) injected ^{3}H-TdR and ^{14}C-uric acid into rats and subsequently gave them acupuncture therapy. They have found that the splenic lymphocyte DNA and RNA system, as well as the immune system, was stimulated.

Electron microscopic studies of skin and lymph nodes of animals after acupuncture showed infiltration of only small numbers of erythrocytes and lymphocytes in the vicinity of the acupuncture needle (12). However, when moxibustion instead of the needle was applied to the skin, a remarkable effect was produced. Large numbers of immunocytes infiltrated the area, including lymphocytes, monocytes, granulocytes, and mast cells. The lymph nodes were enlarged after moxibustion, but not acupuncture.

The acupuncture effect on white cell has also been observed in human subjects. Sixty-six adult patients who were operated on to remove tumors were treated with acupuncture therapy of their inflammatory lesions daily for three sessions. All had a significant increase in leucocytic phagocytosis (27).

J. L. Wu, et al., (22) measured the peripheral blood lymphocyte (PBL) and E-rosette formation cell (E-RFC)in twenty-five patients undergoing acupuncture treatment. Acupuncture therapy significantly increased the ANAE activity in the PBL and also increased E-RFC.

Acupuncture therapy increased the leucocytic count and stimulated IgA production in the small intestine while antagonizing cholera infection (13).

The promotion of leucocytosis by acupuncture can be used to counteract the leucopenia induced by anticancer chemotherapy. In a two-year study, Chen, et al., (4) compared the effects of acupuncture therapy and moxibustion with those of herbal therapy in cancer patients. Among 238 cases of leucopenia, acupuncture and moxibustion therapy produced remarkable improvement in 179 patients (75.2 percent). The leucocyte count was increased by more than 4,000 count/mm^3 6 days after treatment. But in 34 cases treated with herbal medicine, only 5 obtained improvement.

As previously discussed, acupuncture therapy is effective in treating asthma (see chapter 11), so it is not surprising that it is also effective in treating allergy and hypersensitivity. J. A. Gerschman and P. O. Wikstrom surveyed the effectiveness of acupuncture therapy in a dental clinic in Sweden since 1958 and concluded that acupuncture is a valuable alternative therapy, especially in cases involving multiple allergy (7). R. T. Story (20) reported a female patient suffering from allergy for thirty-five years. After acupuncture treatment (daily for ten sessions), she became symptom-free and did not require any medication.

K. Tohya, et al., (21) showed that moxibustion at the acupoint Pishu (B 20) can produce a significant suppressive effect in hypersensitivity. They suggested that the effect is due to suppression of T-cell activity in the spleen, related to cellular immunity.

Forty-five patients suffering from allergic rhinitis were treated with acupuncture and compared to a group treated with antihistaminic medications. Both groups obtained effective relief of symptoms, but the acupuncture therapy seemed more effective and had a more prolonged effect (2).

Q. J. H. Lin, et al., (15) studied six healthy dogs and reported that EAP at the acupoint Zusanli bilaterally produced a higher increase in serum corticosterone level than acupuncture performed at other acupoints. This may be one of the explanations for the effectiveness of acupuncture therapy in allergy and hypersensitivity disorder.

Acupuncture therapy has also been used to treat some types of autoimmune diseases, such as lupus erythematosis. Y. S. Chen and X. Hu (5) reported fifteen such cases treated with acupuncture. Ten patients were clinically cured after six treatments; there was resolution of cutaneous lesions and residual slightly pigmented patches on the skin. Most subjective symptoms disappeared. The other three cases showed a marked improvement.

References

1. Chao, J. H., et al., from All China Society of Acupuncture and Moxibustion. First National Symposium on Acupuncture and Moxibustion and Acupuncture Anesthesia. Beijing: 1979,. p. 312.
2. Chari, P., et al. American Journal of Acupuncture 16:143, 1988.
3. Chen, W. H., et al. Journal of Chinese Acupuncture and Moxibustion 13(2):33, 1993.
4. Chen, W. L., et al. Journal of Chinese Acupuncture and Moxibustion 10(6):1, 1990.
5. Chen, Y. S., and X. Hu. Journal of Traditional Chinese Medicine (in English) 5:261, 1985.
6. Chin, T.F., et al. American Journal of Acupuncture 16:319, 1988.
7. Gerschman, J. A. and P. O. Wikstrom, Swed. Dent. J. 8:225, 1984.
8. Gong, B., et al. Shanghai Journal of Acupuncture and Moxibustion 13(1):34, 1994.
9. Han, J. Journal of Chinese Acupuncture and Moxibustion 13(3):31, 1993.
10. Kao, F. F. and J. J. Kao, eds. Recent Advances in Acupuncture Research. Garden City, NY: Institute for Advanced Research in Asian Science and Medicine, 1979.

11. Kasahara, T., et al. International Journal of Immopharmacology 15(4):501, 1993.
12. Kimura, M., et al. American Journal of Chinese Medicine 16:159, 1988.
13. Kuan, T. K., et al. American Journal of Chinese Medicine 14:73, 1986.
14. Kudo, T., et al. Jpn. J. of Vet. Sci. 49:1009, 1981.
15. Lin, J. H., et al. American Journal of Chinese Medicine 19:9, 1991.
16. Lundeberg, T., et al. Neurosci Letter 128:161, 1991.
17. Malik, V. K., and A. Kumar. Indian Veterinary Journal 68:52, 1991.
18. Min, S. Y. American Journal of Acupuncture 11:237, 1983.
19. Sakic, B., et al. Acupuncture Electro-Ther. Res. 14:115, 1989.
20. Story, R. T. American Journal of Acupuncture 18:123, 1990.
21. Tohya, K., et al. American Journal of Chinese Medicine 17:139, 1989.
22. Wu, J. L., et al. Chinese Medical Journal 98:753, 1985.
23. Yan, W. K., et al. Acta Physiol. Sinica 43:451, 1991.
24. Yang, M. M. P., et al. American Journal of Chinese Medicine 17:89, 1989.
25. Zhao, J. C., and W. Q. Liu. Acupuncture Electro-Ther. Res. 14:1, 1989.
26. Zhao, J. C., and W. Q. Liu. Acupuncture Electro-Ther. Res. 13:78, 1988.
27. Zhou, R. X., et al. Journal of Traditional Chinese Medicine 8:83, 1988.

19

Acupuncture Therapy in Sports Medicine

Recently, interest in acupuncture therapy on sports injury has substantially increased, instead of depending on medication. Coaches and trainers are enthusiastic about it, especially as they want their athletes to get back to work earlier and perform well without side effects. Sports in China didn't receive very much attention until a decade ago when China decided to participate in the Olympic competitions. There are scant reports on the success of acupuncture treatment in sports medicine in the early Chinese literature. Most of the trials are concentrated in laser therapy or moxibustion. (See the Chapter 23.)

It has been reported that Chinese female runners have used acupuncture treatment to improve their physical performance. TENS with a low frequency (2 Hz) stimulation is very popular with athletes competing in swimming, running, or cycling events. Neither TENS nor the acupuncture can be regarded as doping or drugging.

Studies on thirty-six healthy young men showed that acupuncture could significantly increase their maximum performance capacity and physical performance at the anaerobic threshold, a kind of functional improvement in hemodynamic and metabolic mechanism. Such effect was not observed in the placebo group (3).

Reports published in Western medical journals indicate that acupuncture therapy has been considered one of the clinical managements in treating tennis elbow with successful results. E. Haker and T. Lundeberg (5) treated sixty-one patients suffering from tennis elbow epicondylalgia with acupuncture therapy and compared the results on patients treated with other therapeutic techniques, such as low-energy laser, pulsed ultrasound, or steroid elbow band. Steroid elbow band therapy was found to be the best choice, especially in severe cases, in achieving rapid pain relief.

G. Brattberg (1) treated 34 athletes suffering from tennis elbow injury with acupuncture therapy. Twenty-one became completely free of pain, previously they had steroid therapy with ineffective result.

Patients suffering from chronic tennis elbow pain were treated with a single nonsegmental acupuncture stimulation. After one treatment nineteen out of twenty-four patients (79.2 percent) reported pain relief, which lasted, on the average, 20.2 hours (6).

The common complaints of athletes are muscle sprain, back pain, stomach spasm, and general pain. Except in cases of severe ailments that need surgery, coaches very seldom to advise their athletes to take medicine, afraid of interfering with their performance. They usually rely on acupuncture therapy or moxibustion or both. S. C. Fu and C. L. Meng (4) reported on 107 athletes suffering from stomach pain, spasm, and the common cold during the years 1988–90. Acupoint pressuring was applied simply by teaching the individual to use his finger pressure on the acupoints Weishu (B 21) and Pishu (B 20). Their results are summarized as follows:

Seventy-five young athletes suffering from excessive sporting lesions were treated with laser infrared irradiation and acupuncture together. All subjects showed an early remission of acute pain and recovered their functions very quickly (7).

Acupuncture Treatment on 107 chinese Athletes

Type of Ailment	No. of Cases	Cured	Improved
Stomach pain	50	47 (94%)	3
Stomach spasm	15	14 (93.3%)	1
Total	65	61 (93.8%)	4
Common cold	30	29 (96.7%)	1
Influenza	12	8 (66.7%)	2
Total	42	37 (88%)	3

(Table from Fu & Meng (4)).

Other investigators reported the use of acupuncture alternative, TENS, effective in relieving pain in young athletes and obtained an 82 percent effectiveness rate, with those patients returning to full sports activity (2).

References

1. Brattberg, G. Pain 16:285, 1983.
2. Dlin, R. A., et al. International Journal of Sports Medicine 1:203, 1980.
3. Ehrlich, D., and P. Haber. International Journal of Sports Medicine 13:486, 1992.
4. Fu, S. C., and C. L. Meng. Chinese Journal of Sports Medicine 12:61, 1993.
5. Haker, E., and T. Lundeberg. Pain Clinic. 6(2):103, 1993.
6. Molsberger, A., and E. Hille. British Journal of Rheumatology 33:1152, 1994.
7. Piras, S., et al. Med. Sport (Turin) 41:241, 1988.

20
Acupuncture in Veterinary Medicine

In ancient times, people considered their livestock part of their family. When the cattle got sick, a travelling practitioner at the street corner or an experienced neighbor would be called for advice on treatment, and acupuncture was probably the most common and simplest way, to be tried first. The use of acupuncture therapy in husbandry and agriculture has been recorded in the oldest Chinese literature. As early as the Spring-Autumn Period (475–221 B.C.), the famed veterinarian Sun Yang wrote the "Needle Classic," titled "Po-Loh Zhen Chian," which described the use of acupuncture in the treatment of domestic animals. This book is comparable to the *Huang Ti Nei Chian* in using acupuncture for the treatment of human subjects. In the Ming Dynasty (A.D.1368–1644), two Yue brothers, Bon-Yuan and Bon-Han, wrote *The Yuan Han Collection on the Treatment of Cow, Horse and Camel,* which contained specific chapters on the use and technique of acupuncture in treating the animals' illnesses. Figure 20-1 shows the front page of *The Yuan-Han Collection,* which was published during the Chin dynasty.

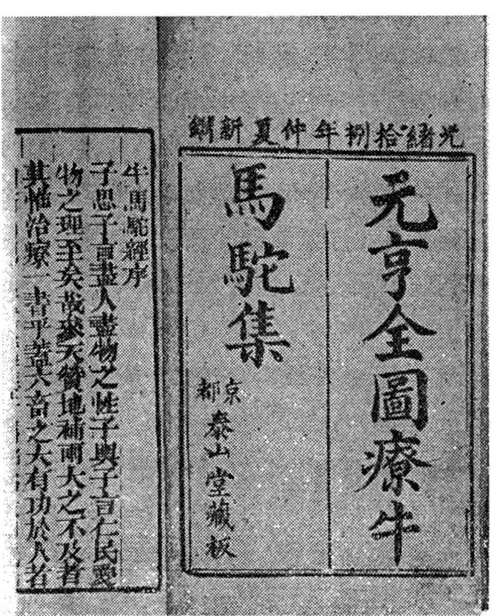
光緒拾捌年仲夏新鐫
元亨全圖療牛
馬駝集
京都
泰山堂藏板

Figure 20-1. The Front Page of the Yuan-Han Collection on the Treatment of Cow, Horse, and Camel

(Published in Kon-su Emperor 18th Year 1890 A.D.)

In the early sixth century A.D., the technique of Chinese acupuncture in veterinary medicine was exported to Japan and adapted, then to Indochina and Arabic countries during the Yuan and Ming Dynasties.

In the early seventeenth century, Gustaf Landgren of Sweden wrote a thesis on acupuncture describing the application of this technique in animals. Acupuncture can do a wonderful job in suppressing pain and strain or in surgery. While the Chinese medical professionals introduced the acupuncture anesthesia in surgical operations in 1957–1958, because of lack of medical supplies and modern facilities, they had to rely on their former training from Western medical colleges and hospitals in practicing their technique on animals and obtained very successful results, especially in gastrectomy and open heart surgery. In 1830, the veterinarian A. Hayne of Vienna applied acupuncture treatment to animals. The technique then spread all over Europe and was widely accepted as one of the treatments for livestock and pets. In 1974, an International Veterinary Acupuncture Society was established in California State, and in 1977 a book called *Veterinary Acupuncture,* by Alan M. Klide and S. H. Kung, was published. The major advantage of acupuncture therapy in veterinary medicine over other methods such as drugs is the lack of side effects and complications. According to a recent article, Chinese veterinarians have treated 15,469 domestic animals with acupuncture for various diseases. An effective rate of 89.2 percent was obtained.

In his review article Y. C. Huang (6) discussed the anatomy and classification of acupoints in animals. In comparison similar to acupoints in human subjects, the acupoints of animals show a higher electrical conductivity and higher concentration of neural and vascular elements as well as mast cells than in the surrounding region of the skin. The location of some acupoints corresponds to the motor points, other to the Golgi tendon organs, but most of the acupoints are associated with meridians and known as meridian points.

R. B. Panzer compared the acupoint location in the horse versus that in the human subject and found either one could achieve the same efficacy in treating many animals' illnesses (21).

Recently, A. M. Klide and B. B. Martin, Jr., have published several observations on the effect of acupuncture in veterinary medicine (12,18,19). Their early report showed that fifteen horses with chronic back pain suffering for from six months to nine years were treated with acupuncture therapy once a week. After an average of 7.9 treatments, thirteen horses (86.7 percent) recovered and returned to work in normal condition. In another try, one milliliter of sterile saline solution was injected into acupoints of nine animals once a week. After nine weeks their pain was alleviated and they could go back into training. Six to twelve months after the treatment they were completely recovered (18). The authors also treated fourteen horses with chronic back pain with laser irradiation (300 μW and 904 nm wavelength) at several acupoints, and ten (71.4 percent) obtained complete relief of their pain and went back to be trained. After one year, nine of the ten horses performed very well, without any suffering or recurrence (19). F. B. Bassut demonstrated that such analgesic effect induced by acupuncture in horses was correlated to an increase of plasma ß-endorphin level in the animal (1).

A. M. Klide (11) reviewed the effects of acupuncture anesthesia in a wide variety of animal species under experimental and clinical circumstance. The advantage included no need to use any depressant and the disadvantages were unfamilar wth this technique and inconsistent results. He did recommend acupuncture anesthesia for surgical operations in geriatric or very sick animals and performed cesarean sections on horses and cows (10).

In goats, EAP anesthesia produces a successful completion of a variety of operations, including laparotomy, rumentomy, cystotomy, ovariohysterectomy and cesarean section. The animals recovered smoothly after operations and showed no complications and no adverse effect on cardiopulmonary parameters (2,3)

In forty-five cases, acupuncture anesthesia was applied to perform casesarean section in cows (20), in which a good relaxation of the uterus was obtained. Comparing this with sixty-eight cows that were under the treatment with chemotherapy of isoxsuprine lactate, it was found that the acupuncture group gave a more superior result to the group with chemotherapy, especially the animals that had longer and retarded deliveries.

J. Kostor and N. Bodurov (14) applied laser acupuncture (HeNe) during the cow's puerperal period by direct radiation on the uterus cervix. They reported there was no change of the animal cardiac activity and EKG was normal, but there was a decrease in the erythrocyte count and Hb level.

J. H. Lin and R. Panzer described the details of acupuncture therapy in treating reproductive disorders in animals, including male, female, and pregnancy complications (17).

Animals, especially house pets, who suffered from neurological disorders such as pain responded to acupuncture therapy faster and recovered more completely than those demonstrating a neurological deficiency consistent with the loss of function. Acupuncture offers a noninvasive alternative when medications were contraindicated or surgery was not an option (9).

Acupuncture therapy on inflammation and trauma of small animals has been found to be very successful. It can stimulate healing of burn tissue or ulcers faster than medication (23).

Acupuncture is also found beneficial in the treatment of musculoskeletal disorders in animals, when analgesics or antiinflammatory medication is ineffective. Acupuncture provides a long-term analgesic effect and increases the circulation to the affected area and produces antiinflammatory effects (25).

F. W. Smith has discussed the neurophysiological basis of acupuncture therapy (27). He interpreted that acupuncture can produce a local effect by stimulating the neuroendocrine system and modulating the electromagnetic energy. The exact mechanism of activation depends on the acupoint selection, type of stimulation, and probably the time of the day the acupuncture is performed.

Thoracolumbar and cervical disc diseases (TLDD and CDD) are often seen in small animals, especially dogs. It has been reported that acupuncture therapy offered a simple and more favorable result than the surgical technique (8). It was also reported that acupuncture therapy is as good as medication in treating the intervertebral disc diseases (24).

A case report showed that a dog suffering from a complicated wobbler syndrome was treated with acupuncture and obtained a remarkable improvement, with an outstanding movement control (29).

In another report, thirty-three horses suffering with aerophagia were treated with acupuncture. Six of them (18.2 percent) were cured, and eight improved (24.2 percent). The overall effective rate was 42 percent (15).

Dogs and cats with chronic respiratory conditions such as allergy and asthma responded to acupuncture therapy very well. In most of the cases acupuncture could reduce the medication dosage (26).

Dermatological disorders, allergy, granuloma, and mite infestation in cats and dogs are also effectively being treated by acupuncture (31).

Several reports have shown the effectiveness of acupuncture therapy in treating preweaning diarrhea in piglets. J. H. Lin, et al., (16) found that acupuncture therapy on piglets' diarrhea was equally as effective as the herbal medication. Table 20-1 summarizes the result as follows.

Hwang reported that acupuncture and moxibustion therapy were more effective in treating preweaning diarrhea of piglets than EAP (5). Later he and his coworkers induced diarrhea experimentally with enteropathogenic *E. coli* in thirty-four piglets and treated them either with EAP

Table 20-1. Acupuncture Therapy in Piglets' Diarrhea

Treatment	No. of Piglets	No. of Diarrhea	Recovery %	Meanday of Diarrhea	Compared to the control
Control	142	111	52.2	3.0 ± 0.6	
Acupuncture*	127	89	79.8	2.0 ± 0.8	$p < 0.01$
Chinese herbs	126	80	85.0	1.8 ± 0.6	$p < 0.01$

* at the acupoint, Changqiang (Du 1).

(From Lin et al. (16))

or traditional manual acupuncture at the acupoints Zusanli and Baihui (Du 20). Eighty percent of the piglets were cured by manual acupuncture, confirmed to be better than EAP (7).

Studies on thirty-two dogs suffering from epilepsy and distemper induced seizure (DIE) have shown that acupuncture therapy effectively suppresses the idiopathic epilepsy and synergistically increases the efficacy of the known carbamazepine antiepileptic activity. However, acupuncture has no effect on suppressing DIE (28).

Klide and his colleagues reported using acupuncture to treat five dogs suffering with intractable idiopathic epilepsy. The dogs were nonresponsive to early medication therapy with antiepileptic agents. The acupuncture was applied on the acupoint along the *du* meridian, Foot Xiao Yang and Foot Taiyang meridians. At the end of treatment, two dogs had a decrease of seizure frequency and three had a decrease of the numbers of seizure and the dose of the drug previously taken (13).

Acupuncture has also been used in avian medicine. M. Partington (22) has presented a descriptive text of currently documented avian acupoints and stated that the application of acupuncture technique in treating birds' illnesses is positive and rewarding.

A. S. Thoressen (30) developed a special diagnostic and therapeutic method to use acupuncture in treating some specific clinical symptoms in veterinary medicine. He claimed there is a 50–60 percent success rate in a single treatment and 75–80 percent success rate after more than three treatments.

References

1. Bassut, E. F. B. Peptides 4:501, 1983.
2. Biharia, A., and A. Kumar. Indian Veterinary Journal 69:1026, 1992.
3. Biharia, A., and A. Kumar. Indian Veterinary Journal 69:891, 1992.
4. Demontay, A. Recl. Medicine Vet. E C. Alfort 162:1371, 1986.
5. Hwang, Y. C. American Journal of Acupuncture 15:361, 1987.
6. Huang, Y. C. Problems in Veterinary Medicine 4(1):12–15, 1992.
7. Hwang, Y. C., and E. M. Jenkins. American Journal of Veterinary Research 49:1641, 1988.
8. Janssens, L. A. Problems in Veterinary Medicine 4(1):107, 1992.
9. Joseph, R. Problems in Veterinary Medicine 4(1):98, 1992.
10. Kline, A. M. Problems in Veterinary Medicine 4(1):212, 1992.
11. Kline, A. M. Vet.-Clin.-North Am.-Small Animal Pract. 22(2):374, 1992.
12. Klide, A. M. Acupuncture Electro-Ther. Res. 9:57, 1984.
13. Klide, A. M., et al. Acupuncture Electro-Ther. Res. 12:71, 1987.

14. Kostor, J., and N. Bodurov. Veterinary Medicine Nanki 24:36, 198.
15. Kuussaari, J. American Journal of Acupuncture 11:363, 1983.
16. Lin, J. H., et al. American Journal of Chinese Medicine 16:75, 1988.
17. Lin, J. H., and R. Panzer. Problems in Veterinary Medicine 4(1):155, 1992.
18. Martin, B. B. Jr., and A. M. Klide. Journal of the American Veterinary Medicine Association 190:1177, 1987.
19. Martin, B. B., Jr., and A. M. Klide. Veterinary Surgery 16:106, 1987.
20. Muxeneder, R., Vien Tieraerztl. Monatschr. 71:320, 1984.
21. Panzer, R. B., American Journal of Chinese Medicine 21:119, 1993.
22. Partington, M. Problems in Veterinary Medicine 4(1):212, 1992.
23. Rogers, P. A., et al. Problems in Veterinary Medicine 4(1):162, 1992.
24. Scavelli, T. D., and A. Schoen. Problems in Veterinary Medicine 1(3): 402, 1989.
25. Schoen, A. M. Problems in Veterinary Medicine 4(1):88, 1992.
26. Schwartz, C. Problems in Veterinary Medicine 4(1):126, 1992.
27. Smith, F. W. Problems in Veterinary Medicine 4(1):34, 1992.
28. Sumano-Lopez, H., et al. Veterinaria (Mexico) 18:27, 1987.
29. Sumano-Lopez, H., et al. Veterinaria (Mexico) 24:339, 1993.
30. Thoressen, A. S. American Journal of Acupuncture 17:160, 1989.
31. Waters, K. L. Problems in Veterinary Medicine 4(1):194, 1992.

21
Side Effects and Mortality

Acupuncture is a relatively safe procedure. Different from drug medication, there are very few adverse reactions or side effects caused by acupuncture. Furthermore, there is no such thing as overdosage on acupuncture. In some cases of surgical operation under acupuncture anesthesia the procedure can last for an hour or longer. However, acupuncture therapy it is not completely flawless; occasionally some adverse reactions or some unforeseen error may occur during the procedure or some side effect, such as infection, show up posttreatment. The most common reaction due to acupuncture is the hyperemia at the site of needle insertion. It is not yet completely understood how it happens, whether it is due to an increased histamine release from the peripheral mast cells or an impurity carried from the needle. Occasionally a kind of autonomic reaction may occur and the patients complain of light headache or syncope, more in males than females, but the incidence is less than 1 percent of the total subjects received the acupuncture treatment.

T. Tanii, et al., (19) described a fifty-three-year-old male who developed a prurigo pigmentosa in his back after he had acupuncture treatment in the last three years. The cause of such an itching skin disease probably is a kind of hypersensitivity to the needle, which was found to contain about 18.12 percent chromium.

Infection

Infection is the most troublsome side effect of acupuncture, especially among the patients receiving acupuncture on the street corner or in the bazaar from the travelling practitioner. Not only can the needle carry invisible microbes from the outside to the body; it also can spread the infection from one already-infected area to another part of the body during the insertion. In ancient times, the Chinese believed that needles made from silver or gold could prevent the contamination by the devil. A change of color on the needle surface would indicate its uncleanness and that it is not fit for operations. There is no evidence to substantiate that a silver or gold needle has less chance of causing infection. It is now well recognized in China and worldwide that thorough disinfection of the needle is a prerequisite for acupuncture practice. Disposable needles are now used generally to prevent infection. In an article by V. Sisco, et al., (17), a special sterilization method adaptable for use in the chiropactic clinics was described. The needle was first treated with dry heat, boiling water, or pressure steam and then soaked in a sodium hypochlorite and 70 percent alcohol solution. Dried heat sterilization of the needle for dental application is reported to be sufficiently safe.

A. J. Norheim (12) reviewed the possible adverse effects caused by acupuncture therapy during the years of 1981–92 and described how there was not one hepatitis infection reported in any Nordic country, then concluded that acupuncture therapy can be considered a fairly harmless form of treatment.

However, in a review article on the risk of acupuncture therapy E. Ernst (3) quoted an extensive list of forty-four categories considered to be contraindications of acupuncture therapy and thirteen different adverse reactions caused by acupuncture. He stated that any blood-borne infectious diseases can be transmitted by reused acupuncture needles. Hepatitis B infection is one of the risks. Three published cases have indicated that acupuncture was the only plausible explanation of an HIV infection.

The most serious infectious disease that can be spread by the needle is the viral infection, especially hepatitis and AIDS. Epidemologically the question has been raised, How great is the risk of getting such an infection through the acupuncture needle? Hepatitis is a contagious disease that has been persistently a dominant infectious disease in China, especially in the southern area. Recently the Department of Public Health in China made a survey of more than ten thousand patients in North China who had received acupuncture therapy more than once. The rate of hepatitis among those individuals was not higher than the rate among the general population in China. In the southern part of China, the hepatitis epidemic is more acute, mainly due to food contamination. There are insignificant data to suggest that acupuncture needles can cause a risk. W. O. R. Phoon (15) reported his finding in Singapore among 6,328 Chinese who previously had acupuncture treatment that only 0.88 percent of them were infected with hepatitis B, the same morbidity rate observed among the general population. Y. P. Zhang, et al., (23) studied the plasma hepatitis B antigen activity (HBAg) of 10,508 Chinese. Among them, 2,905 had acupuncture treatment previously, only 3.9 percent showed a positive HBAg activity, and 7,603 people who previously had no acupuncture treatment showed a 7.7 percent positive HBAg activity. Totally, there is only a 6.7 percent positive rate among the 10,508 Chinese surveyed, such a rate being much lower than what the WHO reports is the occurrence of HBAg positive activity in the general Chinese Population.

On the discussion of the danger and safety in medical practice A. O'Neill reported that about 20 percent of the practitioners in Australia are using acupuncture in their practice. The possible complications and side effects of acupuncture are infections, including AIDS, hepatitis B, and septicemia (13).

Studies on the risk of hepatitis C virus (HCV) infection among the inhabitants of a Japanese endemic area in comparison with the inhibitants of the nonendemic area have shown that the acupuncture needle is positively a cause of such infection (6).

J. H. Lee, et al., (7) reported a case of mycobacterium fortuitum infection in a sixty-five-year-old female at the acupoints on both upper and low extremities, who had had acupuncture treatment in many occasions. The patient showed erythematous to purplish colored nodules and plaques with purulent discharge. After excision and antibiotic treatment she recovered completely without relapse.

Before the industrial revolution in the nineteenth century, Japan generally accepted most Chinese culture and acupuncture was very popular. In the last hundred years the Japanese kept better medical records than the Chinese. Their medical journals have reported several special cases of accidents due to acupuncture treatment. For example, silica granuloma was found in a forty-six-year-old patient who had acupuncture therapy twenty years previously. The granuloma was caused by a gold needle (1). Another report described a metal foreign body found in a patient's kidney and subsequently identified as a broken needle (21). An eighty-four-year-old man had a blackish macule in his left clavicular region, and after examination it was found to be an acupuncture needle localized there for more than ten years (22). In another report two cases of acupuncture accidents involved a fifty-three-year-old man and a sixty-year-old woman. Both had a nodular lesion after acupuncture therapy (9). Histological examination of the lesion showed that the nodule resembled a germinal centerlike structure of the lymph node. T. Isu, et al., (5) reported two cases of spinal cord injury resulting from an acupuncture needle. They involved a delayed myelopathy. Other investigators reported an individual who had a needle remaining in his left renal area after an acupuncture accident (14). A sixty-three-year-old woman had an acupuncture needle implanted in her skin for more than ten years. Electromicroscopic examination of her excised skin showed a deposit of electron-dense particles on the basal lamina of the secretory cells of the sweat glands. X-ray film demonstrated that most of the granules consisted of silver and chloride which came from the materials made for the acupuncture needle (20). E. S. Chiu, et al., (2) showed a chest radiograph of a broken needle in a forty-two-year-old Japanese man who had the needle tip inserted in his subcutaneous tissue for more than four years. Y. Sakei, et al., (16) described a sixty-seven-year-old woman with an embedded acupuncture needle in her paraspinal muscle at the L 1 level. They devised a special neuronavigator system to remove it without any difficulty.

Recently H. Suzuki, et al., (18) reported a case of localized argyria with chrysiasis caused by an implanted acupuncture needle in a forty-one-year-old woman. Electromicroscopic and X-ray studies of the excised tissues showed large amount of silver granulas with selenium and sulfur around eccrine secretory cells, also around blood vessels, lymphates, and nerve fibers. There was a small amount of gold and pigment seen in the surroundings.

Pneumothorax

The other accident due to the acupuncture needle is the pneumothorax, a perforation of the thorax cavity by the needle. H. Nakamura, et al., (11) reported 664 cases of pneumothorax in female patients, several of them resulting from the acupuncture procedure. In another report 4 of 30 cases of pneumothorax were caused by the acupuncture needle (10).

Spinal Cord Injury

H. Gi, et al., (4) reported a case of acupuncture injury of the spinal cord of a forty-five-year-old man who had complained of urinary retention about two weeks after acupuncture treatment. X-ray examination showed there was a broken needle tranversely stabbing through the spinal cord at C_{12} level. There was no motor weakness. After surgical removal of the needle the complaint was relieved.

The Mortality

Recently, H. P. Liu of Inner Mongolia collected twenty-six clinical reports on deaths caused by acupuncture therapy since 1949 (8). Thirty-nine cases included eighteen males, thirteen females, and another eight whose gender was not known. Their age ranged from nine to sixty-four years old. Twenty-nine of the thirty-nine cases received their acupuncture treatment from acupuncturists, one from a nurse, three from other health personnel, four from barefoot doctors, one from an amateur, and one from a Taoist. Most of the thirty-nine people died immediately after the insertion of the needle(s). The average time between the death and the needling was 23.5 hours; the shortest one was within ten minutes.

Autopsy showed that eight of the deaths were due to the damage of CNS, when the acupoint

Feng Chi (G 20) (see Chapter 4, figure 2B) was needled and the needle accidentally went into the brain tissue. Nine people died due to the injury of the heart or aorta, while the acupoint Jiuwei (Ren 15) or Yamen (Du 15) was needled. Fifteen died due to the damage of the lung and trachea; three died due to liver damage. The other four cases were unidentified. The major causes of these accidents were the needle puncturing too deep, resulting in damage of the internal organ; the acupoint not being localized correctly (which happened in twelve of thirty-nine cases), or the electrical stimulation being too strong.

References

1. Cheun, S. I., and W. C. Sun. Journal of Dermatology (Tokyo) 18:92, 1991.
2. Chiu, E. S., et al. New England Journal of Medicine 332:304, 1995.
3. Ernst, E. International Journal of Risk and Safety in Medicine 6: 179, 1995.
4. Gi, H., et al. Neurological Surgery 22(2):151, 1994.
5. Isu, T., et al. Surg. Neurol. 23:255, 1988.
6. Kryosawa K., et al. Gastroenterology 106:1596, 1994.
7. Lee, J. H., et al. Annals of Dermatology 6:69, 1994.
8. Liu, H. P. Shanghai Journal of Acupuncture and Moxibustion 12:135, 1993.
9. Maedi, M., et al. Nishinihon Journal of Dermatology. 49:270, 1983.
10. Marchik, I. K., et al. Likar's Sprava 0(10-12):81, 1993.
11. Nakamura, H., et al. Jpn. J. Chest. Dis. 43:939, 1984.
12. Norheim, A.J. Tidsskrift for den Norshe Laegeforenung 114:1192, 1994.
13. O'Neill, A. Social Sci. Medicine 38(4):497,1994.
14. Pak, K., and T. Tomayozhu. Nishinihon Journal of Urolology 47:539, 1985.
15. Rhoon, W. O., et al. American Journal of Public Health 78:958, 1988.
16. Sakei, Y., et al. Plastic-Reconstructive Surgery 94:1097, 1994.
17. Sisco, V., et al. Journal of Manipulative Physiological Therapy 11:94, 1988.
18. Suzuki, H., et al. Journal of the American Academy of Dermatology 29:833, 1993.
19. Tanii, T., et al. Acta Dermato-Venereol. 71:66, 1991.
20. Tanita, Y., et al. Archives of Dermatology 121:1550, 1985.
21. Yamaguchi, S., et al. Acta Urol. Jpn. 35:165, 1989.
22. Yoshida, N., et al. Nishinihon Journal of Dermatology 50:415, 1988.
23. Zhang, Y. P., et al. Journal of Chinese Acupuncture and Moxibustion 10(4):35, 1990.

22

Acupuncture as a Diagnostic Tool

In traditional Chinese medicine, the practitioners don't use the stethoscope, blood analysis, or any other modern medical equipment to make their diagnosis. Four principles are used to guide them in making a correct diagnosis, which are: "Wang, Wen, Meng, and Qie," meaning, "to observe, to smell, to ask, to touch." The last one, touch, depends upon the skill and experience of the practitioner, using the sphygmological analysis of the pulse to tell the rapidity of the heart function and, from the feeling of the contact, indicate the strength (strong or weak) of the circulation or the condition of the body. Next the practitioner would touch or press a certain acupoint, to see whether there is a *tae qi* sensation by the patient, or a change in the pulse wave. The Chinese acupuncturist claims that each internal organ (Zhan-Fu) communicates through the meridian channel and opens up to the surface by the acupoint.

Although there is no anatomical localization to pinpoint an acupoint or the meridian channel, it has been demonstrated there is a rich lymphatic network surrounding the acupoint, and through this network a venous communication can be established. C. C. Wu, et al., (7) injected the radioactive ^{99}m TeO_4 pertechelate subcutaneously to a patient at the acupoints Kunlun (B 60) and Tai Xi (K 3) bilaterally and recorded the venogram of both sides at intervals of five, eight, eleven, and fifteen minutes. A clear venous flow of the patient's lower extremities could be seen. Thirteen patients suffered from venous thrombosis; an interruption of the deep venous flow could be seen in the venogram. The authors concluded that acupuncture principles could be used as a simple method for the diagnosis of the lower-limb venous diseases, especially in the deep layer. M. F. Chen, et al., (1) have also used such radionucleide technique to study the venogram of their patients.

C. C. Xue (8) reported on ninety-five patients who suffered from various nervous diseases and lost their sensation completely. When they were treated with the acupuncture needle, thirty-nine of them showed an acupuncture-propagated sensation, indicating that their nerve conduction still existed. Therefore, Xue recommended that acupuncture could be used to judge the status of the patient's condition, prognosis, differentiation between organic and functional disorders, index for surgical treatment, and selection of clinical management.

When Nakatani of Japan proposed the Rydoraku Channels theory to explain certain pathological abnormalities of organs (see Chapter 3), he indicated there was a defined variation in conductivity along certain lines of the body, the meridian lines. This can be used for cancer diagnosis. Based on this theory, T. Kobayashi (3) studied 169 patients by measuring their conductivity of Rydoraku lines and found there was an abnormality in the six meridian channels, the pericardium, the heart, the Triple Burner, the spleen, the kidney, and the gallbladder. It reveals a great difference in the abnormality between cancer and noncancerous patients. Such measurement can provide a prognosis on whether the patient under treament is improving or getting worse. Furthermore, the Rydoraku measurement can also make an early diagnosis of microcancer growth, which is significantly different from well-grown cancer tissue or noncancerous tissue. Wm. A. Tider (6) used such a device to detect an early cancer growth even when it was small, by inserting a small electrode into an acupoint.

It has also been reported that the measurement of the electrical conductivity on the acupoint along the lung meridian shows a significant difference between a cancer and a noncancerous patient. Such diagnosis by acupuncture technique is substantiated by the X-ray finding (5).

By using the microscopic bi digital O-ring test method to examine the cellular structure and substances within the cell at the magnified focused projected plane, J. Omura describes the diagnosis of the diseases by localizing specific substances and detecting the specific microbacterial infections and the changes of local chemistry, including blood chemistry, such as glucose, total cholesterol, and uric acid in some arteries or the heart (4).

J. M. Kirilow and K. G. Kostov claim that using an electroaudiovisual method on certain acupoints can provide an exact evaluation of the healing effect on the patients (2).

References

1. Chen, M. F., et al. American Journal of Chinese Medicine 21:221, 1993; Clinical Nuclear Medicine 19:426, 1994.
2. Kirilow, J. M., and K. G. Kostov. Acupuncture Electro-Therap. Res. 19:29, 1994.
3. Kobayashi, T. American Journal of Acupuncture 12:305, 1984; American Journal of Acupuncture 13:63, 1985.
4. Omura, J. Journal of Acupuncture and Electro-Therap. Res. 19:39,1994.
5. Sullivan, S., et al. American Journal of Acupuncture 13:261, 1985.
6. Tider, Wm. A. American Journal of Acupuncture 15:15, 1987.
7. Wu, C. C., et al. Kochsiung Journal of Medical Science (Taiwan) 4:687, 1988; American Journal of Chinese Medicine 22:116, 1994.
8. Xue, C. C. Chinese Medical Journal 98:609, 1985.

23

Alternatives

For thousands of years the Chinese have used acupuncture substantially in the treatment a of variety of human diseases and illnesses of domestic animals, including some intractable ailments. In 300 B.C. moxibustion was developed as an alternative using a moxa burning on the acupoint to replace a needle. In the last three decades the ancient technique of needling and piercing gradually caught up with the rapid progress of science and technology. Curiosity in new knowledge and new methods has pushed us forward to ask how we can make the field of acupuncture become a modern medical science. In this chapter we would like to discuss some techniques being applied as alternatives to acupuncture.

Laser Irradiation

Laser is a concentrated monochromatic light. Different from the light from a lightbulb, it comes from a source, then travels with its photons exactly equidistant in time and space and in only one direction. The first laser system was built around a ruby crystal and produced an intense millisecond beam of pure visible red light that was capable of drilling a deep hole through layers of metal or tissue. Laser has become one of the best weapons and tools in defense, science, and medicine because of its penetration power and accuracy.

The Basic Principle

In an atomic system, there are many allowed energy states. The normal state of an atom is the state of the lowest energy. This state is commonly called the ground state. An atom will emit or absorb radiation only at certain frequencies. These frequencies correspond to the energy separation between the various allowed states such that:

$$E_f = E_i \pm hf$$

where E_f is the final state, E_i is the initial state, f is the frequency of radiation, h is Planck's constant, and ± denotes the absorption and emission, respectively. When light is incident on an atom in its ground state, only those photons with energy hf, which matches the energy separation between the ground state and one of its other allowed states, can be absorbed by the atom. This process is called a **stimulated absorption.** As a result of this absorption of the photon, the atom is raised to various allowed higher energy states called excited states.

Once an atom is in one of its excited states, it will make a transition to a lower energy state with the emission of a photon. The photon energy is equal to the energy separation of the two involved atomic states. This is a **spontaneous emission.** Typically an atom will only remain in an excited state for about 10^{-8} sec.

When an atom is in an excited state, a passing photon of the right energy (equal to the energy difference of the two states involved) will induce the atom to emit a photon and make a transition to the lower energy state. This process is referred to as the **stimulated emission** to distinguish it from the spontaneous emission that will happen if the atom is left on its own. The "stimulation" provided by the passing photon will speed up the emission. The important detail of the stimulated emission is that the two photons that emerge will travel in exactly the same direction with exactly the same energy, and the associated electromagnetic waves are perfectly in phase (coherent).

Let us assume that the atoms in the system are all in the same excited state. When a photon of the right energy passes the "first" atom, it will induce a stimulated emission and result in two coherent photons with the same energy travelling in the same direction. The emitted photons, in turn, will stimulate other atoms to emit photons in a chain reaction. This process will repeat itself many times in the collection of atoms while doubling the number of photons at each step. Eventually an intense beam of photons, all coherent and moving in the same direction, can be built up. This is the underlying scenario of the operation of the laser, an acronym for **L**ight **A**mplification by **S**timulated **E**mission of **R**adiation.

In order to obtain a sustainable laser operation, one has to achieve the condition of **population inversion** with more atoms in an excited state than in the ground state, which can be solved by means of "pumping" the atoms into the excited state by some external sources of energy (an electric pulse or a flash of light). The excited state then decays rapidly by a spontaneous emission into a lower excited state, which is a metastable state. The atom remains in the metastable state for a relatively long time because of the restriction of the selection rule that "forbids" it to make a transition to the ground state. As a photon of the right energy passes by, a stimulated transition (emission) occurs from the metastable state to yet another (lower) excited state, which in turn decays rapidly to the ground state. In this setup, a population inversion is achieved between the metastable state and the ground state while the atom in the ground state cannot absorb at the energy of the lasing transition. Hence we have a workable laser.

The Application

The unique property of a laser is its penetration power. Several laser systems have been developed with varieties of wavelength and intensity since the ruby laser was built. For medical uses we have the Helium-Neon (HeNe) laser, the Argon (Ar) laser, the Neodymium-yttrium aluminium garnet (Nd:YAG) laser, the carbon dioxide (CO_2) laser, and the diode laser with a Gallium arsenide (GaAs) or Gallium-aluminium arsenide (GaAlAs) laser chip. The penetration power of each depends upon its wavelength, the output power and the physical properties of the target tissue when the laser is applied. Figure 23-1 illustrates the difference between five laser systems commonly used in medicine at present.

These five laser systems are used for low-level laser therapy (LLLT) in many medical fields. Mester was the first to introduce the LLLT to heal the "torpid non-healing or slow-to-heal ulcer." The ruby laser was originally applied in ophthalmology and dermatology; although it is still used, it now has mostly been replaced by the Ar laser. The Nd:YAG laser is used for deep vaporisation of tissue mass and also as an incision tool. The CO_2 laser can produce a clean, precise linear and bulk vaporization of the tissue and coagulates the tissue at the surface. The HeNe laser has become one of the most useful laser systems for many diverse medical problems.

Experimental analysis has shown that the GaAlAs diode laser has the greatest penetration power and can run in a continuous wave without overheating. Because the 830 nm beam is well absorbed in subcellular organelles, it can produce the exact effect planned without causing any side effect to the surrounding tissue.

In 1981 the Fourth Congress of the International Society for Laser in Surgery and Medicine was held in Tokyo, Japan. A special session on laser acupuncture was organized. Laser therapy has become one of the best alternatives in acupuncture therapy, simple and effective. It has been widely used to induce analgesia in both China and Japan.

In his book (42), T. Ohshiro especially pointed out the advantage of LLLT in treating sports-related pain by ensuring a quick return to preinjury muscle tone and reduction of inflammation swelling due to injury. He told a story about his first accidental discovery of laser effectiveness in the case of a forty-one-year-old female who suffered from severe intractable postherpetic neuralgia and had been treated 350 times unsuccessfully. The patient received low-level Ar laser irradiation for another purpose, to cure a haemangioma simplex lesion on her sternum. But she received the benefit of relief of the neuralgia pain after the first treatment session. By the time her haemangioma was successful blanched, the postherpetic neuralgia had also resolved.

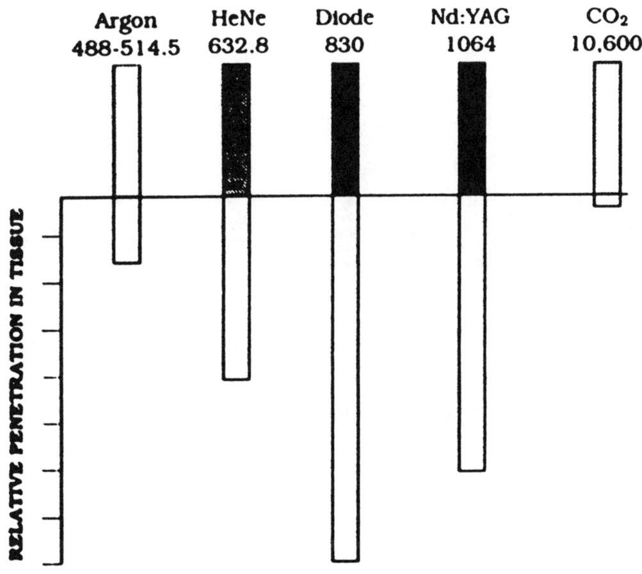

Figure 23-1. The Penetration Power of Five Different Laser Systems

(From Ohshiro (42))

However, the effectiveness of laser acupuncture is very controversial. Several reports described there being no difference between the laser treatment and placebo. For example, E. Haker and T. Lundeberg (13) have treated their patients who were suffering from lateral humeral epicondylalgia with laser beam irradiation at three acupoints: Shousanli (LI 10), Qu Chi (LI 11), and Zhouliao (LI 12). They reported no difference between the laser group and placebo group. G. N. Waylonis, et al., (64) also used low-output HeNe laser irradiation to treat sixty-two patients with chronic and acute myofascial pain for six weeks. There was no difference between the treatment group and placebo group.

But laser irradiation to rats has exhibited an effect on the autonomic nervous system by increasing the sympathetic tone and decreasing the acetylcholinesterase activity. Laser stimulation caused a growth of the membrane potential and increase of the performance capability of the animals, particulary the three-month-old animals (36). Studies on *Drosophila araria* larvae have shown that HeNe laser irradiation (dose 0.3 to 0.5 J/cm^2) would cause an intensive damage as measured by electromicroscopic examination of the midgut cells of the larvae (9).

It has also been found that laser beam irradiation on certain acupoints can cause a remarkable change in the luminescence intensity in hepatic catecholamine and cholinesterase activity in the spinal cord (37). This confirms the early report that laser acupuncture can induce a marked change in activity of cholinergic mechanisms in various areas of the body and spinal cord but has no effect on blood cells.

T. Lunderberg and J. Zhou (35) found that both low-power HeNe laser and GaAs laser applied on certain acupoints could induce an analgesic effect but did not affect the membrane potential of the stretch receptors.

In a double blind study on a group of patients suffering neck and low back pain, HeNe laser therapy increased the skin resistance and reduced the pain (54). HeNe laser therapy can produce pain relief in patients suffering from occupational diseases and increase their ß-endorphin and LEK plasma level (49).

Zhou, et al., (79) reviewed the effectiveness of laser therapy on various illnesses as compared with acupuncture therapy or the combination. The patients suffered shoulder pain, sciatic neuralgia, facial paralysis, arthritis, diarrhea, bronchitis, and infertility. Laser therapy and combination therapy (with acupuncture) gave an average success rate of 90–95 percent, much superior to acupuncture therapy alone (an average of 79 percent success).

T. D. Nikula, et al., treated fifty-six patients with hypertensive diseases by laser and microwave resonance therapy and a positive effect was obtained. They reported that laser therapy can reduce the blood viscosity and peripheral vessel resistance (41).

It has been shown that laser therapy doesn't have a direct effect on the deep tissue, especially HeNe laser irradiation, its penetration power to the skin is poor, only penetrating to 0.4–0.5 mm. deep, and the dermal vascular plexus barrier seems to decrease the penetration (26).

Eighty-three patients suffering of upper-limb edema were treated with acupuncture or a semiconductor laser beam. It was found that the laser acupuncture therapy gave a 44 percent success rate by increasing the fluid discharge and the acupuncture therapy only gave a 20 percent success rate (30).

Two hundred angina pectoris patients were treated with HeNe laser acupuncture. A very good success rate was yielded. The number of attack was reduced, and the patients took smaller amounts of nitroglycerin for prophylaxis. The echocardiogram showed a substantial improvement (18).

T. Mizokani, et al., (39) have used diode laser to treat thirty-two cases of occipital neuralgia. A 81 percent effective rate was obtained. However, for the lower back pain the therapeutic effect of laser therapy is much lower, only 49 percent effective.

One hundred children with scald injury were treated with HeNe laser acupuncture at the acupoints Zusanli, HoKu, Waiguan (SJ 5), Weiz Hong (B 40), Yanglingquan (G 34), and Taixi (K 3) and scanning noncontact over the scald area. The laser acupuncture treatment was carried out for three or four minutes and the scanning for five to ten minutes once a day for a total of five sessions. Eighty-six patients recovered completely from the injury, nine were improved, and four had no effect. After one course of treatment fresh skin appeared to be healing; after a second course of treatment all remainders were healed (16).

Laser acupuncture was also used to treat patients with chronic prostatitis. Both auricular and body acupoints were chosen to receive the laser irradiation. It was claimed to be 89 percent effective (61). Other investigators also reported the using of laser acupuncture in treating chronic prostatitis at the corporal point and obtained an early arrest of pain. The efficacy of the treatment was very satisfactory (3).

One hundred and eleven patients with chronic obstructive bronchitis and asthma were treated with laser acupuncture therapy. The laser beam had a 890 nm wavelength and 1,500 Hz frequency. After the treatment a positive improvement of the bronchial function was observed. The bronchial sensitivity to the sympathomimetic agents was enhanced; the systolic pressure in the pulmonary artery was reduced (73). According to another report, eighty-eight cases of pediatric asthma were treated with HeNe laser acupuncture at the acupoints Feishu (B 13) and Taiyuan (L 9) for two to four minutes each. After six treatments forty-one patients were cured (46.6 percent), and the others were improved (18).

Ninety-six cases of bronchial asthma were treated by CO_2-laser irradiation at the acupoints Tiantu (Ren 22) and Feishu (B 13). A very successful result was obtained, better than the group treated with moxibustion. The pulmonary function of the patients was generally improved after the laser therapy (19).

Twenty-one patients suffering from radicular and pseudoradicular pain syndrome were treated with laser irradiation. Twenty of them (95.2 percent) showed significant relief from their pain (29).

M. Shibuya, et al., (51) treated 310 patients suffering from severe pain with GaAlAs diodide laser pain attenuater (PANALAS-4000) at certain meridian acupoints. The frequency of the laser beam was 5–50 cps. A course of treatment consisted of one to seven treatments per week. At the end of treatment, 175 out of 227 patients (77 percent) showed immediate relief of pain within twenty-four minutes. Another 16 of them (7 percent) showed a such relief of pain within 24 hours after the treatment. The duration of analgesic effect lasted, on the average, two to three days.

To test whether laser acupuncture therapy would affect the muscle strength of the subjects, twelve healthy volunteers were divided into two groups. One group received HeNe laser therapy at the cranial acupoint area, the other group served as control. After four laser treatments the muscle strength of the treatment group increased 12.77 percent higher than that of the control group (55).

Forty-five children suffering from chronic maxillary sinusitis were divided into three groups. One group consisting of eight children was treated with acupuncture therapy, the second group, consisting of nineteen children, was treated with antibiotics, and the other eight were treated with laser acupuncture. It was found that the laser-treated group responded to the treatment much better than the acupuncture group (46).

Low-energy laser was found very useful in treating urolithiasis. A. Nakano, et al., (40) reported thirty-four cases treated with GaAlAs diode laser at the acupoints Shenshu (B 23), Sanyinjiao, and Pangguangshu (B 28). The laser therapy relieved the colic pain immediately, the total effective rate was 59.2 percent, and twelve patients had complete remission (38 percent).

Zhao, et al., (1, p. 141) reviewed the effectiveness of laser acupuncture therapy on 520 patients who suffered from appendicitis, chronic cholecystitis, and acute and chronic pancreatitis. They were irradiated with either CO_2 laser or HeNe laser for ten to twenty minutes at several acupoints. Totally 97 percent were effective. Wang, et al., (1, p. 144) reported 180 cases of rhinitis, pharyngitis, and bronchitis treated with HeNe laser beam at the acupoint HoKu for five minutes. A curative rate of 42.2 percent was obtained. Ye (1, p. 145) treated 197 patients with acute and chronic inflammation of the ear, throat, and nose with laser acupuncture. One hundred and six of them were cured (53.8 percent); only five did not respond to the treatment at all.

HeNe laser irradiation was given to forty-two senior individuals, aged between sixty and seventy-seven years. The acupoint Zusanli was chosen and irradiated for ten minutes once a day. After fourteen sessions the lymphatic enzyme ANAE activity was increased markedly, suggesting an increase of immunity. However, the immunoglobulins IgG, IgA, and IgM levels were not significantly changed (44).

P. P. Si, et al., (52) of the Shanghai Pediatric Clinic treated sixty-three children suffering from neurotic enuresis with HeNe laser irradiation at the acupoints Sanyinjiao, Guanyuan (Ren 4), and Baihui (Du 20), each point for five minutes once a day. After five sessions fifty-six children were cured (88.9 percent) and seven improved. Some of the children did not respond well after five treatments, Zusanli was chosen as acupoint for an extra three sessions of laser therapy for ten to twenty minutes to an hour. They were all substantially improved and the urination frequency returned to normal. L. C. Wang and H. Pan (64) reported their experience with laser acupuncture therapy on enuresis. Fifty children suffering from enuresis were received the HeNe laser for twenty minutes three to four times per week. After ten sessions thirty=eight children were cured (76 percent); only one child had no effect.

Si, et al., applied laser acupuncture therapy to forty-five cases of pediatric deafness at the acupoint Tianrong (SI 17) for ten minutes once a day, totaling ninety sessions. At the end of the treatment six were cured (13.3 percent) and their hearing was recovered. Eight were improved (17.7 percent) (53).

S. K. Me (38) reported his studies on 136 deaf mutes who lost their hearing and speech due to drug toxicity, such as streptomycin, high-fever otitis media, or unspecified illness. He treated them with HeNe laser irradiation at the acupoints HoKu, Baihui (Du 20), Yifeng (SJ 17), and Tai Xi (K 3). Each point was irradiated for five or six minutes, each day three to four acupoints, for a total of forty minutes per day. Some patients might need fifty sessions of treatment. At the end of the treatment 908 cases (72 percent) were cured; their hearing was markedly improved. Another 12 cases had an improvement, and 6 were unchanged.

Four hundred and seventeen cases of pediatric diarrhea were treated with HeNe laser irradiation at the acupoint Zusanli for thirty minutes once a day. After four sessions 328 children were cured, the bowel movements lessened to one or two times a day. Twenty-two were ineffective (4).

HeNe laser acupuncture was used to treated 25 cases of chronic pharyngitis. The beam was directly pointed at the infected area of the pharynx at a distance of 0.5 centimeters. The effective rate was 92 percent. In another twenty-five patients serving as control, treated with regular medication therapy, only fifteen were effective (60 percent) (66).

One hundred and two cases of cervical vertebral disorders were treated with laser acupuncture at the cervical Huatuojiaji (Extra 15). Fifty-nine of them were cured (57.8 percent) and another thirty-four were improved (33.3 percent); 9 failed. It was found that laser therapy was especially effective in those patients who suffered a disorder to the nerve root only and was not effective if the spinal cord also was involved (56).

Walker (62) studied forty-one patients with spastic paralysis due to chronic spinal cord injury over two years. He treated them with HeNe laser irradiation (20 Hz and 1 mV). The clonus was reduced after the therapy, the results similar to that of those who had been treated with electric stimulator.

HeNe laser was also used to treat 74 cases of mastitis at the acupoints Shenshu (Du 12), and Lingtai (Du 10). The low-energy laser beam (15 mW) was pointed at the acupoint at one millimeter distance twice a day. After an average of five sessions they were completely cured. Only 1 patient needed nine sessions of treatment to be completely cured (74).

W. S. Hsu, et al., (20) reported 90 cases of prostate hypertrophy and treated them with HeNe laser needle plus low-frequency electric impulse. The acupoints Huiyin (Ren 1) (midline between the anus and the scrotum) and Shenshu (B 23) were chosen. The laser needle was inserted to five millimeters deep and radiated daily. On the average in six to twelve sessions a curative rate of 83.3 percent was obtained.

A combination of acupuncture and laser acupuncture irradiation was used as an anesthetic technique to repair hernia. X. P. Ka, et al., reported that in thirty-four cases in which Wushu (G 27) and Daju (S 27) were chosen as acupoints, the success rate reached 94.12 percent, not as good as when acupuncture alone was used (90.9 percent) (24).

HeNe laser acupuncture was used in obstetric surgery on 219 women who had abnormal fetal position (1, p. 140). Laser irradiation was given at the acupoints Zhiyin (B 67) of both feet for twenty minutes at a distance of twenty centimeters. After an average one to three treatments 79.5 percent of the women had a corrected position rate. In another 216 cases serving as control (without laser irradiation treatment) only 44 percent had the correction. Under the laser therapy all babies were born healthy and their body weight was normal and the mothers suffered no side effects or reactions during the treatment.

In psychiatrics HeNe laser acupuncture was effective in treating schizophrenia. Y. K. Jia reported twenty-four cases treated with laser therapy at the acupoint Ya Men (Du 15). The result was as good as that for the group who rèceived the antipsychotic drug treatment (22).

HeNe laser acupuncture was used to treat 107 cases of central serous retinitis involving a total of 177 eyes. The acupoints Qiuhou (Extra 7) and Binao (LI 14) were chosen to be irradiated for ten minutes. After one course which consisted of ten treatments, 126 eyes were basically cured (71.2 percent), another 43 eyes were improved (24.3 percent) and 8 failed (32). HeNe laser acupuncture has also been used to treat ninety-seven cases of retinal thrombosis. The needle was inserted into the eyeball, Shenshu (B 23) and Ganshu (B 18), and then irradiated for ten to fifteen minutes once a day. A course consisted of ten treatments; after three days rest a second course could be given. After an average of thirty-five sessions fifty-three patients showed a significant improvement, the obstruction gone. Twelve did not respond to the treatment (33).

Laser acupuncture was also found to be successful in stopping smoking. C. H. Tan, et al., (57) treated 418 male heavy smokers with laser beam at the auricular acupoint for one minute and the intensity was 3 mW, which would give a better result than that for the group treated with body acupuncture.

Using low-intensity HeNe laser acupuncture on acupoint Qu Chi (LI 11) and Touqiaoyin (G 11) it was found the brain circulation was improved after the irradiation, based on the result obtained from the rheoencephalogram. G. F. Zhang, et al, (75) reported that fifty-eight patients with myopia were treated with laser acupuncture. The amplitude of their rheoencephalogram was elevated, and the skin temperature was higher.

Seventy-one patients between twenty-one and forty-six years old suffered from infertility. They were treated with laser therapy. A definite improvement was observed. The spermatozoa density was increased, the number of active mobile spermatozoa was increased, and the number of their degenerative forms was decreased (60).

Table 23-1 lists other clinical data on the effectiveness of laser therapy.

Laser acupuncture has also been practiced in veterinary medicine and found to be effective in relieving pain and strain of the animals being treated (27).

Table 23-1. Clincal Data on Laser Irradiation Therapy

Source	Mode	Acupoint	Diagnosis	No. of Patients	Effectiveness %
Ge (11)	He-Ne Laser	Futu (LI 18) Ermen (Sj 21)	Exopthalmic hyperthyroidism	30	Very effective to lower the high IgG, T_3 & T_4 plasma level and to reduce ^{131}I-uptake.
Chen (5)	He-Ne laser	Sanyinjiao (Sp 6)	Prostate hypertrophy	64	38% were cured and other 55% markedly improved
He (17)	CO_2-laser		Muscular torticollis	154	58% were cured after 10 treatments
Shi (59)	He-Ne laser	Shenque (Ren 8) Zusanli (S 36)	Infantile chronic diarrhea	93	77.4% were cured after 3-5 minute irradiation
Tang (58)	He-Ne laser	Zusanli Sanyinjiao	Acute appendicitis	50	94% short term cured; absence of abdominal mass and tenderness after treatment
Zhang (78)	He-Ne laser	Lingtao (Du 10)	Mastitis	74	100% were cured after 2-9 daily treatments

Moxibustion

Moxibustion is an ancient technique widely applied by professional and nonprofessional Chinese to treat different kinds of illness in conjunction with acupuncture. It is well accepted in Japan and considered to be one of best alternative treatments. In the 1973 evcauation of a Zhou Dynasty tomb in ChiangCha County, Hunan Province, of China, several cloths were found dating back to 300 B.C. in which scripts of moxibustion on arms and legs were described. No acupuncture was mentioned there, indicating that in the early Warring Era moxibustion was very popular and widely used.

An *Atlas of Moxibustion Technique* of the Tang Dynasty (approximately A.D. 700) has been preserved in Dunghuang Grotto which gave another indication how well the ancient Chinese had perfected this medical art.

A Japanese document written a century ago by an emperor's advisor said that moxibustion was effective in curing and preventing illness. Longevity could be obtained when moxibustion was applied at the Zusanli point once a month. Using this treatment a man lived to be more than 174 years old and the ages of his family members were over 100. And the document also described that moxibustion at Feng Chi point would prevent colds and at the Sanyinjiao point would make sexual activity strong.

Literally, the Chinese draw acupuncture and moxibustion together in a name, Zhen Djiu, as an inseparably interchangeable term. Moxibustion uses the same acupoints as acupuncture but stimulates it by thermo-nociceptive mechanism, instead of a needle, probably through the same pathway to the CNS as acupuncture does, and provokes the opioid peptides' release. It is unclear whether the thermoreceptor responds to the moxibustion stimulation the same as to the needle, and would the intensity produced by moxibustion be equally to the twisting or electrical stimulation of the needle. As a statement appearing in ancient Chinese acupuncture literature has described: "Sometimes a disease may not be effectively treated by acupuncture or fails to respond to acupuncture therapy or other medication, but it may be cured by moxibustion . . . " This suggests there is some difference between these two techniques.

The material used in moxibustion is called *AI*, or *moxa*, meaning a "burning herb," from the leaves of *Artemesia vulgaris*, a species of chrysanthemum. The "moxa wool" is made into a form of cone or stick. The moxa-wool cone can be as big as a fava bean or a soybean or as small as a wheat grain. It is placed on a selected acupoint, either directly or indirectly insulated with some medical herbs, even with a piece of ginger or garlic. Quite often some acupuncturist would use a special herb, considered a secret recipe, obtained from his ancestor or mentor.

Figure 23-2 illustrates an example of a moxa cone and how it operates on a patient.

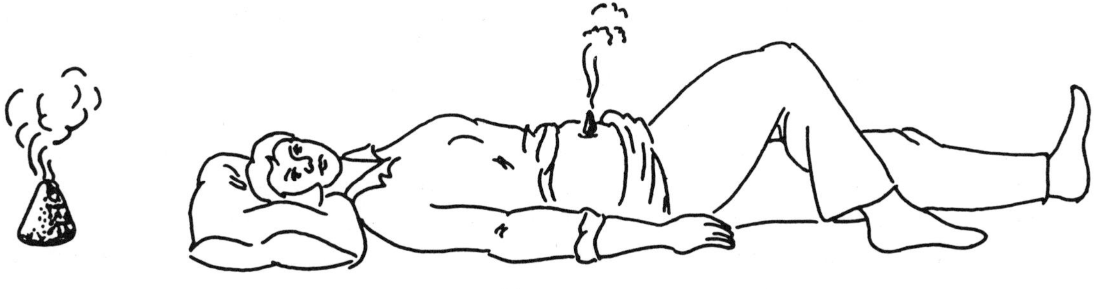

Figure 23-2. Moxibustion Therapy Performed on the Abdomen of a Patient

Figure 23-3 illustrates an example of cupping technique in moxibustion.

A moxa stick is simple to make, rolling the moxa wool into the shape of a cigarette, with a length of twenty centimeters and a diameter of 1.5 centimeters. A burning stick is used directly on the selected acupoint or to warm the needle, which has already been inserted into the point.

The most common application of moxibustion by Chinese practitioners is to induce labor and correct abnormal fetal position. According to the description of an ancient Chinese publication, *The Rule of Classical Medicine,* a moxa cone is placed on the tip of the woman's small toe to cure the puerperal difficulty. In a recent report, 2,069 cases of abnormal fetal position, usually after the seventh month of pregnancy, were treated with moxibustion for fifteen to twenty minutes once a day. The temperature of the moxa cone should be adjusted to a degree tolerable to the patient and

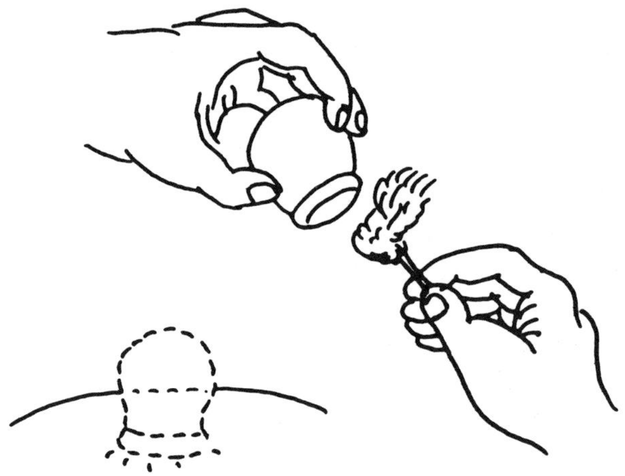

Figure 23-3. Example of a Cupping Technique in Moxibustion Therapy

not cause a pain sensation. After three or four treatments 1,896 women had their fetus in a correct position, the effectiveness rate reaching 90.3 percent (8). The moxibustion technique and the selection of acupoints for various diseases including the indication and contraindication, have been thoroughly reviewed by M. L. Yao (70). According to his experience, moxibustion gave a promising result in the treatment of headache, essential hypertension, sequelae of apoplexy, bronchial asthma, epigastric pain, choleangitis, dysentery, diarrhea, mumps, tuberculosis, dysmenorrhea, leukorrhea, urine retention, impotence, enuresis, scleroderma, leukoderma, dermatitis, and tenosynovitis.

H. Li and F. L. Wang (34) reviewed the literature on moxibustion therapy practiced in China from 1962 to 1992 and reported that moxibustion can increase the immunity, the leucocyte count, and microcirculation. They stated that there are more than twenty kinds of infectious diseases being treated effectively by moxibustion therapy, such as parotiditis tuberculosis, bacterial dysentery, appendicitis, mastitis, epididemitis, tonsillitis, otitis media, and others. The effective rate ranged from 90 to 100 percent. Moxibustion has also been used in the treatment of hypertension, hyperthyroidism, diabetes mellitus, and dermatitis. The results are definitely positive.

Twenty patients who had acute and chronic urinary cystitis, in some cases suffering more than twenty years, were treated with moxibustion at the Guanyuan (Ren 4) point without using any antibiotics. Patients with acute cystitis were cured after one or two treatments and those with chronic cystitis were cured after ten to twenty treatments. The urinary culture was clear from bacteria (77).

In thirty-four cases of acute tonsillitis, moxibustion therapy was applied at the Erheliao (SI 22) acupoint bilaterally. After one treatment twenty-eight (82.4 percent) were cured and another five were improved (59).

H. Zhang, et al., (76) treated 104 cases of lumbar disorders with moxibustion therapy at the C 6 and C 7 vertebrae and HoKu point. Forty-one patients were cured and forty-five showed a marked improvement.

In another report, 82 cases of rheumatoid arthritis were treated with moxibustion. There was a definite improvement of the joint, a decrease of erythrocyte sedimentation rate, and an increase of lymphocyte tranformation rate and E-rosette formation rate. The rheumatic factor became negative after the treatment and the immunoglobin level was back to the normal range (68).

The moxibustion therapy is also used effectively to treat certain dermatitis and decubitus ulcers that usually do not respond well to medication. Moxibustion is applied for twenty minutes and continually for twenty to thirty consecutive sessions. At the end of the treatment the circulation underneath the tissue was improved, and the ulcer was gradually healed.

S. H. Yang, et al., (69) reported that moxibustion has the protective effect on choleangitis induced by chemicals in rats.

Transcutaneous Electrical Nerve Stimulation

TENS is not a Chinese invention. It was in 1858 that Francis first described the relief of pain by electricity in tooth extractions by using galvanic stimulation (25). The technique was gradually modified and became a well-accepted TENS, used by many anesthesiologists and neurologists. It does not need a needle and acupoint selection. The voltage of electricity is relatively higher than what EAP requires. TENS has an advantage in that patients can perform the technique themselves at home. Recently TENS has opened new areas of medical treatments, not only in physical therapy, but also in the treatment of various kinds of pain, in obstetrics for labor induction and delivery, for morning sickness, and for osteogenesis. The details of the TENS technique, clinical application and contraindication have been well discussed in the books written by M. R. Gersh (12) and J. Kahn (24).

Testing high-frequency TENS in healthy people has shown that the dental pain threshold is elevated, though it wouldn't be abolished by the administration of the opiate antagonist naloxone (45).

R. A. Dlin, et al., (10) treated twenty-two young athletes with TENS at the acupoint in the vicinity of pain area. Eighteen patients (81.8 percent) had relief of their pain and returned to full sports activity. Six subjects experienced recurrence of pain after ten days to two months. Further treatment with TENS gave a very good satisfactory result and no adverse reaction was reported.

J. Q. Wang, et al., (63) found there is no significant difference between producing antinociception by EAP or by TENS. Naloxone can block the low-frequency TENS but not the high-frequency stimulation.

C. P. Ledergerber reported that two cases of spinal cord injury involved a lower extremity and urinary bladder paralysis. They were treated with TENS and transcutaneous EAP together. An excellent improvement of their motor and sensory deficit of the extremity as well the bowel and bladder function was observed (31).

J. S. Han, et al., (14) treated thirty-two patients suffering from spinal spasticity with TENS stimulation by using Han's Acupoint Nerve Stimulator (HANS) via a skin electrode placed over the acupoints of the head and leg. They reported that high-frequency (100 Hz) but not low-frequency (2 Hz) stimulation was effective in ameliorating the muscle spasticity. The therapeutic effect lasted for ten minutes in the first treatment and became consolidated after consecutive daily treatments for three months. Such antispastic effect by high-frequency stimulation can be partially reversed by naloxone, indicating it is mediated, at least in part, by endogenous opioid ligand interaction with the kappa opiate receptors, most probably the DYN in the CNS. A similar result was reported by X. Yu (71).

TENS (three to four volts) was applied to the palms of thirty-two patients who suffered from phobia and obsessive compulsive disorders. Eighty percent of them showed an effective improvement. They lost their anxieties and fear within a few minutes (68).

TENS was used to treated forty-four cases of premature heartbeat. Thirty patients (68 percent) showed effective reducing of their heartbeat from an average of 74.12 ± 11.66 beat/minute down to 70.82 ± 9.49 beats/minute (6).

Magnetic Acupuncture

Magnetic acupuncture is an alternative technique that uses a magnetic tablet applied on certain acupoints instead of a needle. In studies of 500 patients with severe pain, Zhou claimed that magnetic acupuncture can elicit a manual acupuncture–like effect to induce analgesia in the patients (79).

S. R. Hsu used a magnetic blunt-tip needle instead of the regular steel or silver needle to treat patients with pain, hypertension, tennis elbow injury, or sprain. He obtained a remarkable result, relieving the patients' pain, lowering the blood presssure, and causing a rapid cure. He stated that the magnetic acupuncture therapy can give a better curative and effective rate to his patients than regular needles (21).

For the patients who are nervous and usually scared at seeing a needle, magnetic acupuncture is probably a good alternative to recommend. Magnetopressopuncture technique has been introduced to sedate children during dental treatment. It was also recommended in inebriated people with particular psychological problems (28).

R. Shapiro used a small magnetic pellet instead of a needle to perform the acupuncture therapy on his patients. He claimed the magnetic pellet technique produced a rapid result and was effective and non-invasive (48).

C. P. Chiang, et al., (7) reported 330 cases of thyroidectomy surgery under magnetic acupuncture anesthesia in combination with narcoleptic agent (Fentanyl and droperidol). The auricular acupoint Shenmen was chosen. It was found that in using magnetic acupuncture anesthetically the effective rate was only 59.5 percent, but the combination of magnetic acupuncture anesthesia and NLA gave an effective rate of 73.7 percent.

The magnetic needle was used to treat prostate hypertrophy. In thirty cases that received such treatment, eleven (36.6 percent) showed a substantial reduction of the size of the gland, four were ineffective, and the others were improved (67).

Qi-Gong

Qi-Gong is a kind of martial art practiced feverishly in China and in Japan. Chinese call the Qi a "gas" or "force" circulated in the body continuously and invisibly, through the twelve pairs of meridians and the two extra meridians. By way of technique and special breathing, Chinese claim that one can bring the Qi together, or concentrate it at certain points of the body, voluntarily, like electrical currents connecting in a series, which can build up from a few mV to a hundred volts (like the electric eel). This concentrated Qi would build into a force big enough to stimulate or can block the meridian channels or the nerve conduction.

Qi-Gong is similar to Western meditation, Indian yoga, or Japanese Zen included in the category of traditional psychotherapy. Inappropriate training can lead to physical and mental disturbance. Physiological effects of Qi-Gong include the change in EEG, EMG, respiratory and heart rate, skin potential, skin temperature and fingertip volume, sympathetic nerve functions, gastrointestinal activity, metabolism, and an endocrine and immunity system. The psychological effect of Qi-Gong are similar to those of a minor episode with LSD or marijuana, which include: motor phenomenon and perceptual changes, warmth or chillness, an itching sensation in the skin, numbness, soreness, bloatedness, relaxation or tenseness, floating, a sensation of rising to the sky or falling or standing upside down or like playing on a swing following respiration and circulation of the intrinsic Qi. Some patients may experience dreamlike illusion, unreality and pseudohallucination. But such phenomena are transcient and will vanish as the Qi-Gong exercise terminates.

What is Qi? How does Qi-Gong work? No one, especially in the Chinese scientific profession, can come out with an explanation. It is difficult to tell whether it is a superstition or a technique difficult to learn and perfect.

Y. Omura, et al., (43) used the Qi-Gong therapy to treat their patients at the acupoints Shimen (Ren 5) and Qihai (Ren 6), below the umbilicus, for ten to twenty minutes each. It resulted in an improvement of their circulation, fall of blood pressure, relaxation of the spastic muscle, and relief of pain and enhanced the general well-being of their patients. Using the bidigital O-ring test to evaluate the effectiveness of Qi-Gong, they studied the patients during Qi-Gong therapy and found there was a significant change from +4 in pre–Qi-Gong state to a −3 and −4 states during Qi-Gong performance, which are very similar to the results accomplished by acupuncture therapy. They also emphasized that such effects can be produced in children who had no knowledge of Qi-Gong nor of medicine. This suggests that Qi-Gong is neither hypnosis nor a psychological placebo phenomenon.

Studies on seven subjects showed that Qi-Gong exercise caused a reduction of electrical conduction in several acupoints, an average of 17–35 percent (47).

Microwave Acupuncture

He, al., (14) treated forty-nine cancer patients with microwave acupuncture therapy and obtained a marked therapeutic effect in their patients. The immunological function was greatly improved. The patient who did not respond well to other medication therapy previously responded more favorably to cancer therapy. The leucopenic effect induced by radiotherapy or chemotherapy was lightened and reduced substantially after the microwave acupuncture treatment.

References

1. All China Society of Acupuncture and Moxibustion Second National Symposium on Acupuncture and Moxibustion and Acupuncture Anesthesia. Beijing: People Health Publisher, 1984.
2. Alliluer, I. G., et al. Klin. Med. (Moscow) 68:54, 1990.
3. Arbulier, M. G., et al. Urol. Nevrol. 0(5):4, 1988.
4. Chao, P. C. Shanghai Journal of Acupuncture and Moxibustion 12(1): 27, 1993.
5. Chen, C.P. New Journal of Traditional Chinese Medicine 25(5):37, 1993.
6. Chen, Y. X., et al. Journal of Chinese Acupuncture and Moxibustion 14(1):3, 1994.
7. Chiang, C. P., et al. Shanghai Journal of Acupuncture and Moxibustion 12(1): 5, 1993.
8. Chien, S. C. The Acupuncture and Moxibustion. Tianjin: Science and Technology Publisher, 1990. p.110.
9. Dimitriadis, V. K., and I. A. Liapis. Acupuncture Electro-Ther. Res. 10:67, 1985.
10. Dlin, R. A., et al. International Journal of Sports Medicine 1:203, 1980.
11. Ge, T. Y., et al. Journal of Traditional Chinese Medicine (in English) 8:85, 1988.
12. Gersh, M. R. Electrotherapy in Rehabititation. Philadelphia: F. A. Davis, 1992, pp. 149–217.
13. Haker, E., and T. Lundeberg. Pain 43:243, 1990.
14. Han, J. S., et al. Chinese Medical Journal 107(1):6, 1994.
15. He, C. J., et al. Journal of Traditional Chinese Medicine 7:9, 1987.
16. He, J. Z. Laser Therapy 2(4): 179, 1990.
17. He, J. G. Journal of Chinese Acupuncture and Moxibustion 10(4):11, 1990.
18. He, S. H., and Y. H. Gor. Journal of Chinese Acupuncture and Moxibustion 11(2): 25, 1991.
19. He, Y. Z. and Z. Q. Liang. Journal of Chinese Acupuncture and Moxibustion 14(1):13, 1994.
20. Hsu, W. S., et al. Journal of Chinese Acupuncture and Moxibustion 11(6):3, 1991.
21. Hsu, S. R. Journal of Traditional Chinese Medicine 8:239, 1988.
22. Jia, Y. K., et al. Journal of Traditional Chinese Medicine 7:269, 1987.
23. Ka, X. P., et al. Journal of Chinese Acupuncture and Moxibustion 11(4):28, 1991.

24. Kahn, J. Principle and Practice of Electrotherapy. 3d. Ed. NY: Churchill Livingston, 1994, p. 107–126.
25. Kane, K., and A. Taub. Pain 1:125, 1975.
26. Kolari, P. J., and O. Qiraksinen. Acupuncture Electro-Ther. Res. 18:17, 1993.
27. Koster, I. and N. Bodurov Vet. Med. Nauki 24:36, 1987.
28. Kozma, A., Rev. Chir. Oncol. Radiol. ORL Oftalmol. Stomatol Ser. Stomatol. 34:151, 1987.
29. Kreczi, T., and D. Klinglev. Acupuncture Electro-Ther. Res. 11:207, 1986.
30. Kuzmina, E. G., et al. Med. Radiol. 35:18, 1990.
31. Ledergerber, C. P. American Journal of Acupuncture 12:149, 1984.
32. Li, G. S. Journal of Chinese Acupuncture and Moxibustion 11(1): 15, 1991.
33. Li, G. S., and G. M. Li. Journal of Chinese Acupuncture and Moxibustion 11(4):7, 1991.
34. Li, H., and F. L. Wang. Journal of Chinese Acupuncture and Moxibustion 13(4):46, 1993.
35. Lunderberg, T., and J. Zhou, American Journal of Chinese Medicine 16:87, 1988.
36. Lupyr, V. M., and N. G. Sergieuko G. Radiobiologi Ya 30:671, 1990.
37. Lupyr, V. M., and N. G. Sergieuko. Fizid. ZH (Kiev) 32:293, 1986.
38. Me, S. K. Journal of Chinese Acupuncture and Moxibustion 11(5):9, 1991.
39. Mizokani, T., et al. Laser Therapy 2:171, 1990.
40. Nakano, A., et al. Nishinihon Journal of Urology 50:845, 1988.
41. Nikula, T. D., et al. Urechebnoe Delo 0(10):32, 1992.
42. Ohshiro, T., Low Reactive Level Laser Therapy. New York: John Wiley and Sons, 1991, p. 215.
43. Omura, Y., et al. Acupuncture Electro-Ther. Res. 14:61, 1989.
44. Pan, Y., et al. Journal of Traditional Chinese Medicine 28(1):50, 1987.
45. Pertovarra, A., and P. Kemppainev. Brain Research 215:426, 1981.
46. Pothman, R., and H. L. Yeh. American Journal of Chinese Medicine 10:55, 1982.
47. Sancier, K. M. Acupuncture Electro-Ther. Res. 19:119, 1994.
48. Shapiro, R. American Journal of Acupuncture 15:43, 1987.
49. Shatskiya, N. N., et al. Gjiena Truda I Profasional NYE Zabolevainya 0(6):25, 1992.
50. Shi, B. P., et al. Journal of Traditional Chinese Medicine 5(2):89, 1985.
51. Shibuya, M., et al. Neurological Surgery 13: 607, 1985.
52. Si, P. P., et al. Shanghai Journal of Acupuncture and Moxibustion 12:16, 1993.
53. Si, P. P., et al. Journal of Chinese Acupuncture and Moxibustion 13(4): 24, 1993.
54. Snyder-Machler, L., et al. Physical Therapy 69:336, 1989.
55. Sopler, D., American Journal of Acupuncture 12:117, 1984.
56. Tan, S. H., et al. Journal of Chinese Acupuncture and Moxibustion 13(3): 15, 1993.
57. Tan, C. H., et al. American Journal of Acupuncture 15:137, 1987.
58. Tang, H., and Y. D. Fu. Journal of Traditional Chinese Medicine 1:43, 1981.
59. Tei, M. T. Journal of Chinese Acupuncture and Moxibustion 14(2):34, 1994.
60. Ticktinskii, O. L., et al. Urol. Nefrol. 0(3):55, 1986.
61. Vazianovx, A. F., et al. Vrach. Delo. 0(2):45, 1991.
62. Walker, J. B. Brain Research 340:109, 1985.
63. Wang, J. Q., et al. International Journal of Neurosci. 65:117, 1992.
64. Wang, L.C., and H. Pan. Journal of Chinese Acupuncture and Moxibustion 11(5):21, 1991.
65. Waylonis, G. N., et al. Archives of Physical Medical Rehabilitation 69:1017, 1988.
66. Wu, K. F. Shanghai Journal of Acupuncture and Moxibustion 12(1): 26, 1993.
67. Wu, Y. S., and W. M. Chen. Shanghai Journal of Acupuncture and Moxibustion 12(1):36, 1993.
68. Yamashita, T., et al. Psychiatria et Neurologia Japonia 93:645, 1991.
69. Yang, S. H., et al. American Journal of Chinese Medicine 21:237, 1993.
70. Yao, M. L. Journal of Traditional Chinese Medicine 5:220, 1985.
71. Yu, Y. Chinese Medical Journal 73(10):593, 1993; 73(10):637, 1993.
72. Yuewei, Z., et al. American Journal of Acupuncture 19:315, 1991.
73. Zamotaev, I. P., et al. Klin. Med. (Moscow) 69:68, 1991.
74. Zhang, W. C., et al. Shanghai Journal of Acupuncture and Moxibustion 12(2):69, 1992.
75. Zhang, G. F., et al., from All China Society of Acupuncture and Moxibustion Beijing: 1979, p. 71.
76. Zhang, H., et al. Journal of Chinese Acupuncture and Moxibustion 14(1):21, 1994.
77. Zhang, L. W. Journal of Chinese Acupuncture and Moxibustion 14(2):50, 1994.
78. Zhang, W.C., et al. Shanghhai Journal of Acupuncture and Moxibustion 12(2):69, 1993.
79. Zhou, L. American Journal of Acupuncture 17:15, 1989.

Index

D

E

F

G

H

Q

R

S

T

U

V

W

Y

Z